A GLOSSARY OF
ANESTHESIA
AND RELATED TERMINOLOGY

A GLOSSARY OF
ANESTHESIA
AND RELATED TERMINOLOGY

SANFORD L. KLEIN, D.D.S., M.D.
Professor and Chairman, Department of Anesthesia
University of Medicine and Dentistry of
New Jersey–Rutgers Medical School
Piscataway, New Jersey
Chief of Anesthesia
Middlesex General–University Hospital
New Brunswick, New Jersey

MEDICAL EXAMINATION PUBLISHING CO.

Klein, Sanford L.
   A glossary of anesthesia and related terminology.

   1. Anesthesia--Dictionaries. 2. Anesthesia--
Terminology. I. Title. [DNLM: 1. Anesthesiology--
Terminology. WO 215 K64g]
RD82.K6   1984   617'.96'0321   83-19331
ISBN 0-87488-973-1

Printed in the United States of America

This book is respectfully dedicated to the memory of
William F. Harrigan, D.D.S., M.D.,
first of the great chiefs with whom I trained.
Without his multiple manifest indulgences I would surely now
be polishing pontics in Passaic.

Contents

Preface

The standard of care in anesthesia practice is becoming increasingly complex at a rate which may not be fully apparent to either the clinician or the student of anesthesia. Having to deliver clinical care on a daily basis tends to inhibit awareness of the differences between anesthesia today and 10 years ago. Even less concern may be devoted to how the specialty may change during the next decade. Similarly, the academician-researcher may be too narrowly focused to recognize the consequences of new techniques and agents.

When I started my anesthesiology training in New York State 10 years ago, three ventilators and five electrocardiograph monitors were available for 11 operating rooms in our university hospital. Diethyl ether, cyclopropane, ethylene, and flurnoxene were used extensively. Monitoring of central venous pressure by a water manometer was considered sophisticated and arterial lines were a clinical rarity. Modern operating rooms in 1985 have at least a two-channel monitor (where three-, four-, five-, or six-channel monitoring is not available). Flammable anesthetics are becoming as obsolete as ocean liners, and oxygen analyzers and disconnect monitors are now, or soon will be, the universal standard of care. In the near future, intraoperative monitoring of the electroencephalogram analyzed by microprocessor will probably become routine. Within the next decade the design of the conventional anesthesia machine should change radically. Electronics will probably adjust flow control, perform startup checks, and help to do everything but "wash the hoses" (come to think of it, that is gone too, due to disposable equipment). Further, we can look toward introduction of the true analgesics and a change in the very basis for the existence of anesthesia as a separate discipline. This may happen within the lifetime of many who are in training today. Anesthesia will become even more technical and will be more involved in intensive care, while in the operating room we will still defend the patient against the consequences of surgery, certainly beyond our current considerations of fluid and electrolytes, blood replacement, and acid-base balance.

This book is written to aid the student, practitioner, and teacher of anesthesiology to cope with the ongoing changes by providing short, concise, and hopefully clear definitions of common anesthesia-related terms, so that what was, what is, and what will be can be appreciated from a common semantic background. It is not meant to be a comprehensive text. Excellent anesthesiology references already exist: Miller; Wollman and Larson. It is meant to aid in understanding a complex field and to be a quick reference when consultation of weightier tomes would be inappropriate. Some attempt has been made to be exhaustive; however, after four years of work the author would not be surprised if a simple everyday term were left out, due to either typographical error, not seeing the forest for the trees, ignorance, or "the word processor did it!" The project has grown considerably, so much so that we have had to delete rather than add in the final stages of preparation. My personal fondness for historical inference and reference has been somewhat curtailed. So too has my predilection for the complicated high-technology devices now becoming so popular.

This text is the responsibility of the author; however, it would never have seen the light of day without the devoted work of Christine Thompson, a terrific laboratory assistant, who self-programmed to a hundred other job descriptions p. r. n. and did them better than very well. Marcia Feinberg and Phyllis Bergman spent too many hours (usually at their own expense) trying to decipher my handwriting and figuring out what I really meant to say rather than what I wrote. Without their devotion and competence a poorer book would have been ready for the publisher five years ago. I would like to personally thank the following: Amy Carter, who was consistently helpful in the production of the final manuscript; Debra Cayler, Judy Carlson, Tamara Hesse, Barbara Kirchner, Susan Tew, and Martha Lubaroff, who wore down many a finger typing and retyping my innumerable drafts; and my colleagues at The University of Iowa for reviewing portions of the manuscript. Mark Stasi and Lynn Griebahn did much of the assembly of word lists without which the job would have been impossible. Jane Vanderbosch and Sharon Schmahl contributed valuable research and Russell Spinelli helped flog the word processor programs through the IBM 370. A special thank you goes to my former work place, The Department of Anesthesia, University of Iowa Hospitals and Clinics, for its unflagging support across many years and many chairmen. Dr. Jeffrey Apfelbaum reviewed the final manuscript and did a fine job catching errors and inconsistencies.

I would also like to thank my wife, Dr. Virginia Klein, not only for putting up with this effort, but also for her help in the dual wilderness of statistics and computer science where I would have been lost forever without her assistance. Lastly, I would like to thank Esther Gumpert, my third editor at Medical Examination Publishing Co. , Inc. , and her predecessors, Howard Granat and Joe Cahn, for their efforts. They all deserved a more prompt and less irascible author.

notice

The author and the publisher of this book have made every effort to ensure that all therapeutic modalities that are recommended are in accordance with accepted standards at the time of publication.

The drugs specified within this book may not have specific approval by the Food and Drug Administration in regard to the indications and dosages that are recommended by the author. The manufacturer's package insert is the best source of current prescribing information.

ABANDONMENT: The refusal, in a medicolegal context, on the part of a physician or dentist to continue caring for a patient without the patient's consent.

ABDOMINAL ELECTROCARDIOGRAPHY: An obstetric technique for determining the fetal electrocardiogram by the application of electrodes to the mother's abdominal wall. Difficulty is encountered due to electric interference from the maternal electrocardiogram and abdominal wall musculature and gross interference from fetal movement.

ABDUCENS: The sixth cranial nerve and the most likely to be affected by a drop in cerebrospinal fluid pressure after a spinal anesthetic. Paralysis of the abducens causes diplopia. See Cranial nerves.

ABLATION: The process of removing material from the surface of an object, usually by **vaporization** or decomposition. Ablation may also mean complete mechanical destruction; cryosurgery is used in the total ablation of a tumor. Ablation-type heat shielding is used on the nose cones of rockets returning to earth.

ABORT: The abrupt termination of an ongoing event.

ABSOLUTE ZERO: The temperature which, according to theory, is the lowest physically possible. This temperature has been closely approached but never reached in practice. In units it is 0 degrees Kelvin, -273.15 degrees Celsius, and -459.67 degrees Fahrenheit.

ABSORBENT CHANNELING: A phenomenon occurring in poorly packed absorbent canisters which can severely affect the proper absorption of CO_2. The cross-sectional area of absorbent to which the gas stream is presented is reduced dramatically by small passageways or channels which course through the absorbent from one end to the other, bypassing the bulk of active absorbent. This can lead to a relatively rapid yet insidious buildup of CO_2 in the gas mixture which the patient breathes.

ABSORBER: See Carbon dioxide absorption.

ABSORPTION: The process by which a substance becomes available to the circulating fluids of the body. The rate of absorption depends on the physical characteristics of the substances being absorbed and the nature of the barriers and membranes between the site of initial deposit and the circulation.

ABSORPTION ATELECTASIS: The phenomenon which occurs when the air passage-way to the alveolus is blocked. If the patient has been breathing air it can be assumed that at the instant of blockage PAO_2 is approximately 100 torr, $PACO_2$ is approximately 40 torr, alveolar pressure of nitrogen is 573 torr, and partial pressure of water vapor is 47 torr. In capillary blood flowing past the alveolus, the partial pressures of nitrogen and water vapor are the same; however, PO_2 is about 40 torr and PCO_2 is about 45 torr. This gives a net positive pressure to the alveolus which will lose gas to the pulmonary blood and gradually collapse. This gradual collapse is splinted by nitrogen which shifts slowly to the alveolus from the blood flowing past it, tending to keep the alveolus open. In any situation where alveolar O_2 has been augmented to take the place of alveolar nitrogen, absorption atelectasis occurs more quickly because the partial pressure difference between alveolar O_2 and capillary O_2 is much greater, and in fact, when a healthy individual breathes 100% O_2, PAO_2 approaches 668 torr, $PACO_2$ is 45 torr, and water vapor is 47 torr. See Atelectasis.

ABSORPTION INDICATOR: A chemical added to CO_2 absorption granules to demonstrate progressive diminution of absorptive capacity. A commonly used indicator is the chemical ethyl violet. As absorption capacity decreases, the indicator changes from white to purple. The deeper the purple, the less absorption capacity is available. It has a critical pH (the pH at which color changes) of 10.3. Absorption indicators are only qualitatively accurate; a purple granule may turn white again when exposed to air due to a limited regeneration of strong base capacity. Any absorption chamber which is color-tinged should be refilled. See Carbon dioxide absorption.

ABS PLASTIC: A class of plastics which is identified as belonging to the acrylonitrile-butadiene-styrene group. They are usually of good rigidity, high impact strength, and fair hardness over a wide temperature range. ABS is a typical plastic used in helmets, luggage, and machine parts, where abrasion resistance is not a prerequisite.

ABUSIVE LEGAL PROCESS (BARRATRY): The use of the courts to harass an individual. Along with defamation, it is grounds for a countersuit in patient-initiated malpractice action.

ACCUMULATION: A phenomenon resulting from repeated drug administrations which are spaced so closely together that neither metabolism nor excretion is fast enough to prevent the drug from increasing in concentration in the body. For example, succinylcholine is a drug which undergoes extremely rapid metabolism in the plasma. However, a fast-running intravenous infusion of succinylcholine can actually cause the plasma concentration of succinylcholine to rise continuously until the infusion is stopped or a plateau is reached (based on an equilibrium between administration and metabolism).

ACCURACY: A measurement or, when applied to laboratory equipment, the specification of the freedom from error of a device. Most often this is expressed as a percentage over a particular range; for example, a 2% error on a scale of 100, in whole numbers, means that 98 may be registered on the machine as 96, 97, 98, 99, or 100, and the machine is operating within design limits.

ACETAMINOPHEN (TYLENOL): An effective alternate drug to the salicylates when analgesic and antipyretic actions are needed. Acetaminophen is a breakdown product of phenacetin. It is well tolerated by the gastrointestinal tract, but overdosage may cause severe hepatic or renal damage or death.

ACETAZOLAMIDE (DIAMOX): A drug which inhibits the enzyme carbonic anhydrase. By inhibiting this enzyme, acetazolamide prevents the combination of H_2O and CO_2 from forming carbonic acid, which then dissociates into hydrogen ion and bicarbonate. It functions as a diuretic and mild antihypertensive agent. The drug at times has found controversial use as a preanesthetic agent for open eye injuries as it is known to decrease intraocular pressure. Acetazolamide interferes with the CO_2 transport mechanism and may, at least transiently, give rise to increased CO_2 tension in the peripheral tissues and decreased CO_2 tension in the pulmonary alveoli.

ACETYLATION: A form of drug metabolism in which an acetyl group, $COCH_3^+$, is added to a drug or other pharmacologically active compound to change its reactivity.

$$(CH_3)_3N^+ - CH_2 - CH_2 - O - \overset{\displaystyle O}{\overset{\displaystyle \|}{C}} - CH_3$$

Acetylcholine.

ACETYLCHOLINE (ACh): A neurotransmitter substance released at autonomic nerve endings by cholinergic neurons. Synthesis of ACh is controlled by the enzyme choline acetyltransferase, which mediates transfer of an acetyl group from acetyl coenzyme A to choline. Following release at cholinergic nerve endings, ACh is rapidly hydrolyzed and inactivated by the enzyme acetylcholinesterase. Acetylcholine produces peripheral vasodilation (flushing of the face, increased skin temperature); stimulates secretion from exocrine glands (sweating, salivation, tearing); causes bronchoconstriction, decreased heart rate, and pupillary constriction; and stimulates gastrointestinal smooth muscle (peristalsis, defecation, urination). See Fig. See Neuromuscular blocking agent, Succinylcholine.

ACETYLCHOLINESTERASE: An enzyme found in red blood cells and nerve terminals which is responsible for the hydrolysis of acetylcholine to choline and acetic acid. Nerve terminal acetylcholinesterase is usually referred to as true cholinesterase. It is also found in the placenta, where its function is unknown. See Pseudocholinesterase.

ACETYLENE (C_2H_2): A colorless gas with a distinct odor, which can explode spontaneously when compressed at room temperature. Its primary use is for welding and cutting metals with flame. It is 92.3% carbon and can therefore be considered nearly gaseous carbon; mixed with O_2 it can reach a torch tip temperature of 3500 degrees Celsius. Employed as a general anesthetic earlier in this century, acetylene was discontinued because of its combustibility and because better anesthetics were developed.

ACETYLSALICYLIC ACID (ASPIRIN): One of a series of salicylates which are usually taken orally as an analgesic, an antipyretic, and/or an anti-inflammatory agent. In small doses, it also causes inhibition of platelet aggregation and prolongation of bleeding time; it is therefore a significant preoperative drug.

ACID: A substance which, according to the Bronsted-Lowry definition, tends to dissociate and release hydrogen ions (H^+) when in solution. The substance itself may be either positively or negatively charged or neutral.

Acid-Base Balance: (I) Acid-base normal values.

	Range	Average
Hemoglobin	12. 5 - 16. 0 gm%	
pH arterial	7. 35 - 7. 45	7. 4
PCO_2	34 - 45 mmHg	40 mmHg
Total CO_2 (plasma)	23 - 33 mmol	28 mmol
Bicarbonate (plasma)	22. 8 - 27. 5 mEq/L	24 mEq/L
Buffer base (whole blood)	43 - 47 mEq/L	
Base excess	-2. 5 - +2. 5 mEq/L	

Acid-Base Balance: (II) Effect of alterations in CO_2 and HCO_3^- on acid-base equilibrium.

PCO_2		Metabolic Acidosis / Respiratory Acidosis	Respiratory Acidosis	Metabolic Acidosis / Respiratory Acidosis
Increase ↑ Normal ↓ Decrease		Metabolic Acidosis	Normal	Metabolic Alkalosis
		Metabolic Acidosis / Respiratory Alkalosis	Respiratory Alkalosis	Metabolic Alkalosis / Respiratory Alkalosis

Normal

Below ←——————— HCO_3^- ———————→ Above

ACID-BASE BALANCE: A general term for the way in which the body maintains its hydrogen ion concentration (pH) despite the constant production of cationic end products by metabolic processes. The acid-base status is ensured in three major ways: (1) maintenance of a large buffering capacity, (2) manipulation of the volatile acid (carbonic acid), and (3) elimination of excess acid or base (over a period of a few days) by the kidneys. See Fig. See Acidemia, Alkalemia, Buffer, Buffer base, Carbon dioxide transport, Henderson-Hasselbalch equation, Metabolic acidosis, Metabolic alkalosis.

ACID-BASE COMPENSATION: The adaptive response made by the body to adjust to a primary disturbance in acid-base equilibrium. A primary disturbance is a change from the normal caused by a nonphysiologic or pathologic process which precedes any body adaptation to the disturbance. The initial rapid response is due to changes in ventilation which alter $PaCO_2$ (the secondary disturbance) so as to return hydrogen ion concentration to normal. For example, in the patient with metabolic acidosis, ventilation increases allowing the CO_2 to be exhaled and arterial pH to return to normal. The slower response, completed in a number of days, occurs when the kidney either excretes more acid or conserves more bicarbonate to oppose the primary disorder. See Acid-base balance, Henderson-Hasselbalch equation, Metabolic acidosis, Metabolic alkalosis.

ACID CITRATE DEXTROSE ANTICOAGULANT: See Blood storage, Blood types.

ACIDEMIA: A condition existing when the arterial blood pH is less than 7. 35 or hydrogen ion concentration is above the normal range of 35-45 nEq/L.

ACIDOSIS: A physiologic condition which would cause acidemia (pH < 7. 35) if not compensated by respiratory or metabolic changes. See Acid-base balance, Metabolic acidosis, Respiratory acidosis.

ACRYLIC CEMENT: See Methylmethacrylate.

ACTION POTENTIAL (SPIKE POTENTIAL): A change in the electric state of a nerve membrane (the critical part of nerve impulse transmission). During the action potential, the polarity of the inside of the nerve membrane (relative to the outside) changes from approximately -60 mV to approximately +40 mV because of an influx of sodium ions. The electric change of the membrane from negative to positive is referred to as depolarization. Repolarization occurs when the sodium is transferred back to the outside of the membrane. Large nerve fibers can depolarize and repolarize at a rate of 1000 times/sec. See Fig.

ACTIVATED CHARCOAL: A material which is nearly pure amorphous carbon. Its unique properties are due to its incredible internal surface area. Depending on its method of manufacture and the source from which it comes (which can range from petroleum and coal to peach pits and coconut shells). it can be designed to trap molecules of a particular size. Canisters of activated charcoal are commonly used to remove halogenated hydrocarbons from operating room air. The binding of material to activated charcoal can, to a certain extent, be reversed by heating.

ACTIVATED CLOTTING TIME (ACT): A blood test to determine the adequacy of heparinization for cardiopulmonary bypass patients. A blood sample is drawn into a special test tube that contains a magnet. The tube is then placed in an incubator-timer device, such as Hemachron (International Technidyne Corporation), where it is warmed. The time is noted from the start of the drawing of the blood sample until the machine detects changes in position of the magnet as it is moved by fibrin strand formation. With proper heparinization the ACT should approach infinity.

ACTOMYOSIN: The combination of actin and myosin, two proteins found in muscle cells. It is the longitudinal shortening of these two proteins as they interdigitate with each other which is responsible for muscle contraction. See Fig.

ACTUAL BICARBONATE: See Carbon dioxide total in blood.

6

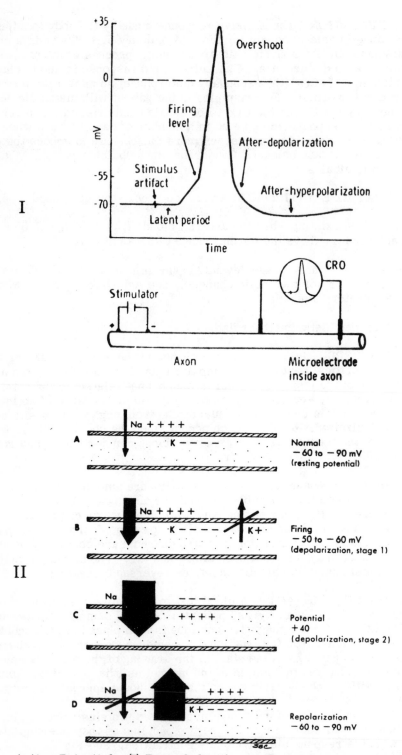

I

II

Action Potential: (I) Recorded with one electrode inside and one electrode outside the cell membrane. (II) Ionic shifts across the cell membrane which cause changes in electric potential.

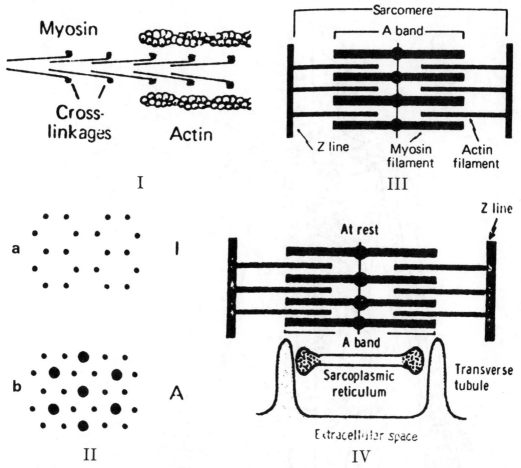

Actomyosin: (I) Arrangement of actin and myosin filaments in skeletal muscle. (IIa) Cross-section through the I band. (IIb) Cross-section through the lateral portion of the A band. (III) Detailed structure of myosin and actin. (IV) Muscle contraction Ca^{2+} ions (black dots) are normally stored in the cisterns of the sarcoplasmic reticulum. The action potential spreads via the transverse tubules and releases Ca^{2+}. The actin filaments slide on the myosin filaments and the Z lines move closer together. Ca^{2+} is then pumped into the sarcoplasmic reticulum and the muscle relaxes.

ACUPUNCTURE: The ancient Chinese system of medical therapy based on stimulation of the skin at previously designated points, usually by needles, to treat disease. It has generated considerable enthusiasm recently as a means of anesthesia. Widely conflicting claims for efficacy and effectiveness have been voiced. Some evidence exists that the effects of acupuncture are caused by central nervous system release of endorphins. See Fig.

ACUTE INTERMITTENT PORPHYRIA: See Porphyria.

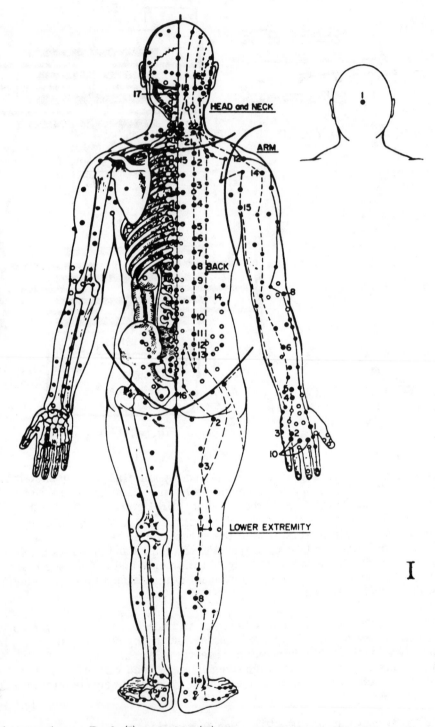

Acupuncture: Back (I) and side (II) views of the body showing various points for the application of acupuncture. (Index of selected points shown on page 10.)

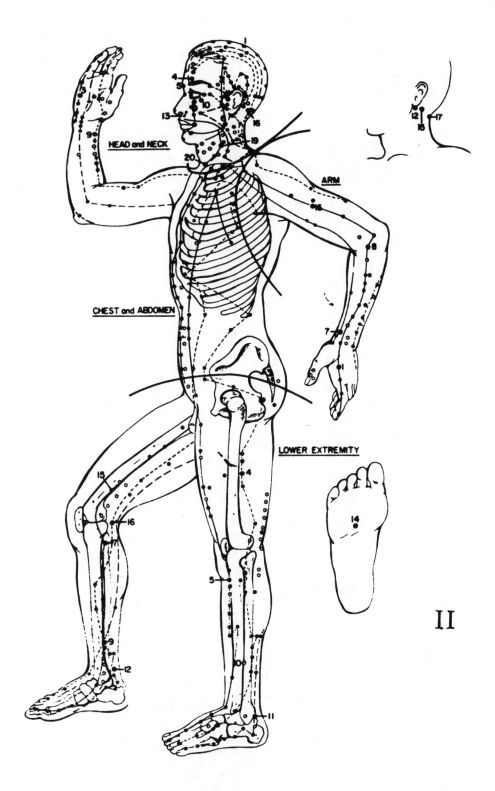

HEAD and NECK

ARM

CHEST and ABDOMEN

LOWER EXTREMITY

II

Head and Neck

1. Vertex — hyakue, pai hui (GV20)
2. Supraorbital — yohaku, yang-pei (GB14)
3. Temporal — taiyo, tai-yang
4. Mid-eyebrow — bichiyu, chien
5. Glabella — Indo, yin-tang
6. Inferior Masseter — kyoshiya, chia-che (S3)
7. Infratemporal — Gekan, hsia-kuan (S2)
8. Median canthus — seimei, chang-ming (B1)
9. Midinfraorbital — shiyokyu, cheng-chi (S4)
10. Lateral infraorbital — kyugo, chiu-hon
11. Superior tragus — jimon, erh-men (T21)
12. Posterior earlobe — eifu, I-feng (T17)
13. Infranasal — jinchiyu, jen-chung (L1)
14. Lateral oral angle — chiso, ti-ts'ang (S7)
15. Inframastoid — Imei I-mong
16. High lateral trapezius — Fuchi, fengs-chi (GB31)
17. C1-C2 — Amon, ya-men (GV15)
18. Para C1-C2 — Tenchyu, tien-chu (B10)
19. Lateral thyroid — jingei jen-ying (S9)
20. Supra Sternal — tentotsu, t'ien-t'u (CV22)
21. C7-T1 — Daizui, ta-ch'ui (GV14)
22. Para C7-T1 — Chizen

Chest and Abdomen

1. Midsternum — danchyu, shan-chung (CV17)
2. Subxyphoid — кyubi chiu-wei (CV15)
3. Sub Breast — nyukon, Ju-keng (S18)
4. Midepigastrium — chyukan, chung-wuan (CV12)
5. Lateral umbilicus — tensu, t'ien-shu (S25)
6. Upper hypogastrium — kikai, chi-hai (CV)
7. Low hypogastrium — kangen, kuan-yuan (CV4)
8. Lower hypogastrium — chyu kyoku, chung-chi (CV3)
9. Suprapubic — kyoku kotsu chu-ku (CV2)
10. Lateral inguinal — Iho

Back

1. para T2-T3 — fumon, feng-men (B12)
2. para T3-T4 (lung) — haiyu, fei-yu (B13)
3. para T5-T6 (heart) — shinyu, hsin-yu (B16)
4. para T7-T8 (diaphragm) — kakuyu, ke-yu (B17)
5. para T9-T10 (liver) — kanyu, kenye (B18)
6. para T10-T11 (gallbladder) — tanyu, tanyu (B19)
7. para T11-T12 (spleen) — hiyu, p'i-yu (B20)
8. para T12-L1 (stomach) — Iyu, wei-yu (B21)
9. para L2-L3 (kidney) — jinyu, shen-yu (B23)
10. para L4-L5 (colon) — daichyoyu, ta-chang-yu (B25)
11. para L5-S1 — Kangenyu kuan-yuan-yu (B26)
12. para S1-S2 (small bowel) — shyochyoyu, hsiao-ch'ang-yu (B27)
13. para S2-S3 (bladder) — bokoyu, p'ang-k'uang-yu (B28)
14. Lateral L2-L3 — shishitsu chih-shih (B47)
15. T3-T4 — mumei
16. Posterior anal — chyokyo, ch'ang-ch'iang (GV1)

Upper Extremities

1. First dorsal web — gokoku, ho-ku (L14)
2. Fourth dorsal web — chyushyo, chung-chu (T3)
3. Fifth lateral metacarpal — kokei, hou-chi (SI3)
4. Dorsal distal forearm — gaikan, waikuan (T5)
5. Dorsal low forearm — shiko, chih-kou (T6)
6. Dorsal upper forearm — shitoku szu-tu (T9)
7. Radial styloid process — letsuketsu, lieh-ch'uen (L7)
8. Lateral cubital crease — kyokuchi, chu-ch'ih (LI11)
9. Volar distal forearm — naikan, neikuan (P6)
10. Inter M.P. joint — hachija, pa-hsieh
11. Finger tip — jissen, shih-hsuan

Acupuncture: Index of selected points.

ACUTE LABORATORY: A laboratory (operating room, blood gas, intensive care) usually staffed around-the-clock to deliver accurate quantitative evaluations of patient samples in a time which is only slightly longer than the analysis apparatus cycle time and the administrative bookkeeping time combined. Reasonable objectives of an acute laboratory are the determinations of blood gases, serum electrolytes, ionized calcium, serum glucose, fluid osmotic pressures, hemoglobin, and hematocrit. As an example, semiautomated analyzers for blood gas measurement usually cycle in 2 or 3 min. Therefore, an acute laboratory can reasonably be expected to report on every blood gas specimen received in under 5 min.

ACUTE TOXIC ENCEPHALOPATHY: See Reye syndrome.

ADAPTATION: See Nociceptor.

ADAPTOR: A specialized form of connector joining two or more components which are otherwise physically incompatible.

ADDICTION: A pattern of behavior characterized by compulsive and undeniable use of a drug by self-administration for pharmacologically, physically, or socially unacceptable reasons.

ADDISON ANEMIA: See Anemia.

ADENOHYPOPHYSIS: See Hormone.

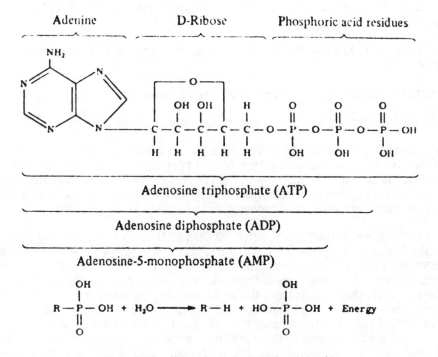

Hydrolysis of energy-rich phosphate bonds

Adenosine Triphosphate: Adenosine triphosphate, its subunits, and the basic chemical reaction for energy release.

ADENOSINE TRIPHOSPHATE (ATP): A ubiquitous, labile compound, present in all cells of the body, which provides energy for many of the body's biochemical reactions. ATP can function as an energy transfer molecule because the two phosphate molecules of ATP are joined to adenosine monophosphate by "high-energy bonds," i.e., making or breaking this molecular bonding requires a large amount of energy, in this case 8000 cal. See Fig.

ADENYL CYCLASE: An enzyme activated in many combinations of hormone and receptor sites which in turn causes the conversion of cytoplasmic adenosine triphosphate (ATP) into cyclic 3',5'-adenosine monophosphate (cAMP). See Receptor/receptor site.

ADIABATIC: Occurring without loss or gain of heat. Anesthetically, adiabatic processes occur during the expansion and compression of a gas. In the adiabatic compression of a gas, no heat is added from the surroundings during compression. However, the temperature of the gas rises according to the following ratio: final temperature/initial pressure X final volume/initial volume. This relationship, which is seen in regulator accidents, occurs when high-pressure O_2 is admitted to a regulator which has been inadvertently oiled. The gas already in the regulator is compressed very rapidly in an adiabatic process. As it is compressed, its temperature rises, surpassing the ignition temperature of the oil, causing a fire which will then be O_2-fed.

ADRENAL CORTEX: See Corticosteroid.

ADRENALIN: The term used by the British Pharmacopoeia for epinephrine. See Epinephrine.

ADRENERGIC BLOCKING AGENT: See Autonomic nervous system, Receptor/receptor site.

ADRENERGIC DRUG: See Autonomic nervous system.

ADRENERGIC NERVOUS SYSTEM: See Autonomic nervous system.

ADRENOCORTICAL STEROIDS: The collective term for the steroid hormones synthesized and secreted by the adrenal cortex. (They are all derivatives of cholesterol.) The two classes of steroids are the corticosteroids (with 21 carbons, C_{21}) and the adrenal androgens (with 19 carbons, C_{19}). The corticosteroids are subclassified into mineralocorticoids and glucocorticoids. See Corticosteroid.

ADULT RESPIRATORY DISTRESS SYNDROME (ARDS): A symptom complex with many etiologies that is typified by severe hypoxia, increasing hypercapnia, interstitial infiltrates and edema, microemboli, alveolitis, and, as the disease progresses, frank filling of the alveoli with fluid and the appearance of alveolar hyaline membranes. Pathophysiologically, the most striking phenomenon observed is the severe reduction of lung compliance or "stiff lung," which is due to the interstitial infiltrates, filled alveoli, and an increase in absolute lung water. Stiff lung increases the work of breathing. The functional residual capacity progressively decreases, ventilation/perfusion mismatch increases, and alveolar dead space increases. Treatment is aimed toward immediate relief of the hypoxic condition, usually requires mechanical ventilation, and is often accompanied by positive-end expiratory pressure, while acid-base derangements caused by hypoxia and hypercapnia are brought under control. See Infant respiratory distress syndrome, Surfactant.

ADVERSE REACTION: A reaction which is not desired following administration of a drug.

AEROBIC: Requiring the presence of O_2 to exist or grow.

AEROBIC METABOLISM: The degradation of food molecules and subsequent energy production carried out in the presence of abundant O_2. From aerobic metabolism of glucose the body gains 38 ATP molecules/glucose molecule metabolized. The net efficiency of this reaction is 44% with 56% of the total energy available released as heat. The end products are CO_2 and H_2O. When O_2 is not available, many body tissues can continue some energy production via anaerobic metabolism.

AEROSOL: A suspension of discrete particles in air.

AFENTANYL: See Fentanyl.

AFFERENT: Going toward or moving toward the center. For example, afferent sensory nerves from the skin return information to the central nervous system. Afferent and efferent (going or moving away from the center) depend on the point of reference.

A FIBER: See Nerve fiber, anatomy and physiology of.

AFIBRINOGENEMIA: A marked deficiency in the blood fibrinogen levels, encountered most dramatically in disseminated intravascular coagulation. See Disseminated intravascular coagulation.

AFTERGLOW: See Persistance.

AFTERLOAD: A determinant of cardiac output. It represents the ventricular wall tension during ejection and is affected by impedance, left ventricular size and shape, wall thickness, stroke volume, and ejection rate. Afterload is related to myocardial O_2 consumption.

AGGLUTININ: See Blood types.

AGGLUTINOGEN: See Blood types.

AGONIST: A pharmacologic agent or physiologic product which causes a clearly defined biologic response. Its biologic effect is proportional to the number of receptor sites it occupies on the cells for which it is targeted.

AIR: The mixture of gases which make up the atmosphere in which life on Earth exists. For the purposes of anesthesia, three components of air are important: N_2 (which makes up 78.08% of air), O_2 (20.94%), and CO_2 (0.03%). The remainder of the gases which make up air are primarily argon, neon, helium, krypton, xenon, and radon in total amounts of less than 1%.

AIRCO, INCORPORATED: A large company with many subsidiaries, among which is the Ohio Medical Products Division. This subsidiary company is responsible for many medical products, including compressed gases, and is located in Madison, Wisconsin.

AIR EMBOLUS: The presence of air in the circulation. This is not a natural occurrence and is almost invariably seen, albeit rarely, in trauma cases and as a potential problem in certain surgical cases. It can occur in any procedure in which a negative intrathoracic pressure is communicated to the periphery by means of a large vein. The most common example occurs when the cervical veins are exposed during a sitting cervical laminectomy, and the negative pressure can draw air in from the atmosphere surrounding the surgical wound. This air will pass centrally very quickly to the right side of the heart. If the air volume is high enough, and it occupies the right atrium and/or the right ventricle and right outflow tract, it can completely block the right side of the heart, precipitating failure. It may, in other circumstances, pass out of the right side of the heart, get far into the periphery of the lungs, and cause a block by preventing blood flow to large segments of the lungs. In this situation, a severe ventilation/perfusion abnormality would result with possible disastrous consequences to the patient. Air can also traverse a patent foramen ovale and embolize to the systemic arteries.

AIR ENCEPHALOGRAPHY: A neuroradiologic technique in which the ventricles of the brain are outlined by the withdrawal of cerebrospinal fluid and the injection of air below the dura, usually by lumbar puncture. It is significant to anesthesiologists because, since the air can rarely be drawn out effectively, the residual volume of remaining air will grow appreciably if the patient is subjected to an anesthetic with N_2O. See Nitrous oxide.

AIR EQUIVALENT: A measurement of the efficiency of a material to absorb radiation expressed as the thickness of the layer of air which causes the same amount of absorption.

AIR MONITORING: A type of air sampling for waste anesthetic gases in an operating room to determine leaks in the high-pressure gas supply side of the anesthesia machine. It is done when the room is empty and a long enough time has elapsed for N_2O to equilibrate in the room air. When functioning flowmeters on the low-pressure side of the machine are turned off, any N_2O that is detected is from the high-pressure side. This type of monitoring is most conveniently done in the morning just before surgery begins.

AIR PRODUCTS COMPANY: A worldwide chemical and related equipment manufacturer based in Allentown, Pennsylvania. It is one of the major suppliers of medical gases in the United States.

AIR SAMPLING: The intermittent or continuous monitoring of waste anesthestic vapors in the operating room. Considerations of air sampling include not only the type of instrument used to obtain the sample, but the timing of the sample, the location to be sampled, and the gas to be detected. The conventional procedure monitors the air within the breathing zone of the anesthetist sampling before, during, and after anesthetics are administered. An average inhaled concentration is obtained by continuous sample collection and storage in a gas-tight bag. Determination of the concentration of anesthetic vapor gives a "time-weighted average."

AIRWAY; AIRWAY MANAGEMENT: The maintenance of the functional integrity of the air passageways from their anatomic beginning in the nose and mouth through the multiple divisions of the pulmonary tree to the alveolus. In common usage, airway refers to only the upper airway, which ends at the trachea. Lost airway refers to the blockage of part of the anatomic air passageways. Maintenance of·an open airway is one of the most basic reflex responses. This reflex is severely attenuated by general anesthesia. See Cardiopulmonary resuscitation.

AIRWAY RESISTANCE: See Resistance, airway.

ALBUMIN: A serum protein produced by the liver; one of the major determinants of serum osmolarity. Normally the body contains about 5 g albumin/kg weight. It is available in various proprietary preparations, such as plasma protein precipitate, Plasmanate, or 25% albumin, and is used as a volume expander following blood loss. It is a human serum protein and therefore expensive. When appropriately heat-treated it does not transmit the hepatitis virus.

ALCOHOL: The oldest known sedative drug. Medical use includes intravenous administration to stop labor. It markedly potentiates all central nervous system depressants, especially the benzodiazepines.

ALCOHOL NEURITIS: The intense burning pain which occurs following incomplete destruction of a nerve by an injection of alcohol for neurolysis.

ALCURONIUM: A nondepolarizing, competitive muscle relaxant related to curare. See Neuromuscular blockade, assessment of; Neuromuscular blocking agent.

ALDACTONE: See Spironolactone.

ALDOMET: See Methyldopa.

Aldosterone.

ALDOSTERONE: A potent, naturally occurring steroid. It acts on the kidney and plays an important role in the regulation of sodium and potassium balance in the body. Aldosterone, a mineralocorticoid, is excreted by the adrenal cortex and acts to conserve sodium. Antialdosterone agents are often used in the control of hypertension. See Fig.

ALGESIMETER: A device used to measure a subject's sensitivity to pain produced by precise pricking with a sharp point.

ALGOGENIC SUBSTANCE: A substance which is released upon noxious stimulation of the skin or viscera and either excites or sensitizes nociceptors. Known algogenic substances include serotonin, bradykinin, and prostaglandin E.

ALGORITHM: A set of directions, rules, and procedures for solving a particular problem or accomplishing a particular process. For example, both the series of internal directions which would allow a blood gas machine to calculate base deficit from blood sample values and the series of steps used to deliver contaminated material to Central Sterilizing are algorithms.

ALKALEMIA: A condition of the blood in which the pH is greater than 7.44 or the hydrogen ion concentration is below the normal range of 36-44 nEq/L.

ALKALI RESERVE: A derived value for the buffering capacity of the blood which corresponds to actual bicarbonate. An archaic means of reporting acid-base status. See Carbon dioxide total in blood.

ALKALOSIS: A pathophysiologic condition which would cause alkalemia (pH > 7.44) if not compensated by respiratory or metabolic changes. See Acid-base balance, Metabolic alkalosis, Respiratory alkalosis.

ALLANDER AIR CURTAIN: A sophisticated high-technology operating room air filtration system. The Allander air curtain provides large flows of slowly moving air originating from vents in the ceiling over the operating table. The intent is to sweep contaminated particle-laden air down and away from the operative site. The return ducts for the air curtain are located low in the operating room walls. All recirculated air goes through a HEPA filter. Air is recirculated at a rate of 100-400 changes/filter. See HEPA filter.

ALLEN TEST: A clinical test performed at the wrist to determine the patency of the radial and ulnar arterial blood supply to the hand. The patient is asked to make a tight fist thereby expressing the blood from the hand. The examiner compresses the ulnar and radial arteries at the wrist and the patient then opens the hand. Compression is maintained on one vessel while the other is released. The procedure is repeated to test the second artery. If flow to the hand is shared by the radial and ulnar arteries, color should return to the palm and fingers in roughly equal time when supplied by one vessel only. If, however, one vessel dominates supply, the color will return only when this vessel is released, with the hand remaining white when the noncontributory vessel is released. This test is used to determine if artery catheterization at the wrist is likely to result in ischemia of the hand. As an example, if the Allen test shows that the ulnar artery does not significantly contribute to the blood supply of the hand, catheterization of the dominant radial artery at the wrist would have an increased risk of ischemic damage to the hand.

ALLERGEN: An agent which induces an allergic response.

ALLERGIC RESPONSE: An inappropriate, apparently self-destructive response to an innocuous stimulus to an organism. It can range from respiratory discomfort by contact with various pollens to respiratory and cardiovascular collapse in severe reactions to, for example, penicillin. Allergic responses are mediated in part through the immune system. See Allergen, Bradykinin, Histamine.

ALLODYNIA: The perception of pain when a nonnoxious stimulus is applied to normal skin.

ALL-OR-NONE LAW: A principle relating to the functioning of nervous tissue which states that there is no partial response to a stimulus. If the stimulus is strong enough, the nervous system responds with a maximum action potential or it does not respond at all. The similarity to binary systems (in which the signal state is either 1 or 0, positive or negative) is apparent.

ALLOSTERIC INHIBITION: The distortion of the three-dimensional configuration of the active sites of enzymes which causes them to function less than optimally. By nonspecifically binding close to the active sites on enzymes, anesthetic molecules may cause allosteric inhibition which may, in turn, be part of the mechanism of action of anesthetics.

ALLOY: A material which is not a pure element but which exhibits metallic properties. At least one major component of the alloy must be a metal. For example, amalgams are alloys which have the metal mercury as one component; steels are alloys of iron and carbon.

ALPHA BLOCKER: See Autonomic nervous system, Receptor/receptor site.

ALPHADOLONE: See Althesin.

ALPHA-ENDORPHIN: See Endorphins.

ALPHANUMERIC DISPLAY: A visual representation of letters and numbers on an electronic device. See Fig.

ALPHA PARTICLE: The nucleus of a helium atom containing two protons and two neutrons. A stream of alpha particles is called an alpha ray(s) and is the result of the breakdown processes of certain radioactive nuclei. Alpha particles are relatively large, can travel only a few centimeters in air, and can be stopped by such materials as paper or skin. They remain quite dangerous, however, because the stoppage of an alpha particle requires the transfer of a large amount of energy to the material stopping the particle. Alpha particles can pose a significant health hazard.

ALPHAPRODINE (NISENTIL): A meperidine-like narcotic used frequently in obstetrics for pain relief and as a substitute for meperidine or morphine in balanced anesthesia technique. It was formerly used in combination with a narcotic antagonist as a general anesthetic, with or without N_2O. See Narcotic.

ALPHA RECEPTOR: See Receptor/receptor site.

ALPHAXOLONE: See Althesin.

ALTERNATING PULSE: See Pulsus alternans.

ALTHESIN: A combination of two steroids, alphadolone and alphaxolone, administered as a short-acting intravenous anesthetic. It is a clear, colorless, isotonic solution of neutral pH. The drug is used clinically in England, but is available only for research purposes in the United States. It can cause anaphylactoid-type reactions. Cremophor El is the solvent for althesin which may, in part, be responsible for the severe allergic reactions.

ALUMINUM (Al): An element with an atomic weight of 26.97, a specific gravity of 2.70, and a melting point in excess of 658 degrees Celsius. It is resistant to corrosion and a number of chemicals. It can be attacked by alkalis and hydrochloric acid. After O_2 and silicon, it is the most abundant element. By various alloying processes it can be made into a material with good conductivity, about two-thirds that of copper, high tensile strength (on the order of 20,000 lb/in^2, and a good strength-to-weight ratio.

ALVEOLAR AIR, ALVEOLAR GAS: The percent contribution of the gases which make up the air filling the ideal alveolus at sea level. Of a total of 760 mmHg, the

18

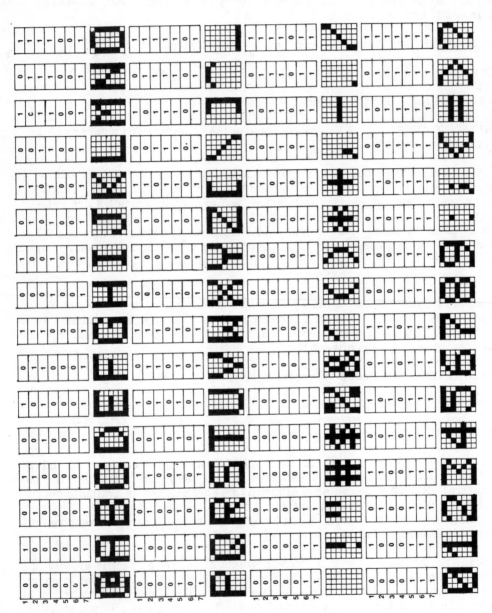

Alphanumeric Display: Elements of an alphanumeric display using a surface with five elements across and seven elements down (35 total) to present the alphabet, numbers, and some simple symbols. Along with each character is the binary code which commands the appropriate elements of the surface to be on or off to show that character.

partial pressure of N_2 is 563 mmHg, the partial pressure of water vapor at 100% humidity is 47 mmHg, and the PCO_2 (which can be assumed to be normal arterial CO_2 tension) is 40 mmHg. Subtracting these three values from a total of 760 mmHg leaves 110 mmHg as the alveolar O_2 tension. Alveolar O_2 tension, however, is exquisitely sensitive to ventilation/perfusion (V/Q) ratios. In one extreme situation, the V/Q abnormality known as shunt occurs when no gas exchange between alveolar gas and the blood takes place. Alveolar O_2 tension rises toward its inspired tension of 159 mmHg partial pressure (21% of 760). In the V/Q abnormality dead space (the other extreme), no ventilation of the affected alveoli takes place, and the gas in the alveoli ultimately comes into equilibrium with the blood flowing past it such that the PO_2 approaches 40 mmHg and the PCO_2 approaches 45 mmHg. See Absorption atelectasis, Alveolar air equation, Ventilation/perfusion abnormality.

ALVEOLAR AIR DIAGRAM (OXYGEN-CARBON DIOXIDE DIAGRAM; RAHN AND FENN DIAGRAM): A complex graphic representation of the interrelationship of O_2 saturation and CO_2 content which combines all of the O_2 and CO_2 dissociation curves. The former varies with the changing PCO_2 (Bohr effect) and the latter varies with the O_2 saturation (Haldane effect).

ALVEOLAR AIR EQUATION; ALVEOLAR GAS EQUATION; ALVEOLAR PARTIAL PRESSURE OF OXYGEN EQUATION: A mathematic method for determination of mean alveolar partial pressure of oxygen (PAO_2). The formula depends on knowing the partial pressure of oxygen inspired (PIO_2). It assumes that (1) the partial pressure of inspired carbon dioxide ($PICO_2$) is zero, (2) arterial partial pressure of carbon dioxide ($PaCO_2$) is a good representation of alveolar carbon dioxide partial pressure ($PACO_2$), (3) nitrogen partial pressure is not changed by ventilation since nitrogen is not metabolized and therefore is at a steady state, (4) the respiratory quotient R is either measured or can be assumed to be 0.8, and (5) the partial pressure of water vapor at 37 degrees Celsius and 47 mmHg is constant in the alveoli so that FIO_2 is 760 mmHg (at sea level) - 47 = 713 mmHg. Under these conditions,

$$PAO_2 = FIO_2\,(713) - PACO_2 \left[FIO_2 + \frac{1 - FIO_2}{R} \right]$$

The expression in brackets is a correction for R, since the volume of O_2 consumed per minute is greater than the volume of CO_2 produced.

ALVEOLAR-ARTERIAL CARBON DIOXIDE DIFFERENCE: The difference in CO_2 tension found in the alveolus vs. arterial blood. This difference is rarely greater than 1 mmHg, as CO_2 is rarely affected by V/Q abnormalities or diffusion block in the lung. See Alveolar end capillary difference.

ALVEOLAR-ARTERIAL OXYGEN DIFFERENCE (PAO_2 - PaO_2): A measurement in millimeters of mercury which describes the inequality between PaO_2 and PAO_2 in normal young individuals breathing room air. The PaO_2 is approximately 97 mmHg. At the same time, the normal average PAO_2 is about 101 mmHg. The difference between the two, approximately 4 mmHg, is known as the alveolar-arterial O_2 difference. The difference gets larger as age increases, reaching 20-25 torr in the elderly. The alveolar-arterial O_2 difference also increases with larger percentages of inspired O_2. The difference is explained by the fact that not all arterial blood has been exposed to the alveoli. See Alveolar air, alveolar gas; Alveolar air equation; Alveolar and capillary difference; Shunt; Ventilation/perfusion abnormality.

ALVEOLAR CELL TYPES: The five distinct cell types identified in normal alveoli. Type 1 pneumocytes are flattened, pavement-like cells. Type 2 pneumocytes are rounded cells which contain granules. They synthesize pulmonary surfactant, which is vital in decreasing the fluid tension at the fluid-air interface of the alveoli, thereby facilitating full expansion of the alveoli. The remaining types are brush cells, alveolar macrophages (foreign particle scavengers), and mast cells, which secrete heparin, histamine, and serotonin. Alveoli are lined by one cell layer of epithelium (septal cells) attached to a basement membrane which separates the alveoli from the underlying endothelial cells of the capillaries.

ALVEOLAR CONCENTRATION CURVE: A graphic display of the relationship between the fractional alveolar (F_A) and inspired (F_I) anesthetic concentration as a function of time. The approach of F_A to F_I varies inversely with blood solubility of the agent: the greater the solubility, the lower the alveolar concentration. The alveolar concentration, however, immediately rises regardless of the solubility. This is due to the fact that at the initiation of anesthesia, the alveolar concentration is zero and is low after the first several breaths. The difference between the alveolar to mixed venous anesthetic partial pressures is small and, therefore, does not allow for any significant uptake of the anesthetic agent. During the first 1-2 min, however, the alveolar concentration increases, which in turn increases the partial pressure difference allowing for increased uptake of the anesthetic depending on its solubility.

ALVEOLAR CONCENTRATION OF ANESTHETICS: The percentage of alveolar gas which is anesthetic vapor. The concentration of anesthetic vapor or gas in the alveolus depends on the following variables: concentration at which it is delivered, rate and depth of ventilation of the alveolus, and rate at which it diffuses across the alveolar membrane and enters the arterial blood. Since there is rarely a diffusion barrier preventing the passage of anesthetics into the blood, the last variable is based on the solubility of the agent in the blood. The more soluble the anesthetic agent, the greater the amount that will enter the blood in a fixed period of time without raising its partial pressure appreciably. The greater the amount entering the blood, the less left in the alveolus. The less left in the alveolus, the lower the alveolar tension, or concentration, of the agent. Paradoxically, then, highly soluble agents take much longer to induce anesthesia than poorly soluble agents. (Low alveolar partial pressure $\rightarrow$ low arterial partial pressure $\rightarrow$ low brain partial pressure $\rightarrow$ little anesthetic effect.)

ALVEOLAR DEAD SPACE: The volume of air within unperfused alveoli which does not take part in inspiratory exchange. This is of little significance in the healthy individual. See Anatomic dead space, Ventilation/perfusion abnormality.

ALVEOLAR DIFFUSION MEASUREMENT: See Diffusion.

ALVEOLAR END CAPILLARY DIFFERENCE: The potential difference between the partial pressures of gases in the alveolus and in the capillary exiting the alveolar capillary interspace. Under normal circumstances, the difference between the PO_2 of the alveolus and the PO_2 of the capillary is so small as to be undetectable. However, when diffusion is disrupted and the transfer of O_2 across the alveolar membrane is slowed, the PO_2 of the capillary blood may not reach the PO_2 of the alveolar gas in the time available for O_2 transfer. In this case, a diffusion block is said to exist. With CO_2, which is 20 times as diffusible as O_2, little diffusion block occurs, even under extreme circumstances. See Fig.

ALVEOLAR GAS EQUATION: See Alveolar air equation.

ALVEOLAR MACROPHAGE: See Alveolar cell types.

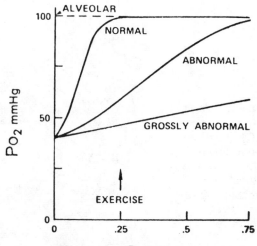

Time in Capillary – sec

Alveolar End Capillary Difference: Graph showing the effect of a barrier to O_2 transport across the alveolar membrane. The X axis is blood transit time in the capillary; the Y axis is capillary PO_2. Exercise lowers transit time to about 0.25 sec. If diffusion is normal then there is still enough time for capillary PO_2 to equilibrate with alveolar PO_2.

ALVEOLAR PARTIAL PRESSURE OF OXYGEN EQUATION (MEAN ALVEOLAR PAO_2): See Alveolar air equation, Respiratory exchange ratio.

ALVEOLAR PLATEAU: The period occurring during end expiratory N_2 analysis when N_2 content is nearly uniform. The gas measured at this time is considered pure alveolar gas. See Single breath test.

ALVEOLAR VENTILATION: The portion of tidal volume which reaches the alveoli and is involved in gas exchange in the lung. If alveolar ventilation is halved, the $PACO_2$ is doubled. See Alveolar dead space.

ALVEOLAR VESSELS: A network of capillaries traversing through lung septa that plays an integral role in diffusion of gases.

ALVEOLUS: The terminal air sac of the lung in which gas exchange occurs between alveolar air and pulmonary capillary blood. There are approximately 300 million alveoli in the healthy human lung. Approximately 0.3 mm in diameter, the alveoli have a combined surface area between 50 and 100 m^2. In any disease process which tends to destroy the septa between alveoli, the surface area becomes tremendously diminished. The alveolar wall separating blood from gas is less than 1 μm thick. See Fig. See Diffusion.

AMBU BAG: See Ambu resuscitator.

AMBU RESUSCITATOR (AMBU BAG): One brand of self-inflating bag for resuscitation purposes which has almost become a generic term. The bag is usually sold in combination with a nonrebreathing valve. In one modification an O_2 reservoir is added to the tail of the bag to increase inspired O_2 concentration. See Breathing bag.

Alveolus: Electron micrograph
showing the alveolus, pulmonary
capillary interface (C), erythrocyte (EC), alveolar epithelium
(EP), interstitium (IN), capillary
endothelium (EN), fibroblasts
(FB), basement membrane (BM),
and plasma. The long arrow
shows the diffusion path for O_2.

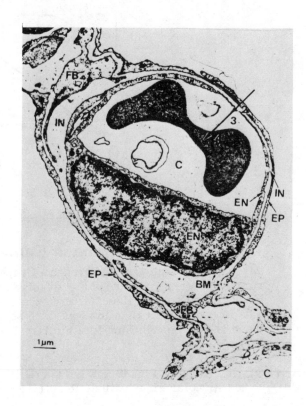

AMBU VALVE: See Nonrebreathing valve.

AMERICAN ASSOCIATION OF NURSE ANESTHETISTS (AANA): A professional organization founded in 1931, with a membership of over 19,000 registered nurses
(RNs) who have received between 1 and 2 years of post-RN training in the administration of anesthesia and who have passed a nationally administered qualifying examination. RNs who have met these qualifications are designated as Certified Registered Nurse Anesthetists (CRNA). Nurse anesthetist training programs are at
least 18 months long and may last up to 27 months. There are some schools which
grant a bachelor's or master's degree in addition to the certificate in anesthesia.

AMERICAN BOARD OF ANESTHESIOLOGY (ABA): The certifying board for specialists in anesthesiology. Originally (1937) an affiliate of the American Board of Surgery, the advisory board for medical specialties of the American Medical Association (AMA) approved the establishment of the ABA as a separate major board in
1941. Individuals who are certified by the ABA are designated as diplomates in anesthesiology. Certification is established by passing the board examination to become a diplomate but the requirements also include 12 months of post-MD/DO clinical training in an area other than anesthesiology and 24 months of training in clinical anesthesia. The applicant must then complete a specialized year, devoted to research and/or advanced clinical practice, as a fellow. Prior to 1985, in lieu of
this specialized year the candidate must have substituted 2 years of practice in
the field of anesthesiology. Eligible candidates must pass a written examination
which qualifies them to take an oral examination. As of early 1982, the ABA has
certified approximately 10,000 diplomates.

AMERICAN DENTAL SOCIETY OF ANESTHESIOLOGY: An organization with the purpose of bringing together dentists in the United States who are especially interested in anesthesiology. The organization, which furthers research in dental anesthesia and pain control, is based in Chicago.

AMERICAN MEDICAL ASSOCIATION (AMA): A national organization, founded in Philadelphia in 1847, which represents the medical profession. The AMA acknowledges Dr. Nathan Smith Davis as its founder because of his early work in organizing the association. Currently, the AMA has approximately 226,000 members from the approximately 440,000 physicians in the United States.

AMERICAN NATIONAL STANDARDS INSTITUTE (ANSI): An organization which evolved from the merger in 1918 of five leading engineering societies with segments of the Departments of War, Navy, and Commerce. It provides a voluntary unit for coordinating the development of engineering and related standards. (ANSI has developed extensive standards for anesthesia equipment.) Based in New York City, it comprises the nation's trade, technical, professional, consumer, and labor groups, and is a private, nonprofit organization which operates in the public interest and in close cooperation with the federal government.

AMERICAN SOCIETY OF ANESTHESIOLOGISTS (ASA): The national organization which represents anesthesia and traces its origins to the Long Island Society of Anesthetists formed in 1905. It became the New York Society of Anesthetists in 1911. The number of regional societies of anesthesia continued to multiply until December 1936 when the American Society of Anesthetists, representing a nationwide constituency, was organized. In 1945 the American Society of Anesthetists became the American Society of Anesthesiologists. The ASA began the 1980s with over 17,000 members and is the sixth largest specialty group in American medicine. It is based in Chicago.

AMERICAN SOCIETY OF DENTAL ANESTHESIOLOGISTS: An organization comprising dentists who have had at least 2 years of training in clinical anesthesia from an accredited anesthesia program. Formed in 1980, it is based in San Bernardino, California.

AMERICAN STANDARD COMPRESSED GAS CYLINDER VALVE OUTLET CONNECTIONS: A safety system which applies to large gas cylinders, i.e., sizes F, M, G, H, and K. Since tanks of these sizes do not use yokes and connections are made by direct piping to their valves, the gas cylinder valve outlet connections are made in 12 different combinations of diameter and number of threads per inch. The threads can vary, being right-handed or left-handed and internal or external. This safety system is used between the valves of the cylinder and the regulator; the Diameter Index Safety System (DISS) is used on the low-pressure side of the regulator. Although these systems all rely, in part, on differences in threading, they cannot be interchanged.

AMETHOCAINE: An alternate name for the local anesthetic tetracaine. See Tetracaine.

AMICAR: See E-Aminocaproic acid.

AMIDONE: See Methadone.

AMIGEN: A brand name for preparations of protein hydrolysates (a sterile solution of amino acids and short-chain polypeptides) for parenteral feeding (hyperalimentation), administered through a large central vein. Amigen is commonly used in the postoperative period when patient nutrition is hampered due to inability to feed orally. It is physically incompatible with many other drugs and solutions. Other brand names are Aminosyn and Travasol.

AMIKACIN (AMIKIN): A semisynthetic aminoglycosidic antibiotic related to streptomycin. It is used for serious gram-negative infections. It may be implicated in enhancing neuromuscular blockade.

AMINO ACID SOLUTIONS: See Amigen.

E-AMINOCAPROIC ACID (AMICAR): A drug used to inhibit plasminogen activators and plasmin. It is helpful in treating bleeding disorders in which hemorrhage occurs due to premature lysis of clots. See Disseminated intravascular coagulation, Hemorrhage, Primary fibrinolysis.

AMINOGLYCOSIDES: A class of antimicrobial antibiotic agents primarily used to treat gram-negative infections. In addition to the class leader, streptomycin, neomycin, gentamicin, kanamycin, tobramycin, amikacin, and paromomycin are useful aminoglycosidic agents. Adverse side effects include significant ototoxicity and nephrotoxicity. See Fig. See Antibiotic, Streptomycin.

AMINOPHYLLINE: A soluble salt of the xanthine compound theophylline. Its major effect is the relaxation of bronchial smooth muscle and stimulation of the myocardium. It is used in anesthesia primarily to treat bronchial constriction.

AMITRIPTYLINE: See Tricyclic antidepressant.

AMNIOTIC FLUID EMBOLISM: A catastrophic event in which amniotic fluid enters the maternal circulation. It involves the rupture of the membranes or a tear at the placental margin. The syndrome produced by this condition is a combination of mechanical blocking of the pulmonary vessels by the particulate matter in the amniotic fluid and an anaphylactic reaction to the foreign substances in the fluid. There is a sudden decrease in blood return to the heart, a sharp rise in pulmonary vascular resistance, and marked (to extreme) ventilation abnormalities. Part of the syndrome may be caused by the high concentration of various prostaglandins in the amniotic fluid. Aside from the immediate cardiovascular problems, amniotic fluid embolism can lead to extreme cases of disseminated intravascular coagulation. Amniotic fluid embolism is fatal in approximately 50% of cases. See Disseminated intravascular coagulation.

AMOBARBITAL: See Barbiturate.

AMPERE (AMP, A): A unit of electric current in the standard international (SI) system. It defines 1 amp as that current maintained in two parallel conductors, 1 m apart in a vacuum and of negligible cross-section, which will produce between the conductors a force equal to 2×10^{-7} newton/m of length. An older and approximately equivalent definition of ampere is a current of 6.25×10^{18} electrons/sec past a single point in a circuit or 1 ampere = 1 coulomb/sec.

Aminoglycosides.

Generic Name (Trade Name)	Spectrum of Activity	Comments
Streptomycin SO₄ IM	Fairly broad spectrum of activity. It is used in the treatment of tuberculosis and infections caused by G⁻ microbes, including tularemia and bubonic plague.	Streptomycin, like all the aminoglycosides, is generally bactericidal in action, especially in larger doses. It is most notably effective against G⁻ rods. Side effects include ototoxicity, a generally reversible nephrotoxicity, and, rarely, neuromuscular blockade which can lead to respiratory paralysis. This blockade is most likely to occur if an aminoglycoside is given soon after the administration of general anesthesia or of neuromuscular blocking agents. Streptomycin can also cause allergic reactions, eosinophilia, and optic nerve dysfunction. Rapid bacterial resistance occurs.
Kanamycin (Kantrex) IM IV PO	Fairly broad spectrum. It is used in the treatment of infections caused by G⁻ microbes. Pseudomonas is not sensitive to kanamycin.	Kanamycin is related to streptomycin but resistance is slower to develop. It is ototoxic, nephrotoxic, and can cause eosinophilia as well as neuromuscular blockade.
Gentamicin (Garamycin) IM Topical	Broad spectrum. It is the drug of choice for many serious G⁻ bacillus infections. Effective against many Pseudomonas species.	Gentamicin is ototoxic, though this is mostly vestibular as opposed to auditory. It can also produce neuromuscular blockade, GI upset, headache, proteinuria, acute renal insufficiency, and tubular necrosis.

26

Aminoglycosides (continued)

Generic Name (Trade Name)	Spectrum of Activity	Comments
Tobramycin (Nebcin) IM IV	Closely related to gentamicin and effective against Pseudomonas.	Side effects similar to gentamicin.
Amikacin (Amikin) IM IV	Similar to gentamicin.	Side effects similar to gentamicin.
Neomycin (Neosporin) IM Topical	Broad spectrum.	The toxic effects of neomycin include nerve deafness, renal damage, and possible neuromuscular blockade.

AMPHETAMINE: A class of powerful central nervous system drugs which stimulate alpha and beta receptors peripherally. They have been used orally as antidepressants and fatigue suppressants. Parenterally, they have been used acutely in hypotensive crisis. Because of their severe abuse potential the amphetamines have fallen into disfavor. Preoperatively, **chronic** abusers of amphetamines and amphetamine-like compounds may exhibit disordered thinking, inappropriate behavior, and extreme wasting due to an appetite suppression effect. They are prone to possible cardiovascular collapse under anesthesia.

AMPLIFIER: A device which takes an input signal such as light, sound, or current flow and outputs it higher in magnitude. This is usually accomplished by using the variations in the input signal to control the variations in the output signal. In physical terms, the input signal can be viewed as the control function on a floodgate or a stream. A strong input raises the gate and the stream output rises. The reverse also occurs. Changes in the stream flow exactly mirror changes in the gate position. This term is most often used in relation to electric or electronic systems. See Operational amplifier.

AMPLIFIER, CLASS A, CLASS AB, CLASS B, CLASS C, CLASS D: A designation concerning the way amplifiers operate. A class A amplifier is relatively inefficient but has a very low degree of distortion. A class D amplifier is efficient but greatly distorts the input signal. An inverse relationship exists between efficiency and distortion throughout the series. Expensive high-fidelity systems tend toward class A operation. They reproduce the signal correctly but use a lot of power in doing so. Telephones tend toward class D operation, giving only fair voice duplication but using little power.

AMYGDALA: A bilateral ovoid mass of gray matter located in the anterior part of the temporal lobes of the brain. In humans, it appears to be associated with the more violent emotions.

AMYOTROPHIC LATERAL SCLEROSIS (ALS): A motor neuron disease characterized by progressive muscle weakness and wasting due to the degeneration of corticospinal tract neurons and brain stem and spinal cord anterior horn motor cells. ALS affects twice as many males as females with the peak incidence between 50 and 60 years of age. Death usually occurs within 5 years. ALS patients may exhibit an exaggerated response to nondepolarizing muscle relaxants and they may become hyperkalemic when depolarizing muscle relaxants are administered. Variants of ALS are progressive spinal muscular atrophy, a less severe disease with much longer survival, and progressive bulbar palsy, a more severe disease which affects the muscles innervated by the cranial nerves and corticobulbar tracts. Death occurs within 3 years and is frequently due to respiratory problems.

AMYTAL: See Barbiturate.

ANACROTIC NOTCH: A notch in the ascending limb of the pulse-pressure tracing usually only seen if the sample site is close to the aortic valve. It is believed to represent the junction of the pulse-pressure wave with the slower but larger fluid movement wave. See Pulse-pressure tracing.

ANAEROBIC: Having the capacity to exist or grow with little or no O_2.

ANAEROBIC METABOLISM: The degradation of and energy production from food molecules without the presence of O_2. This type of metabolism is very low in recoverable (non-heat-producing) energy because it only forms two molecules of ATP/ molecule of glucose. The end products of anaerobic glucose metabolism are pyruvic acid and hydrogen ions. These two products combine to form lactic acid, which can be reconverted to glucose or directly used for energy when O_2 is again available. The brain has a very limited ability to function anaerobically. The heart has essentially no anaerobic capacity, but it can directly use lactic acid for energy very efficiently. This mechanism provides a margin of safety for the heart during heavy exercise. See Aerobic metabolism.

ANALEPTIC: A drug or agent which acts to increase central nervous system activity. See Pentylenetetrazol.

ANALOG: A physical variable representing either a physiologic parameter or a numeric value. A thermometer filled with mercury is an analog device in that temperature is represented by the expansion of the volume of mercury along a scale.

ANALOG COMPUTER: A fundamental computer class which operates on the principle that both input and output are continuously changing quantities. This is distinct from the digital computer, which represents each input as a number and then manipulates the number by the rules of mathematics. In the analog computer, problem variables are translated into equivalent electric or mechanical circuits as analogs for the physical phenomena under investigation.

ANALOG-TO-DIGITAL CONVERTER (ANALOG-TO-DIGITAL CONVERSION): A device designed to take a continuous quantity or value and convert it into a discrete quantity or value. It is most frequently used in medicine to convert physiologic data (e.g., heart rate, blood pressure) into discrete binary numbers for use on a digital computer. See Binary code.

ANASARCA: See Edema.

ANATOMIC DEAD SPACE (V_D): The portions of the respiratory tract (from the nose and mouth to the terminal bronchioles) which do not participate in gas exchange and in which two-way flow exists. In healthy individuals, anatomic dead space usually is calculated as 2 ml/kg. A 70-kg man has a dead space of 140 ml/tidal volume under normal conditions. See Alveolar dead space, Physiologic dead space, Ventilation/perfusion abnormality.

ANATOMIC SHUNT: See Shunt.

ANECTINE: See Succinylcholine.

ANEMIA: A condition in which there is a reduction, below normal, in the number of circulating erythrocytes and/or in the quantity of hemoglobin. Anemias may be classified on the basis of etiology: (1) excessive blood loss, (2) deficient red cell production (erythropoiesis or bone marrow inhibition), (3) excessive red cell destruction, and (4) decreased production together with increased destruction of red cells. Anemias can be acquired or congenital. Thalassemia (Cooley, Mediterranean) is a congenital type in which there is a decreased rate of production of one polypeptide chain of hemoglobin. In pernicious anemia (Addison anemia), a type of anemia with a strong familial component, there is a lack of secretion of intrinsic factor, a constituent of normal gastric juice. This condition does not allow for normal absorption of vitamin B_{12} which is vital for normal red cell formation. An example of acquired anemia is hemolytic anemia, a progressive, often rapid, destruction of red cells which can be a catastrophic consequence of mismatched blood transfusion or a result of various poisons or toxins.

ANEMOMETER, HOT-WIRE (HOT-WIRE RESPIROMETER): A device for measuring the volume of moving gas. It works by the following principle. The wire is placed in an airstream. A constant voltage is applied across the ends of the wire. With no movement of the airstream, a known current flows through the wire (depending on its resistance) and heats the wire to a known temperature. The continuous heating of the wire is balanced by heat transfer from the wire to the nonmoving air around it. As the air around the wire begins to move, its ability to cool the wire rises in proportion to its velocity past the wire. Within reasonable limits, the drop in temperature of the wire can be read as air velocity. Alternately, the change in electric resistance of the wire, which occurs as it cools, can also be interpreted the same way.

ANEROID: Functioning without a fluid. An aneroid gauge for measuring blood pressure does not contain mercury.

ANESTHESIA, AWARENESS DURING (RECALL): The phenomenon of a patient who has undergone a general anesthetic recalling single or multiple events occurring during anesthesia. Several reports have indicated that the problem of recall is increased in N_2O/O_2/narcotic relaxant techniques. Although careful evaluation can usually show some incidence of recall irrespective of the general anesthetic technique, most studies show recall to be on the order of 1-2%. Dreams, hallucinations, and unpleasant sensations connected with the anesthetic period have been reported to occur 2-20% of the time, depending on the situation and the anesthetic technique employed. Anecdotal reports exist of patients who were assumed anesthetized but were actually paralyzed and awake during a prolonged surgical procedure. They suffered for hours from the pain of the operation but were totally incapable of doing anything about it and subsequently became mentally disturbed. These reports are difficult to verify.

ANESTHESIA CHART: A record of anesthesia that is ongoing, on-line, and in "real time." Harvey Cushing, the famed neurosurgeon, and Ernest Amory Codman, a surgeon, are credited with introducing the first record of the vital signs, pulse and respiratory rate, during anesthesia while they were still sophomore medical students at Harvard in the early 1890s. The modern anesthesia chart records not only vital signs, but also a description of induction procedures, gas flows as necessary, and all other monitored modalities. A number of attempts have been made through the years to automate this charting procedure. It is interesting to note that anesthesia is one of the few areas of personal service in which the practitioner is expected to write up his or her work and perform it simultaneously. See Fig.

ANESTHESIA CIRCUIT FILTER: A passive device which filters any particulate matter (e.g., bacteria, dust) circulating within the breathing circuit.

ANESTHESIA DOLOROSA: A pain sensation in an area of the body known to be anesthetized.

ANESTHESIA FOUNDATION: An organization dedicated to the advancement of anesthesiology. Established under the sponsorship of the American Society of Anesthesiologists in 1956, it is a nonprofit foundation that uses its available funds to provide financial assistance to needy anesthesiology residents. It promotes programs to encourage medical students and young physicians to consider a career as an an-

30

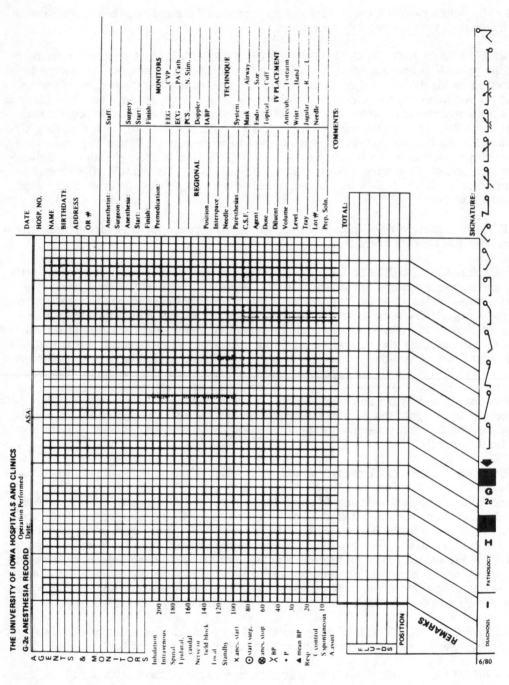

Anesthesia Chart: Anesthesia chart used at The University of Iowa Hospitals and Clinics (front view).

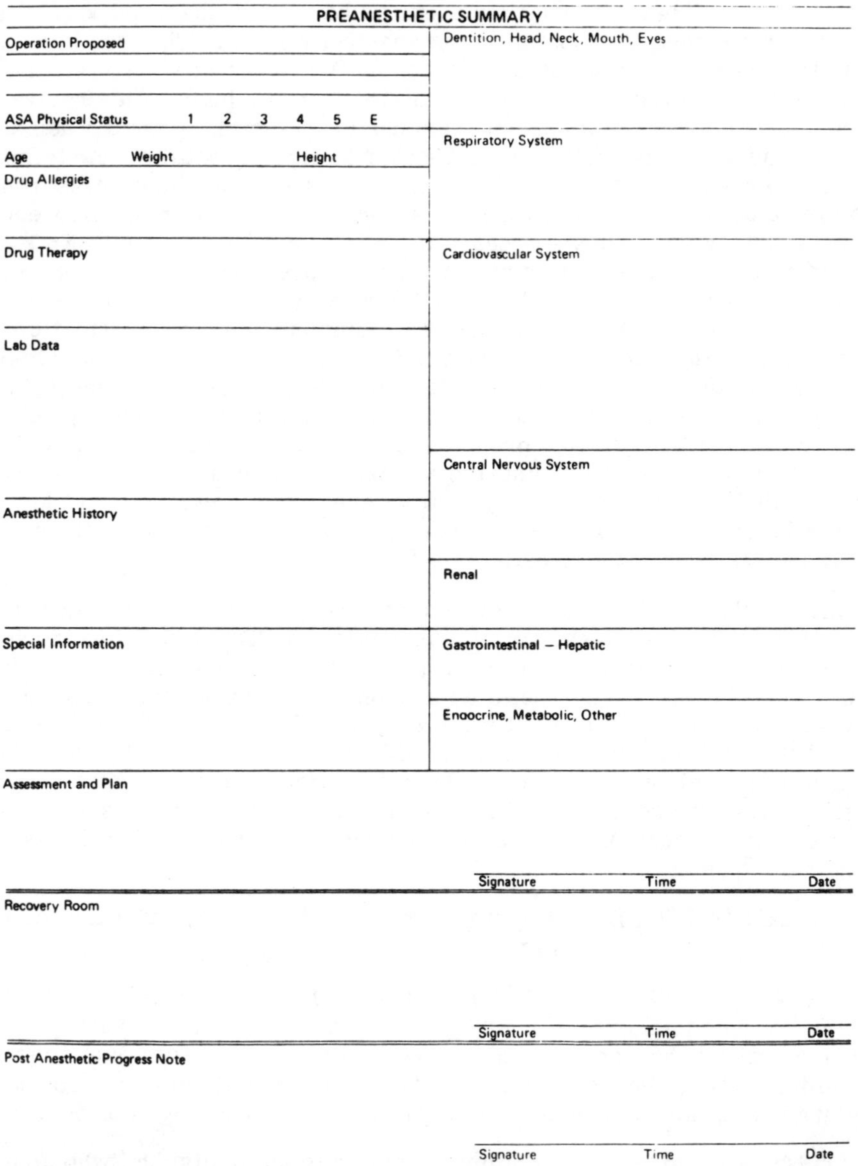

PREANESTHETIC SUMMARY

Operation Proposed	Dentition, Head, Neck, Mouth, Eyes
ASA Physical Status 1 2 3 4 5 E	Respiratory System
Age Weight Height Drug Allergies	
Drug Therapy	Cardiovascular System
Lab Data	
	Central Nervous System
Anesthetic History	
	Renal
Special Information	Gastrointestinal — Hepatic
	Endocrine, Metabolic, Other

Assessment and Plan

Signature	Time	Date

Recovery Room

Signature	Time	Date

Post Anesthetic Progress Note

Signature	Time	Date

Anesthesia Chart: Anesthesia chart used at The University of Iowa Hospitals and Clinics (back view).

esthesiologist. It also supports educational programs and research related to anesthesiology and preserves and recognizes the American heritage of anesthesiology.

ANESTHESIA, GENERAL (COMPONENTS OF): See General anesthesia.

ANESTHESIA MACHINE, CONTINUOUS FLOW: See Continuous flow anesthesia machine.

ANESTHESIA, PRESSURE REVERSAL OF: An unusual phenomenon, discovered in the laboratory, which may give insight into the mechanism of action of anesthetics.

As a generality, very high hydrostatic pressures have been observed to increase the amount of anesthetic needed to maintain the anesthetic state. This has been demonstrated on tadpoles immobilized by ethyl alcohol. When the pressure is raised high enough, on the order of tens to hundreds of atmospheres, the tadpoles revive and begin to swim about. The same phenomenon has been shown on newts when anesthetized by halothane or pentobarbitol and subjected to high pressures. A striking demonstration of the pressure reversal of anesthesia is seen when high pressures reverse anesthetic depression of chemiluminescence. The relationship between hydrostatic pressure and anesthesia appears to be biphasic, at least with N_2O. When administered at a 70% concentration at atmospheric pressure, N_2O is not an anesthetic; while keeping the concentration of N_2O constant and raising pressure to approximately 2 atmospheres, N_2O becomes a complete general anesthetic. As seen experimentally in mice, if the pressure is raised further, particularly by the addition of helium, the relative partial pressure of N_2O must be increased in order to maintain the same level of anesthesia. The complex interrelationship between the anesthetic effect and increased pressure is being used as a research tool to investigate the mechanism by which anesthetics exert their effects. One theory proposes that anesthetics act by expanding critical areas of the cell membrane to produce the anesthetic effect. Elevated pressures reverse this action on the cell membrane and therefore reduce the anesthetic effect.

ANESTHESIA SYSTEM, CLOSED: A system, in strict definition, in which the patient rebreathes all expired gases with the exception of CO_2, which is absorbed. Oxygen taken up by the patient is restored by a continuous low O_2 inflow to the breathing system. Closed systems are the most economical in conserving fresh gas supplies. Clinical practice usually requires the inflow of more than the estimated 250 ml of O_2 that the adult human requires per minute plus replacement of any O_2 or anesthetic agent which might escape from the patient through the skin or through open body cavities. The excess O_2 provides a margin of safety. Closed-system techniques also eliminate much of the load on the scavenger systems used to dispose of waste anesthetic gases.

ANESTHESIA SYSTEM, OPEN: A system, in strict definition, in which the patient rebreathes no expired gas. See Fig.

ANESTHETIC ADMINISTRATION, SUBJECTIVE EFFECTS OF: A catchall phrase which applies to the complaints of anesthetists concerning increased fatigue, difficulty in concentrating, headache, nausea, and feeling of disequilibrium connected with the administration of anesthesia. The fact that these effects are reported is one of the arguments for scavenging waste gases in the operating room.

ANESTHETIST: A generic term commonly applied to any individual who administers anesthesia.

ANGEL DUST: See Phencyclidine.

ANGINA PECTORIS: The pain, arising from relatively hypoxic myocardium, resulting from a relative mismatch of myocardial oxygen demand and oxygen supply. It is usually described as "crushing" or "constricting." Worsened by exercise, it is usually treated by nitroglycerin, which appears to work both by dilating the coronary arteries and by decreasing afterload. Nitroglycerin can be administered either sublingually or by dermal paste or patch. An anesthetically significant angina variant is unstable angina, which occurs at rest and is not necessarily relieved by nitroglycerin. It often exacerbates to an infarction.

Anesthesia System, Open: Comparison of the various anesthesia gas delivery system nomenclatures.

	Insufflation	Nonrebreathing Valves	T-piece	Magill and Mapleson B, C, & D Systems	Open Drop	Circle System	To and Fro
Dripps	Insufflation	Open	Semi-open	Semi-open	Semi-open	Semi-closed Closed	Semi-closed Closed
Collins	Open	Semi-closed nonrebreathing	Open (no exp. arm) Semi-open (with exp. arm)	Semi-closed partial rebreathing nonrebreathing	Open Semi-open if towels added	Semi-closed partial rebreathing Closed	Semi-closed partial rebreathing Closed
Adriani	Insufflation	Semi-closed nonrebreathing	Semi-closed (if no air dilution)	Semi-closed	Open	Semi-closed Closed	Semi-closed Closed
Conway	Open	Semi-closed nonrebreathing	Semi-closed rebreathing Semi-open (low gas flow and short exp. limb)	Semi-closed rebreathing nonrebreathing	Semi-open with occlusive packing	Semi-closed absorption Closed	Semi-closed absorption Closed
Moyers	Open	Semi-open	Open (no exp. limb) Semi-open (with exp. limb and high fresh gas flow)	Semi-open (high fresh gas flow) Semi-closed (low fresh gas flow)	Open Semi-closed with towels or thick mask	Semi-closed Closed	Semi-closed Closed

Anesthesia System, Open (continued)

	Insufflation	Nonrebreathing Valves	T-piece	Magill and Mapleson B, C, & D Systems	Open Drop	Circle System	To and Fro
			Semi-closed (with exp. limb and low fresh gas flow)				
Wright	Open		Semi-closed without absorption Semi-open (if exp. limb occluded during inspiration)	Semi-closed without absorption	Open Semi-open with occlusive packing	Semi-closed with absorption Closed	Semi-closed with absorption Closed
McMahon	Open	Open	Open Semi-closed	Open Semi-closed	Open Semi-closed	Semi-closed Closed	Semi-closed Closed

ANGIOGRAPHY: The radiographic visualization of blood vessels following the injection of radiopaque dye. The technique is useful as a diagnostic aid in cerebrovascular attacks, coronary artery disease, and myocardial infarctions.

ANGIOTENSIN: An extremely potent vasoconstrictor hormone which exists in the circulation as a precursor molecule and is activated by the enzyme renin. Renin, in turn, is released by the kidney in response to decreased blood supply.

ANGSTROM: A unit of measurement of wavelength equal to one ten-billionth meter (10^{-10} m).

ANILERIDINE (LERITINE): A meperidine-like narcotic drug used as a morphine substitute. See Narcotic.

ANION: A negatively charged ion. The principal anions in the body are Cl, HCO_3^-, PO_4^{2-}, and SO_4^{2-}.

ANION GAP (UNMEASURED ANIONS): The difference between the quantity of measured anions and measured cations in the blood. Serum is electrically neutral with an equal number of anions (-) and cations (+). The major cations measured in the laboratory are sodium and potassium; the major anions are chloride and CO_2 (as HCO_3^-). The sum of sodium plus potassium is always greater than the sum of bicarbonate and chloride. The missing unmeasured anions (anion gap) are nonvolatile organic and inorganic acids such as sulfates and phosphates (HPO_4^-). The anion gap is usually 12 ± 2 mEq/L. A low anion gap (< 10 mEq/L) is rare and occurs in situations in which abnormal unmeasured proteins replace sodium as serum cations (e.g., IgG myeloma). An increased anion gap is found in bromism (elevated serum Br^- seen in overdose of proprietary over-the-counter medications). Other significant increases in anion gap occur when metabolic acidosis is caused by ketone bodies, excessive lactate, or salicylate overdose.

ANOXIA: A condition in which there is not enough oxygen. It is also called O_2 deficiency and is used interchangeably with hypoxia.

ANTACID: A compound which is given orally to neutralize stomach acid. Aluminum hydroxide and magnesium trisilicate are two often used ingredients of antacids. Unfortunately, because of the unpredictability of gastric mixing, antacids cannot be relied on 100% to neutralize all available stomach acid.

ANTAGONISM: The pharmacologic effect seen when two or more drugs administered concurrently produce an effect which is less than the sum of their individual actions. Often the drugs compete for the same receptor site thereby interfering with drug activity. See Potentiation, Summation, Synergism.

ANTIANALGESIC: A drug or preparation which appears to lower the pain threshold, i.e., it seems to make a standard stimulus more painful. This phenomenon is most often seen with sedatives, hypnotics (barbiturates), and phenothiazines and appears in doses below those which produce unconsciousness.

ANTIANXIETY: See Fig. See Anxiety.

ANTIBIOTIC: A compound used to fight infectious diseases. Multiple subclasses and molecules exist. Almost without exception, the first of any series of antibiotics was discovered in nature and then, through chemical manipulation, multiple

Antianxiety Agents.

Generic Name (Trade Name)	Structure	Comments
A. Benzodiazepines		The benzodiazepines are widely used antianxiety drugs having anticonvulsant properties. They are also used as skeletal muscle relaxants (particularly diazepam). They do not produce significant extrapyramidal or autonomic side effects. They are pharmacologically similar to the barbiturates but are not as likely to produce physical dependence and tolerance, and are less lethal when taken in very large dosages. Side effects include fatigue, ataxia, paradoxical excitement, nausea, rash, and altered libido. The differences between the benzodiazepines include half-life, pain on injection, tendency to accumulate, and the route of degradation and elimination.
Chlordiazepoxide (Librium)	$NHCH_3$; C_6H_5 ; Cl ; N, O	
Diazepam (Valium)	CH_3 ; O ; N ; C_6H_5 ; Cl	
Oxazepam (Serax)	OH ; O ; H ; N ; C_6H_5 ; Cl	
Clorazepate (Tranxene)	OH ; OH ; COOH ; H ; N ; C_6H_5 ; Cl	
Lorazepam (Ativan)	O ; H ; OH ; Cl ; H ; N ; N ; Cl	

37

Prazepam (Verstran)

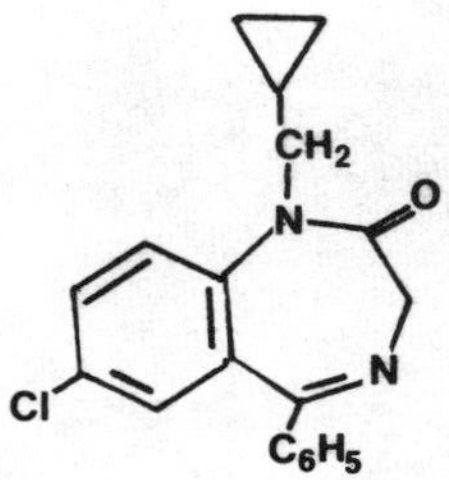

Nitrazepam (Mogadon)

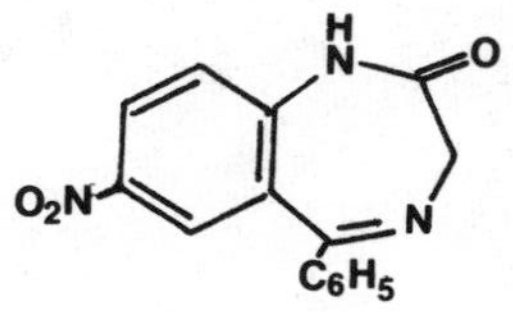

Flurazepam HCl (Dalmane)

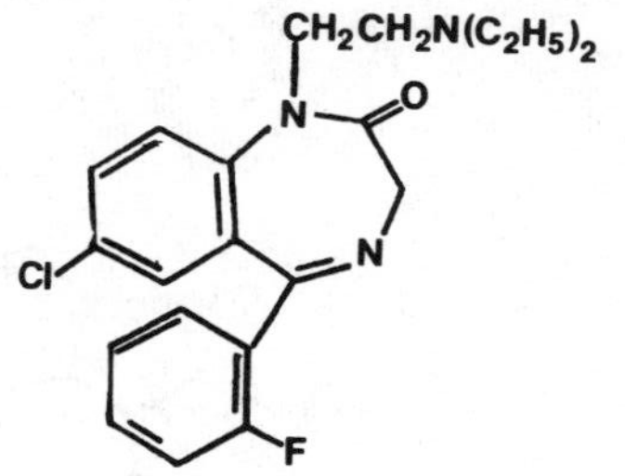

Flurazepam HCl is considered a sedative hypnotic. It has some advantages over barbiturates in that it does not immediately suppress REM sleep and causes very little rebound REM upon its discontinuation. It does not induce hepatic microsomal enzymes and has a very high therapeutic index and low addiction potential.

Midazolam

A new water-soluble, short half-life benzodiazepine which may assume significance as an induction agent.

Triazolam (Halcion)

A new short-acting benzodiazepine used as a hypnotic.

Antianxiety agents (continued)

Generic Name (Trade Name)	Structure	Comments
B. Butyrophenones		
Droperidol (Inapsine)	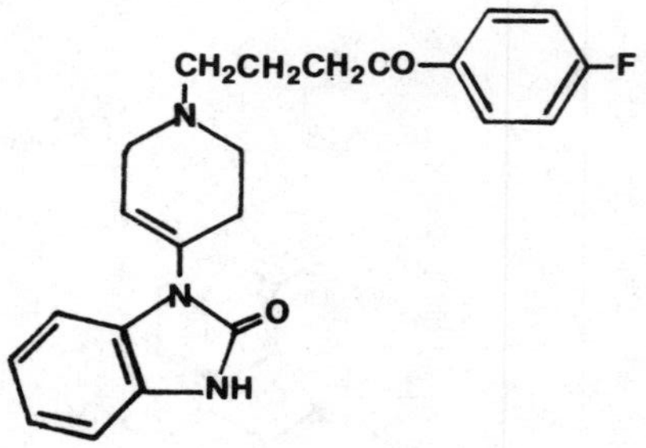	Used at times as a preoperative anti-anxiety drug, droperidol is most commonly used in conjunction with fentanyl (Sublimaze), a narcotic analgesic. This combination (Innovar) is used to produce neuroleptanesthesia. The droperidol produces calmness and drowsiness. It also reduces the incidence of postoperative nausea and vomiting.

Antibiotics: Anti-G⁺ pharmacologic agents.

Generic Name (Trade Name)	Spectrum of Activity	Comments
Erythromycin (Erythrocin) Estolate (Ilosone) Various other salts PO IM IV	G⁺ cocci, many G⁺ bacilli, <u>Mycoplasma pneumoniae</u>, and others.	All of the erythromycins have either a bacteriostatic or bactericidal mode of action, depending on the drug concentration and the nature of the microorganism against which it is used. Side effects include fever, eosinophilia, skin eruptions, and false increases of the SGOT. IM injections often produce pain that lasts for several hours. IV infusion is likely to be followed by thrombophlebitis. Some preparations can cause cholestatic jaundice.
Lincomycin (Lincocin) PO IM IV	Similar to erythromycin though somewhat less broad. It is not structurally related to erythromycin, however.	Lincomycin is used in the treatment of infections caused by bacteria resistant to penicillin and erythromycin. It is very effective in the treatment of chronic osteomyelitis. Side effects include severe diarrhea and potentially fatal pseudomembranous colitis.
Clindamycin (Cleocin) PO IM IV	Related to lincomycin, it generally has a broader spectrum of activity than lincomycin or erythromycin.	Severe diarrhea and pseudomembraneous colitis are possible side effects. The latter can be fatal.

Antibiotics: Anti-G$^+$ pharmacologic agents (continued)

Generic Name (Trade Name)	Spectrum of Activity	Comments
Vancomycin (Vancocin) IV	Similar to erythromycin.	Vancomycin is used in the treatment of severe infections caused by cocci. Side effects include permanent deafness, fatal uremia, macular rashes, and anaphylaxis.
Spectinomycin (Trobicin) IM	Similar to erythromycin plus some G$^-$ microbes.	Spectinomycin is used in the treatment of acute gonococcal infection. Side effects include nausea, fever, chills, urticaria, and blood dyscrasias.
Bacitracin Topical	A number of G$^+$ cocci and bacilli.	Formerly, bacitracin was used parenterally in the treatment of infant pneumonia and emphysema caused by Staphylococcus. In this form, it shows a high degree of nephrotoxicity. It is available as an ointment for the treatment of both skin and eye infections.

Antibiotics: Antifungal agents.

Generic Name (Trade Name)	Spectrum of Activity	Comments
Amphotericin B (Fungizone) PO IV Topical	Spectrum includes species of Histoplasma, Cryptococcus, Candida (except tropicalis), Coccidioides, Torulopsis, Rhodotorula, Blastomyces, some Aspergillus, and Sporotrichum.	Amphotericin B is fungistatic at normal doses. It is quite toxic and adverse effects include chills, fever, vomiting, and acute hepatic failure. The majority of people show a decrease in renal function. Renal impairment may become permanent. It is poorly absorbed orally and is quite unstable, thus requiring the preparation of a fresh solution for each injection.
Flucytosine (Ancobon) PO	Spectrum includes species of Cryptococcus, Candida, Torulopsis, Aspergillus, and Sporotrichum.	Flucytosine is well absorbed from the GI tract and readily passes into the cerebrospinal fluid and aqueous humor. Adverse effects include bone marrow depression and GI disturbances. It can be used in patients with renal impairment.
Griseofulvin (Fulvicin-U/F) PO	Spectrum includes species of Microsporum, Trichophyton, and Epidermophyton.	Griseofulvin is fungistatic. Serious adverse reactions to it are rare, though headache, GI disturbances, blood dyscrasias, renal and hepatic effects, and some nervous system effects do occur.
Nystatin (Candex) PO Topical	Spectrum includes species of Candida, Cryptococcus, Epidermophyton, Trichophyton, Blastomyces, and Histoplasma.	Nystatin is fungicidal and fungistatic. GI absorption is low. Side effects include mild GI disturbances.

congeners were created. For example, streptomycin, a natural product of yeast, has led to the discovery or partial synthesis of neomycin, kanamycin, gentamicin, tobramycin, etc. The physical as well as chemical incompatibilities of antibiotics must be kept in mind when they are injected intravenously. A number of antibiotics, prepared as sodium or potassium salts, may also affect the body's electrolyte balance. See Fig.

ANTICOAGULANT: A drug which interferes with the clotting process and causes bleeding to be prolonged. Two major types of anticoagulants exist. The first type, of which parenteral heparin is the only clinically available drug, works directly at multiple levels of the clotting mechanism but most directly in preventing the conversion of prothrombin to thrombin. The second type, the coumarin derivatives (usually given orally), depresses synthesis in the liver of various coagulation factors, particularly factors II, VII, IX, and X. Coumarins antagonize vitamin K, which is needed for the synthesis of these factors. Heparin is used for rapid anticoagulation. In surgery it is most often used in cases of extracorporeal circulation in which

Anticoagulants: Factors which can affect the action of the coumarin class of anticoagulants.

Increases Anticoagulant Action	Decreases Anticoagulant Action
Antibiotics	Vitamin K excess in poly-
Alcohol*	vitamin mixtures
Chloral hydrate*	Antihistamines
Anesthetics	Corticosteroids
Sulfonamides	Diet high in vitamin K
Quinine	(vegetables, fish, and
Propylthiouracil	fish oils)
Prolonged hot weather	Mineral oil
Prolonged narcotics	Barbiturates
Phenylbutazone	Alcohol*
Oxyphenbutazone	Chloral hydrate*
Anabolic steroids	Griseofulvin
Phenyramidol	Glutethimide
Clofibrate	Cholestyramine
Dextrothyroxine	Ethchlorvynol
Salicylates in excess of	Coumarin underdosage
1 gm/day	Unreliable prothrombin
Drugs affecting blood	determination
elements	
Hepatotoxic drugs	
Dietary deficiencies	
vitamin C	
protein	
choline	
cystine	
Coumarin overdosage	
Unreliable prothrombin	
determination	

* Increased and decreased prothrombin time responses have been reported.

prevention of coagulation is essential. It is also used in microvascular surgery where anticoagulants are assumed to prevent clotting in the microvascular circulation. Heparin can be directly antagonized by the drug protamine (a fish protein). Coumarin derivatives can be reversed in two ways: (1) by vitamin K, which requires 6 hr to increase liver production, and (2) by fresh frozen plasma. See Fig.

ANTIDEPRESSANT: See Tricyclic antidepressant.

ANTIDIURETIC HORMONE (ADH) (VASOPRESSIN): A hormone of the posterior pituitary which regulates free water clearance by acting on the distal nephrons of the glomeruli. As secretion of the hormone increases, urinary volume decreases and electrolyte concentration of the urine rises. In higher concentrations (greater than that required for antidiuresis), vasopressin causes contraction of smooth muscles in the vasculature, particularly in capillaries and venules. See Diabetes insipidus, Inappropriate antidiuretic hormone syndrome.

ANTIEMETIC: A pharmacologic agent used to prevent nausea or vomiting (emesis). The most commonly used agents for this purpose are antihistamines or phenothiazine derivatives. Two characteristics of antiemetics are noteworthy: (1) The antiemetic effect is not usually the primary effect of the drug. (2) Since antiemesis is not an absolute, what appears to be an adequate dose of an antiemetic may not prevent vomiting.

ANTIFUNGAL AGENT: See Antibiotic.

ANTIHISTAMINE: A pharmacologic substance which is a competitive antagonist of endogenous histamine. The classic antihistamines, e.g., diphenhydramine, antagonize the effects of histamine at H_1-receptors which are located in the smooth muscle of the intestines, blood vessels, and bronchi. H_2-receptors, significant primarily in the gastric parietal cells, are only blocked by the newer antihistamines like cimetidine. H_1-blockers are not completely effective at routine clinical dosages. Central sedation is often an unwanted side effect. See Fig. See Histamine.

ANTILIRIUM: See Physostigmine.

ANTIOXIDANT: A material added to a compound to retard oxidation and deterioration. It is found primarily in rubber and other organic products.

Antihistamines: H_2-antagonist.

Prototype Generic Name (Trade Name)	Structure	Comments
Cimetidine (Tagamet)		Available in oral and parenteral forms, it can decrease gastric secretion by 50% and can cause CNS dysfunction, constipation, and diarrhea. It is becoming more popular as a preoperative premedicant.

Antihistamines: H_1-antagonists.

Prototype Generic Name (Trade Name)	Structure	Comments
A. Alkylamines Chlorpheniramine (Chlor–Trimeton)		The alkylamines are among the most potent of the H_1 antagonists while they also show a low incidence of drowsiness. They show strong anticholinergic effects.
B. Ethanolamines Diphenhydramine (Benadryl)		The ethanolamines are potent antihistamines which possess anticholinergic, antiemetic, and sedative properties. Diphenhydramine is used as an antiparkinsonism agent as well as being widely used parenterally for moderate to severe allergic reactions.
C. Ethylenediamines Pyrilamine (Neo-Antergan)		The ethylenediamines show some incidence of drowsiness as well as occasional dizziness. GI upset is common.

D. Phenothiazines

Promethazine (Phenergan)

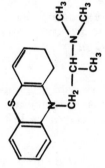

The phenothiazines can have many side effects, including extrapyramidal effects, orthostatic hypotension, and endocrine changes. Promethazine has been advocated for the treatment of motion sickness, for relief of nausea and vomiting, and for sedation.

E. Piperazines

Cyclizine (Marezine)

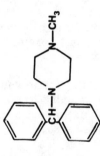

The piperazines are used in the treatment of motion sickness and for relief of postoperative nausea and vomiting. They show a relatively low incidence of drowsiness.

F. Miscellaneous

Cyproheptadine (Periactin)

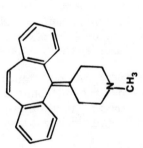

Cyproheptadine has antiserotonin, anticholinergic, and sedative properties. It can cause some degree of epigastric distress.

ANTIPSYCHOTIC AGENTS: The pharmacologic products, also known as major tranquilizers, that are used to treat severe psychotic illness, such as schizophrenia. The major classes of antipsychotic agents are phenothiazines, thioxanthenes, and butyrophenones. See Fig. See Droperidol, Phenothiazines.

ANTISIALAGOGUE: An agent which prevents salivation. It was classically used as a premedicant particularly when diethyl ether, a potent sialagogue (promoting salivation), was to be administered. With the newer, more modern general anesthetics, the practice of prescribing antisialagogues prior to anesthesia has been questioned. The most commonly used antisialagogues are atropine, scopolamine, and glycopyrrolate.

ANTISTATIC MATERIAL: A substance which cannot accumulate electrons because of its inherent molecular makeup. Most surfaces can be made antistatic by proper coatings. See Capacitor.

ANURIA (ANURESIS): The condition in which there is absence of excretion of urine. Clinically, however, anuria is said to exist when less than 100 ml of urine is excreted daily by the average adult.

ANXIETY: A subjective feeling of uncertainty and/or apprehension which appears detached from, or out of proportion to, an apparent cause. Anxiety produces physiologic changes such as hypertension, tachycardia, muscle tremors, sweating, and gastrointestinal disturbances. A patient is frequently premedicated prior to surgery in an effort to lessen anxiety. See Antianxiety.

AORTIC INSUFFICIENCY: A condition in which the aortic valve is variably incompetent and a regurgitant stream from the aorta is added to the normal ventricular filling from the left atrium. In attempting to adapt to aortic insufficiency, the left ventricle increases in wall thickness and chamber size.

AORTIC STENOSIS: A narrowing of the cross-sectional area of the aortic valve. It is primarily an obstruction to ventricular emptying causing a tremendous increase in the pressure work the left ventricle must produce to maintain cardiac output. The area of the normal adult aortic valve is approximately 3 cm^2; the symptoms of stenosis may begin when this area falls below 1 cm^2. The left ventricular wall thickens but the heart chamber remains the same size. This thick wall is very vulnerable to ischemic insult.

AORTOCAVAL SYNDROME: A group of circulatory deficiencies seen in the pregnant patient near term and possibly also seen in the grossly obese, patients with ascites and patients with abdominal masses. The enlarged uterus in the supine patient can partially occlude (1) the aorta (aortic compression) decreasing flow to the uterus and lower body or (2) the inferior vena cava (inferior vena cava syndrome) decreasing blood return to the heart, thereby diminishing cardiac output (supine hypotensive syndrome). Tilting the patient to the left minimizes the compression. A mechanical uterine displacer (Kennedy displacer) may also be used.

APEX ACCELEROMETRY: A technique which determines the rate of change in velocity of heart muscle during ventricular contractility. This measurement of acceleration is correlated with aortic blood acceleration which, in turn, is a reflection of cardiac contractility.

APGAR SCORE: A scoring system for evaluating the condition of a newborn infant. The five factors that determine the Apgar score are heart rate, respiratory effect,

Antipsychotic agents.

Prototype Generic Name (Trade Name)	Structure Substitutions	Comments
A. Phenothiazines	General Structure	All phenothiazines can produce atropine-like effects (though pupil dilatation and tachycardia are uncommon), postural hypotension, lowering of body temperature, and various endocrine effects. They are not physically addicting.
Aliphatic Derivatives Chlorpromazine (Thorazine)	$R_1 = CH_2-CH_2-CH_2-N(CH_3)_2$ $R_2 = -Cl$	The class leader of the phenothiazines, chlorpromazine can produce moderate extrapyradimal effects and severe sedative effects. It has antiemetic properties.
Piperazine Derivatives Fluphenazine (Permitil)	$R_1 = -CH_2-CH_2-CH_2-N$⟨⟩$N-CH_2-CH_2OH$ $R_2 = -CF_3$	Fluphenazine can produce severe extrapyramidal effects, mild hypotension, and mild sedative effects.
Prochlorperazine (Compazine)	$R_1 = -CH_2-CH_2-CH_2-N$⟨⟩$N-CH_3$ $R_2 = -Cl$	Prochlorperazine can produce severe extrapyramidal effects, mild hypotension, and moderate sedative effects. It also has antiemetic properties.
Piperidine Derivatives Thioridazine (Mellaril)	$R_1 = -CH_2-CH_2$ $R_2 = -SCH_3$	Thioridazine produces mild extrapyramidal effects, moderate hypotension, and severe sedative effects.

Antipsychotic agents (continued)

Prototype Generic Name (Trade Name)	Structure Substitutions	Comments
B. Thioxanthenes		The thioxanthenes are less potent than the phenothiazines though their efficacy is the same.
Chlorprothixene (Taractan)	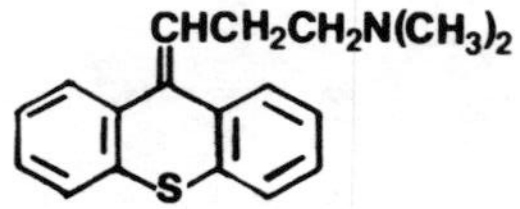 CHCH₂CH₂N(CH₃)₂	Chlorprothixene has moderate extrapyramidal effects, moderate to severe hypotensive and sedative effects, and has antiemetic properties.
Thiothixene (Navane)	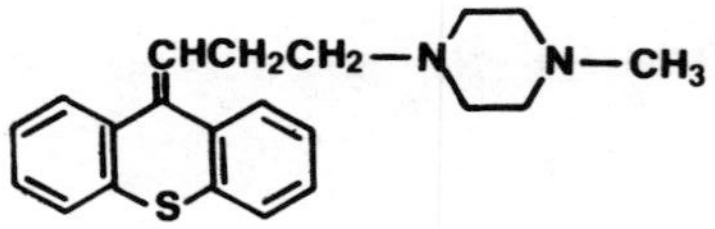	Thiothixene can cause severe extrapyramidal effects, mild hypotension, and mild sedation. It has antiemetic effects.
C. Butyrophenones		
Haloperidol (Haldol)	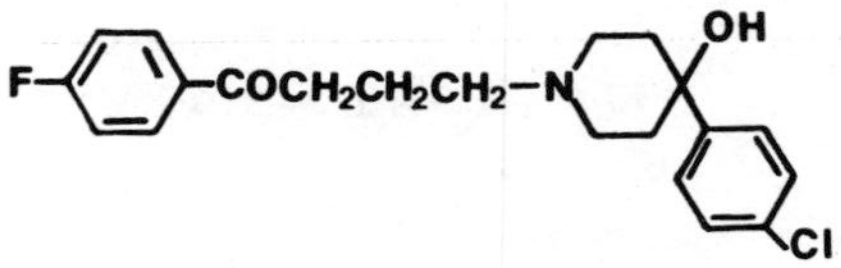	Haloperidol can produce severe extrapyramidal effects, mild hypotension, and mild sedation.
D. Dibenzoxazepines		
Loxapine (Loxitane)	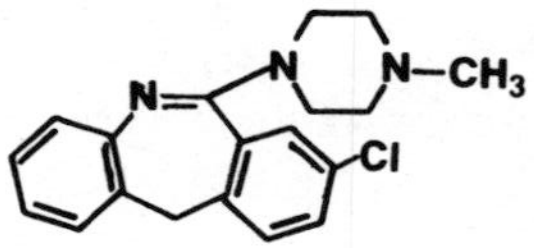	Loxapine can produce severe extrapyramidal effects, mild hypotension, and mild sedation.
E. Dihydroindolones		
Molindone (Moban)	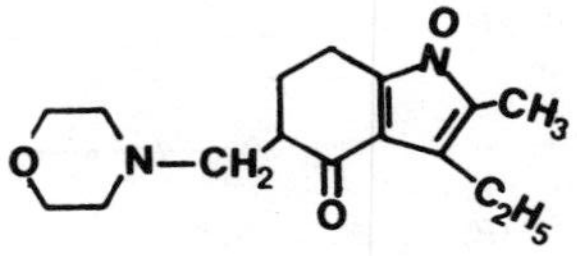	Molindone can produce moderate extrapyramidal effects, mild hypotension, and moderate sedation. It also has antiemetic properties.

Apgar Score.

SIGN	0	1	2
HEART RATE	Absent	Slow (< 100)	> 100
RESPIRATORY EFFORT	Absent	Weak Cry; Hypoventilation	Good; Strong Cry
MUSCLE TONE	Limp	Some Flexion of Extremities	Well Flexed
REFLEX IRRITABILITY	No Response	Some Motion	Cry
COLOR	Blue; Pale	Body Pink; Extremities Blue	Completely Pink

muscle tone, reflex irritability, and color. Since all five factors are rated on a scale of 0-2, the best possible score is 10, the worst 0. Usually, active efforts at resuscitation are required in infants with an Apgar score below 5. Taken at both 1 and 5 min after delivery, the score appears to correlate well with long-term outcome. A mnemonic for APGAR is: Appearance, Pulse, Grimace reflex irritability, Activity, Respiration. See Fig.

APNEA: The absence of respiration.

APNEIC OXYGENATION (DIFFUSION RESPIRATION; APNEIC DIFFUSION OXYGENATION): A physiologic finding pertaining to respiration. A healthy patient denitrogenated by 100% O_2 can maintain arterial O_2 saturation while paralyzed and apneic if left connected to the O_2 source. Experimentally, periods of apnea from 30-55 min have been tolerated in humans. The maintenance of hemoglobin saturation has been ascribed to the mass movement of O_2 down the trachea following the pressure gradient from the reservoir bag (760 torr PO_2) to the cells (40-60 torr PO_2). Carbon dioxide builds up because its pressure gradient in the reverse direction is much less. This limits the technique because pH can fall to very low levels. The concept of apneic oxygenation is the basis for ventilating respirator patients with 100% O_2 before suctioning.

APOMORPHINE: A chemical derivative of morphine used primarily to induce vomiting. After subcutaneous administration, nausea, salivation, and vomiting occur within a few minutes. Since, like morphine, it can produce central nervous system depression, it must be used with care in the already unconscious patient. (Precautions must be taken for securing the airway to prevent aspiration.)

APPARENT DEATH: A state of complete interruption of all bodily processes from which the patient can be restored or resuscitated to independent function.

ARACHNOIDITIS: The inflammation of the arachnoid, which is the membrane located between the dura mater and the pia mater, covering the brain and spinal cord. It is separated from the pia mater by the subarachnoid space. Arachnoiditis is one of the most feared complications of spinal anesthesia as the inflammation can become adhesive and strangle nerve trunks or the spinal cord itself. See Arachnoiditis, chronic adhesive.

ARACHNOIDITIS, CHRONIC ADHESIVE: A pathologic condition in which congestion and thickening of the dura mater occur along with adhesions to the spinal cord and nerves. In advanced forms the cord, nerve, and blood vessels are strangulated. This condition can occur as a result of nonspecific, relatively minor spinal cord injuries and may be caused anesthetically by the inadvertent injection of toxic or contaminated materials during a spinal cord nerve block. See Arachnoiditis.

ARAMINE: See Metaraminol.

ARCHIMEDES PRINCIPLE: The principle stating that a body floating in a fluid displaces a weight of fluid equal to its own weight.

AREA UNDER THE CURVE (AUC): The area bounded by the X and Y axes and the plotted curve of information points. A numeric value can be given to this area by cutting and weighing the AUC or by the mathematic techniques of trapezoidal rule or integration. The AUC is useful in comparing the metabolism of two drugs if plasma levels (X) and time of sampling (Y) are known.

ARFONAD: See Trimethaphan.

ARGON: An inert gaseous element found in the atmosphere. It is obtained commercially by the differential fractionalization of liquid air. The gas has been used experimentally in studies of anesthetic potency.

ARMORED ENDOTRACHEAL TUBE: An endotracheal tube usually made out of latex or, more recently, Silastic which has a stainless steel or nylon spring incorporated into the wall to prevent kinking. These tubes follow the shape of the airway in even the most unusual positions and almost invariably require a stylet for placement because of their extremely flexible nature. See Endotracheal tube.

ARNOLD-CHIARI DEFORMITY: A congenital anomaly in which the tonsils of the cerebellum and the medulla oblongata protrude through the foramen magnum into the

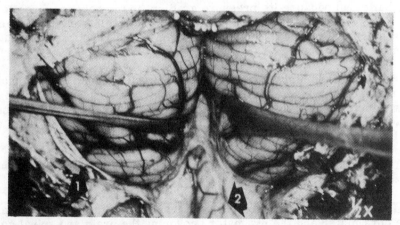

Arnold-Chiari Deformity: Gross specimen of the Arnold-Chiari malformation. Note thickened meninges (1) and the abnormally low cerebellar tonsils (2) projecting into the cervical canal.

spinal canal. This blocks the cerebrospinal fluid outflow from the fourth ventricle and causes hydrocephalus. See Fig.

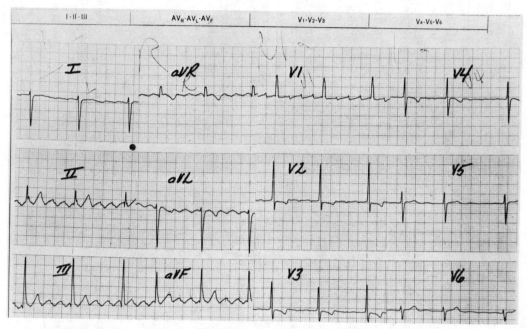

Arrhythmia: A 12-lead ECG showing classic atrial flutter (not necessarily seen in all the leads of the ECG).

ARRHYTHMIA: An irregularity of the heartbeat or the pulse rate. The normal rhythm can become irregular due to heart disease, anoxia, or catecholamine stimulation. See Fig. See Atrial fibrillation, Atrial flutter, Electrocardiogram, Ventricular fibrillation.

ARTERIAL BLOOD PRESSURE: The pressure of the blood on the walls of the arteries. This pressure is contingent on the force of contraction of the heart, the elasticity of the arterial walls, and the volume and viscosity of the blood. Sampling site, sampling technique, and equipment used also cause variation in the absolute value of the arterial pressure obtained. This pressure is measured in terms of millimeters of mercury above atmospheric pressure. As a measurement it is considered one of the "vital signs." In the supine patient, arterial pressure measured in the leg is between 10 and 20 torr higher than arterial pressure measured in the arm. This is due, in part, to a complex resonance phenomenon in the aorta in which each new pressure wave is reinforced by echoes in the fluid column caused by the preceding waves. The numeric value of "normal" resting blood pressure in adults is controversial. It is generally accepted, however, that diastolic pressures above 90 torr and systolic pressures above 160 torr are abnormal and require investigation. See Fig. See Central venous pressure, Diastolic pressure, Hypertension, Hypotension, Mean arterial pressure, Systolic pressure.

ARTERIALIZATION FOR BLOOD SAMPLING: A procedure done when direct puncture of an artery for a blood sample is contraindicated or impossible, particularly in infants. It entails heating a skin site to maximize its capillary blood flow. This

Arterial Blood Pressure: Methods of determining blood pressure.

Method	Equipment Needed	Technique	Advantages and Disadvantages
Auscultation	1. Inflatable bladder with attached pressure gauge (blood pressure cuff and sphygmomanometer).	1. Cuff is wrapped snugly around upper arm and inflated by air pressure to a pressure high enough to collapse artery through entire cardiac cycle. Stethoscope head is placed over distal artery segment and pressure is slowly released. A distinctive rushing sound is heard over the artery as the cuff pressure drops below systolic pressure. These sounds continue changing in quality until the pressure is so low that the artery is open during all the cardiac cycle. These sounds then disappear. The sounds are called Korotkoff sounds (frequency range approximately 4 to 50 hz).	1. Cuff width should be 20% greater than the diameter of the arm (1/3 circumference). a) A cuff too wide gives false low readings. b) A cuff too narrow gives false high readings. 2. Technique is more accurate for systolic than diastolic measurement. 3. Confusion can occur because Korotkoff sounds are often "lost" for three or four heart beats after they are first heard and with cuff pressure still dropping. This poorly understood phenomenon is called the "auscultatory gap." 4. Sounds may be too low to be heard during periods of low pressure.
Oscillation (Oscillotonometrics)	1. Inflatable bladder with attached pressure gauge (blood pressure cuff and sphygmomanometer).	1. As above, except movement of pressure gauge needle is observed. For oscillations with artery completely occluded, these movements are small. As blood first spurts past the deflating	1. Most accurately done with a double cuff apparatus (Riva-Rocci). 2. Not easily done consistently by different examiners. 3. The concept is easily automated by electrically transducing the

Method	Equipment	Technique	Comments
		cuff, oscillations increase. This point is regarded as systolic pressure. The point at which oscillations are maximal is considered mean pressure. Diastolic pressure is poorly perceived by this method.	cuff pressure oscillations (Dinamapp^{tm}).
Palpation	1. As above.	1. As above, except a palpating finger is placed over a distal artery and the first pulse felt is considered the systolic pressure.	1. The most straightforward method. 2. Diastolic endpoint not ascertainable.
Photoelectric	1. As above.	1. A light source and photocell replaces the palpating finger (usually placed on wrist or finger).	1. Detects change in light transmitted from skin surface by color change of each pulse beat.
Doppler Ultrasound	1. Blood pressure cuff and pressure gauge and Doppler Ultrasound crystal receiver.	1. As above, except that Doppler technique is used to detect distal arterial wall movement instead of a palpating finger.	1. The Doppler device is technically sophisticated and relatively expensive. 2. Ascertaining diastolic pressure requires even more sophisticated electric equipment and repeatability is open to question.
Arterial Puncture	1. Percutaneous catheter directly cannulating an artery interfaced to a transducer via a fluid path.	1. The arterial pressure is interfaced to a fluid path which affects the output of a pressure transducer proportionally.	1. An invasive technique with known morbidity. 2. Inherently very accurate but open to many technical problems such as clotting, kinking, or air bubbles in the catheter or electronic drift of equipment.

Arterial Blood Pressure (continued)

Method	Equipment Needed	Technique	Advantages and Disadvantages
Very Low Frequency Sound (Infrasonde)	1. Cuff and electronic stethoscope.	1. Automated apparatus which detects Korotkoff sounds too low in frequency to be heard.	1. Most accurate at low pressures (pediatrics).

is followed by a skin stick. The rapidly flowing blood, not having time to equilibrate with the tissue as to PO_2, PCO_2, and pH, will approximate arterial blood in these parameters. The pH is the most accurate determination obtained from this type of sampling.

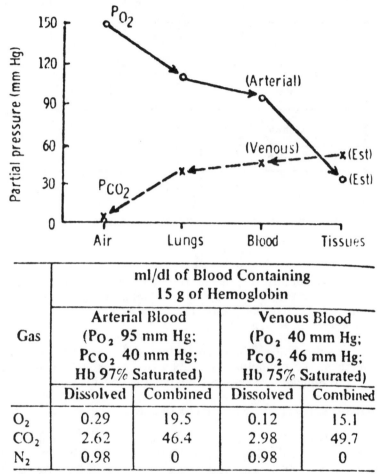

	ml/dl of Blood Containing 15 g of Hemoglobin			
Gas	Arterial Blood (P_{O_2} 95 mm Hg; P_{CO_2} 40 mm Hg; Hb 97% Saturated)		Venous Blood (P_{O_2} 40 mm Hg; P_{CO_2} 46 mm Hg; Hb 75% Saturated)	
	Dissolved	Combined	Dissolved	Combined
O_2	0.29	19.5	0.12	15.1
CO_2	2.62	46.4	2.98	49.7
N_2	0.98	0	0.98	0

Arterialization of Blood: Gas content of blood.

ARTERIALIZATION OF BLOOD: The process by which venous blood receives O_2 from the alveolar gas and in turn gives up CO_2 in the lungs. See Fig.

ARTERIAL PRESSURE DETERMINATION BY PALPATION: A system based on palpating an artery proximal to which a blood pressure cuff is inflated and slowly deflated, with the pressure of the cuff being monitored by a gauge or mercury column. The systolic pressure is read when the first pulse is felt. Systolic measurements are usually slightly lower than those determined by listening for Korotkoff sounds. The cuff adds a resistance drop which lowers the pressure distal to it. Diastolic pressures are not obtainable. See Arterial blood pressure.

ARTERIOLE: The final branches of the arterial system just proximal to a capillary. The walls of arterioles contain smooth muscle capable of contracting sufficiently to completely cut off flow. They can also dilate to several times their normal size.

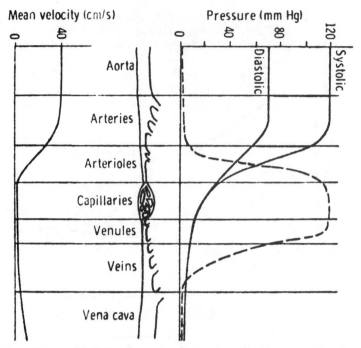

Arteriole: Diagrammatic representation of changes in velocity and pressure as blood flows through the systemic circulation. The dashed line indicates the total cross-sectional area of the vessels; 4.5 cm^2 in the aorta to 4500 cm^2 in the capillaries.

They are the major source of vascular resistance and account for 60-70% of total peripheral resistance. Well supplied with alpha receptors, they are a primary site of action for norepinephrine and its antagonists. See Fig.

ARTERIOVENOUS CAPILLARY: See Microcirculation.

ARTIFICIAL HIBERNATION: A drug-induced state of dormancy characterized by reduced metabolism, muscle relaxation, and a twilight sleep resembling narcosis. High doses of phenothiazines and narcotics are used. This theoretically renders the patient insensitive to pain without gross alteration of the vital signs. However, in practice, achieving this state (without overshoot to cardiovascular or respiratory collapse) is extremely difficult. See Lytic cocktail.

ARTIFICIAL PNEUMOTHORAX: The deliberate introduction of air (under sterile conditions) into the pleural cavity to collapse the lung. An obsolete treatment for tuberculosis to "rest the lung."

ARYEPIGLOTTIC FOLDS: See Laryngospasm.

ASA PHYSICAL STATUS CLASSIFICATIONS: See Physical status classifications, ASA.

ASBESTOS: A fibrous mineral composed of combinations of silicon, magnesium, and O_2. Because of its heat resistance and acoustic dampening properties, it has been extensively used in the manufacture of fabrics, paper, insulating boards, and wall covering.

ASPHYXIA: A state which denies a normal supply of O_2 to the blood. It is synonymous with suffocation. In the practice of anesthesia, the most common cause of asphyxia is airway obstruction.

ASPIRATION: The introduction of any foreign matter into the trachea and upper airways. The aspiration of stomach contents remains one of the most serious complications of anesthesia. It is usually brought about by the reflux of material up the esophagus and the obtundation of the airway reflexes which normally seal the upper airways against reflux. Aspiration pneumonitis (Mendelson syndrome) results when the material actually reaches the bronchioles. The severity of injury depends primarily on the pH of the gastric contents. (Other factors are volume, particulate matter, and bacterial count.) Above a pH of 2.5, little injury occurs beyond that caused by airway closure by solid or liquid blockage. Below a pH of 2.5, however, there is direct toxic injury to the lining of the air passageways, causing an immediate exudation of fluid, bronchospasm, and severe ventilation/perfusion abnormalities.

ASPIRIN: See Acetylsalicylic acid.

ASSAULT: A seemingly violent attempt or willful offer (with violence or force) to do harm to another person, without actually doing the harm threatened. This is one of the grounds for malpractice suits. See Battery.

ASSISTED BREATHING: See Ventilation, assisted.

ASSOCIATION OF UNIVERSITY ANESTHETISTS: An organization formed to promote and discuss research in teaching anesthesia. First organized in Philadelphia in 1953, its membership is open to anesthesiology faculty members in medical schools or in affiliated teaching hospitals located in the United States and Canada.

ASTHMA: A disease characterized by various degrees of bronchial constriction, thickened secretions, increased work of ventilation, wheezing, and impaired gas exchange. The duration of an asthmatic attack may be from a few minutes to many hours, in which case it is referred to as status asthmaticus. The latter may be severe enough to threaten life. Attacks appear to be triggered by airway irritation, which can be environmental (airborne pollen) or iatrogenic (anesthetic vapors). An asthmatic attack is a feared complication during the induction of anesthesia.

ASYSTOLE: The lack of cardiac contraction; standstill of the heart.

ATRACURIUM: A nondepolarizing muscle relaxant of intermediate duration of action. It is a distant derivative of d-tubocurarine.

ATELECTASIS: A collapse of the adult lung caused by bronchial obstruction or external compression. This collapse may affect only a lobe (lobar atelectasis) or a specific segment (segmental atelectasis) of the lung. The blockage may be due to bronchial exudate, foreign bodies, tumor, lymph nodes or aneurysms compressing the bronchi, or bronchial distortions. Atelectasis may also be brought about by loss of surfactant such that the fluid lining of the alveoli develops a significant surface tension and literally pulls the alveoli in on themselves. Patchy atelectasis is a term used to describe small, diffuse, radiopaque areas seen in a chest x-ray which represent collapsed alveoli. Primary atelectasis describes a lung which has not expanded at birth. See Fig.

ATELECTASIS, ABSORPTION: See Absorption atelectasis.

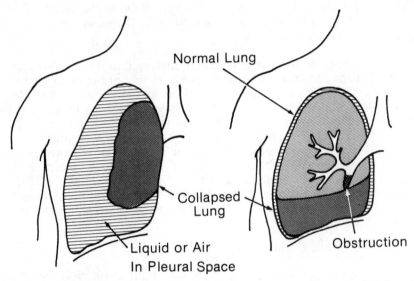

Atelectasis: Atelectasis produced by external compression (left) and bronchial obstruction (right).

ATELECTATIC SHUNT: See Shunt.

ATIVAN: See Benzodiazepine.

ATMOSPHERE: The gaseous medium which envelops the earth. At sea level, it exerts a uniform pressure equal to 760 mmHg.

ATOMIC NUMBER: See Nucleus, atomic.

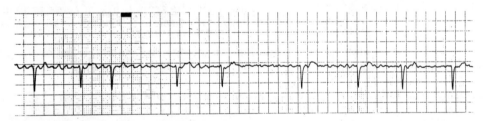

Atrial Fibrillation: Rhythm strip.

ATRIAL FIBRILLATION: A cardiac arrhythmia in which the atria randomly contract at a very high rate. See Fig.

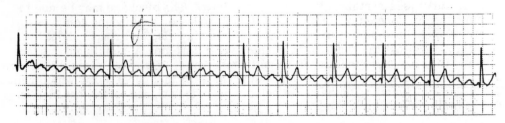

Atrial Flutter: Rhythm strip.

ATRIAL FLUTTER: A cardiac arrhythmia in which the atria contract at a very rapid but regular rate, ranging from 200 to 300 times/min. See Fig.

ATRIAL SEPTAL DEFECT (ASD): A congenital heart anomaly characterized by a patent atrial septum. ASDs are described according to their position in the septum and their embryologic origin. Secundum defects are in the area of the fossa ovalis and result from failure of the septum secundum to develop. Ostium primum defects occur in the lower portion of the septum. Other less common ASDs occur as well. Frequently infants and children will have minimal or no symptoms; however, surgical correction is recommended during childhood. See Endocardial cushion defect, Ventricular septal defect.

ATRIOVENTRICULAR BUNDLE: See Heart, conduction system of.

ATRIOVENTRICULAR NODE: See Heart, conduction system of.

$$H_2C \longrightarrow CH \longrightarrow CH_2 \qquad \qquad CH_2OH$$

$$NCH_3 \qquad CH - O - \overset{\overset{O}{\|}}{C} - CH$$

$$H_2C \longrightarrow CH \longrightarrow CH_2 \qquad \qquad C_6H_5$$

Atropine.

ATROPINE: A naturally occurring alkaloid originally prepared from the belladonna plant (deadly nightshade). As an anticholinergic, atropine (in large doses) blocks the parasympathetic-mediated vagal effect on the adult heart causing tachycardia in the range of 115-120 (increased sympathetic nervous system activity can further increase heart rate), inhibits salivary secretion causing mouth dryness and difficulty in swallowing, and decreases gastric secretion and gastrointestinal motility. In very small doses it may incite central vagal stimulation, causing bradycardia. In large, nonpharmacologic doses, it can cause central nervous system excitation and frank seizure activity. At any dosage, its effects are of short duration. See Fig.

AUTOLOGOUS: Coming from one's self. For example, in an autologous blood transfusion a patient is given his or her own blood w hich had been withdrawn and stored up to 1 month earlier. Autologous blood is used therapeutically in cases of spinal headache. See Epidural patch, Spinal headache.

AUTOMATED ANALYSIS INSTRUMENT (SEQUENTIAL MULTIPLE ANALYZER: SMA 1260; SMA 660): A device which determines on a single serum sample levels of electrolytes, enzymes, cholesterol, or inorganic ions. Usually the tests are based on reaching a particular color intensity after appropriate chemical reactions with a small portion of the sample. The exceptions to this are those tests which require ion-specific electrodes. The SMA 1260 can run 12 tests/sample, 60 samples/hr.

AUTOMATED CELL COUNTER: A device which determines a precise count of a desired cellular element in a sample of blood. Usually, the sample is pretreated to destroy rather than count all unwanted cellular elements. Two types of automated cell counters exist. The electro-optical counter (e.g., Technicon Autocounter) utilizes a photomultiplier tube to detect light bounced from cells. The voltage pulse machine (e.g., Coulter counter) counts cells as they change electrolyte conductivity by moving between two electrodes immersed in that electrolyte.

AUTOMATIC BASELINE CENTERING: An electronic modality (available on oscilloscopic displays of the electrocardiogram) in which the machine centers the trace on its screen without the intervention of the operator.

AUTONOMIC NERVOUS SYSTEM: That part of the central nervous system which controls the involuntary functions of the body, including the regulation of the heart, blood vessels, smooth muscles, and many glands. The autonomic nervous system consists of two parts which balance and antagonize each other, the sympathetic and parasympathetic systems. Because sympathetic nervous system activity is mediated by the release and uptake of the hormones epinephrine, norepinephrine, and

Autonomic Nervous System: (I) Selected actions of the autonomic nervous system.

Site of Effector Cells	Activation of Sympathetic Division (Thoracolumbar) Tends to:	Activation of Parasympathetic Division (Craniosacral) Tends to:
Heart	Increase rate and output	Decrease rate and output
Coronary arteries	Dilate	Dilate
Blood vessels in nose, salivary glands, and pharynx	Constrict	Dilate
Cutaneous vessels	Constrict	
Bronchi	Dilate	Constrict
Gastrointestinal motility and secretion	Decrease peristalsis and muscle tone; constrict sphincters	Increase; relax sphincters
Glycogenolysis by the liver	Increase	
Glands	Decrease secretion	Increase secretion
Sweat glands	Increase (some authorities classify this as parasympathetic function)	
Pupil of eye	Dilate	Constrict
Ciliary muscles	Lessen tone, eyes accommodate to see at a distance	Contract ciliary muscle, eyes accommodate to see near objects
Mental activity	Increase	

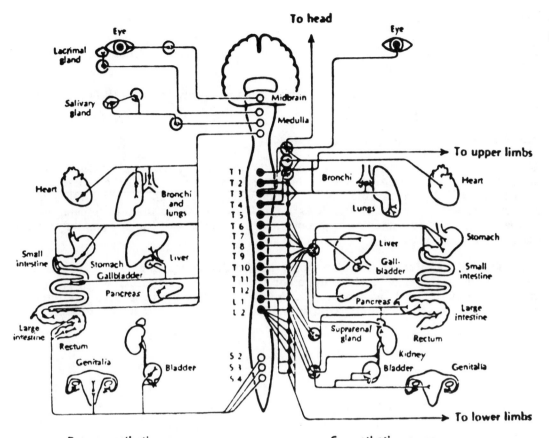

Parasympathetic nerves   Sympathetic nerves
Autonomic Nervous System: (II) Autonomic innervation of various organs.

related adrenergic hormones, it is sometimes called the adrenergic nervous system. (Two apparent exceptions, the sweat glands and the adrenal medulla, while activated by the sympathetic nervous system, are controlled by acetylcholine release.) Since parasympathetic nervous system activity is mediated by the release of acetylcholine, it is also known as the cholinergic nervous system. See Fig. See Central nervous system, Cranial nerves, Receptor/receptor site.

AUTOREGULATION: The ability of tissue, in relation to circulation, to maintain constant blood flow despite variations in mean arterial blood pressures. Normal cerebral circulation offers the most striking example of autoregulation in that the cerebral blood will remain unchanged between mean arterial pressures of 60 to at least 160 torr. The kidney also autoregulates at a range of 10-15 torr higher than the brain. In hypertensive individuals, the range of autoregulation rises. All halogenated hydrocarbon anesthetics increase cerebral blood flow (CBF) and abolish cerebral autoregulation. Hypercapnia increases CBF and overrides autoregulation, whereas hypocapnia decreases CBF but also overrides autoregulation. See Cerebral blood flow, Intracranial pressure measurement.

AVERAGE: A value which is typical of or represents a set of values. In common usage, it is identified with the arithmetic mean or the sum of all the values in a set divided by the number of values within that set.

AVERTIN: See Rectal anesthesia.

AVOGADRO NUMBER: The number of molecules contained in 1 mole of substance. It is expressed as 6.02×10^{23}.

AXON: The part of a neuron that transmits impulses away from a cell body. See Action potential, Depolarization.

AXOPLASM: The cytoplasm of a nerve axon.

AYRE T-PIECE: An apparatus used to modify standard anesthesia equipment in pediatric cases. The prime purpose of the Ayre device is to prevent the pediatric patient from expending excessive energy, which would be the case if the valved adult circuit were used. Many modifications of the Ayre T-piece system have been made. At the same time, by supplying high flows, nonrebreathing of expired gas may be accomplished. See Figs.

AZEOTROPE: A mixture of two or more volatile liquids which cannot be separated by distillation. Halothane and diethyl ether form an azeotrope which was used as a general anesthetic. It is no longer utilized since only slight differences in clinical effect were observed when compared with either agent alone and it was a flammable mixture.

Ayre T-Piece: (I) Modifications to the T-piece.

Name	Shape*	Patient Limb Diameter	Expiratory Limb Diameter	Dealers	Comment
Ayre T-piece	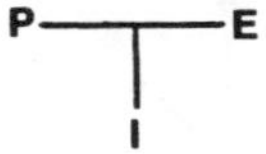	10 mm or 12.5 mm	10 mm or 12.5 mm	Dupaco Foregger	
Bissonnette	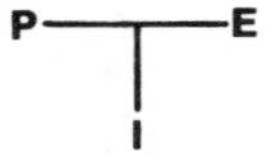	15 mm	Small 3/8" Large 1/2"	Dupaco Foregger	To facilitate attachment to endotracheal tube.
T-piece mask	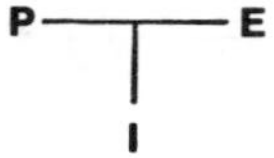	25 mm OD	10 mm	Dupaco	Can accommodate mask or endotracheal tube.
Summers T-tube	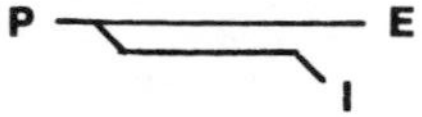	15 mm ID	15 mm OD	Dupaco	Fresh gas flow directed toward patient by shape of inlet tube.
Norman mask elbow (Norman elbow)	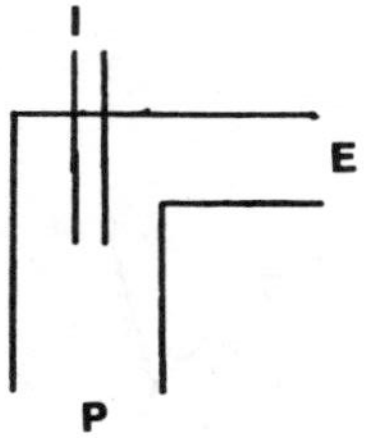	22 mm OD 15 mm ID	15 mm OD	Dupaco	Gas inlet ends 9/16" above mask fitting, reducing dead space. Fresh gas feed blows jet of gas into the mask. Dead space with a 3 L/min flow is 0.2 ml.
Fletcher T-tube	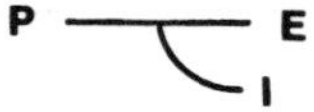	15 mm ID	15 mm ID	Dupaco	Fresh gas inflow tube is bent 90° after leaving tube.
Washington T-tube	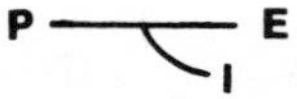	15 mm ID	15 mm OD	Dupaco	Used with male-female sequence of fittings.

Ayre T-Piece (I) (continued)

Name	Shape	Patient Limb Diameter	Expiratory Limb Diameter	Dealers	Comment
Rabbit ears	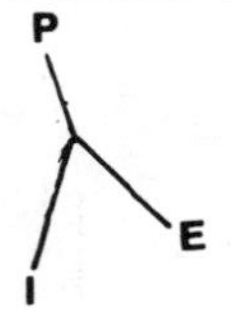	15 mm ID	3/4 or 7/16" OD	Anesthesia Associates	
Magill connection	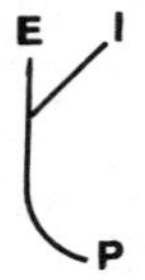	4 mm OD and 2.5 mm ID or 5 mm OD and 3 mm ID		Anesthesia Associates	Fits endotracheal tube. Patient end 90° to Y.
Keets modification of Hanks–Rackow elbow (Keets type Hanks–Rackow elbow)	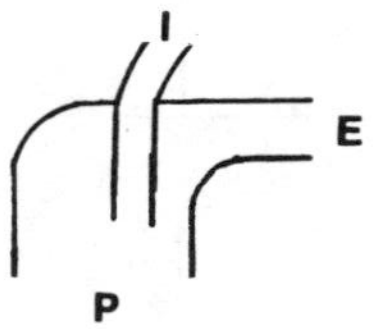	22 mm OD 15 mm ID	15 mm OD	Anesthesia Associates	Modified to blow a jet of gas into the mask. Fresh gas inlet at side or top.
Hanks–Rackow elbow with side inlet	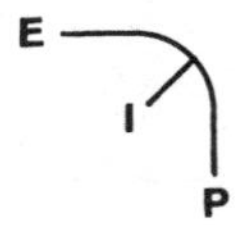	22 mm OD 15 mm ID	15 mm OD	Anesthesia Associates	Gas inflow tube does not extend into lumen at side or top.
Neoprene modified Ayre T-tube	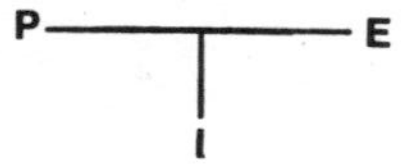	22 mm OD 15 mm ID	15 mm OD	Anesthesia Associates	

NRPR elbow (Non-rebreathing pressure relieving elbow) (Hustead Elbow)	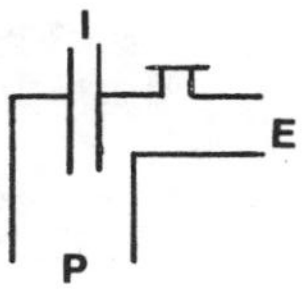 15 mm ID 22 mm OD	15 mm ID 22 mm OD	Puritan-Bennett Corporation	Modified to blow a jet of fresh gas into the mask. Bag can be connected directly to elbow. Pressure relief outlet on top of elbow. Dead space with a 3 L/min flow is 0.2 ml.

*P, patient limb; E, expiratory limb; and I, fresh gas inlet limb.

Ayre T-piece: (II) Modifications to the expiratory limb of the T-piece system.

Equipment	Functional Analysis	Reference
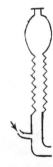 Double-ended bag is fitted to the expiratory limb. The open end of the bag is fitted with an adjustable tap. Corrugated tubing is often used between the T-piece and bag.	Bag allows breathing to be assisted or controlled and spontaneous breathing to be monitored. The tap is adjusted so that intermittent pressure applied to the bag expels the amount of gas required to maintain the equilibrium of the system.	Jackson-Rees G: Anaesthesia in the newborn. Br. Med. J. 2:1419-1422, 1950.
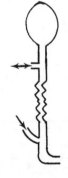 Two T-pieces are used: one at the patient end and one between the reservoir tube and the bag.	If fresh gas flow is delivered to the proximal T-piece, the system functions similar to the Jackson-Rees modification. To control respiration, the anesthesiologist's thumb is put over the sidearm of the distal T-piece. This system may also be used as a Magill system if fresh gas flow is delivered to the distal T-piece.	Baraka A, Brandstater B, Muallem, M, et al.: Rebreathing in a double T-piece system. Br. J. Anaesth. 41:47-53, 1969.
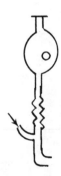 The bag contains two exits-flap valve on bag and an adjustable tap.	For assisted or controlled ventilation, the adjustable tap is closed and the flap valve is covered by the anesthesiologist's thumb during inspiration.	Davenport HT, Pereze E: Infant anesthesia set. Anesthesiology 21:776, 1960.

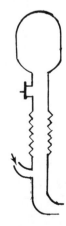

Georgia valve is attached proximal to the breathing bag. Bag is closed ended.

During spontaneous respiration, the valve remains open. When the breathing bag is compressed, the sudden increase in pressure closes the valve.

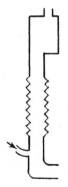

Nonexpansile hose leading to ventilator is attached to expiratory limb of the T-piece.

Ventilator supplies positive pressure during inspiration.

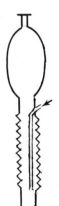

The fresh gas inflow tubing is incorporated inside the exhalation limb.

Manual compression of the bag may be used, or a respirator can be attached for controlled or assisted ventilation.

Freifeld S: Modification of the Ayre T-piece system. Anesth. Analg. 42: 575–577, 1963.

Kuwabara S, McCaughey TJ: Artificial ventilation in infants and young children using a new ventilator with the T-piece. Can. Anaesth. Soc. J. 13:576–584, 1966.

Munson ES, Eger EI: Controlled ventilation in the newborn. Anesthesiology 24:871–872, 1963.

Smith C: Controlled ventilation employing a modified Ayre's technic. Anesth. Analg. 44:842–845, 1965.

Bain JA, Spoerel WE: A streamlined anaesthetic system. Can. Anaesth. Soc. J. 19:426–435, 1972.

Ayre T-Piece (II) (continued)

Equipment	Functional Analysis	Reference
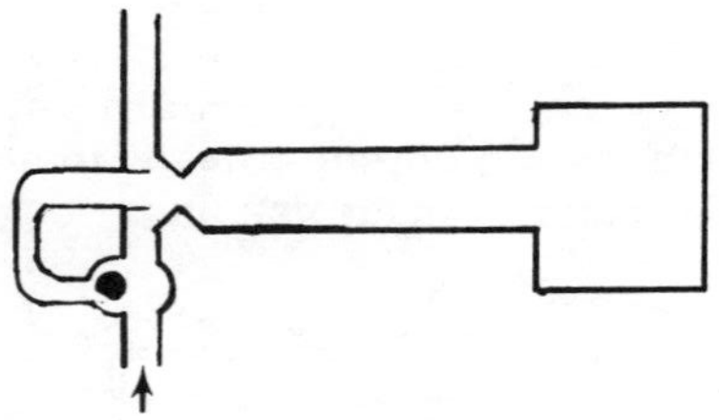 Fresh gas flow is divided into portions: one going directly to the patient, the other into the Venturi-shaped outlet. Position of stopcock determines relative flow to each.	The flow through Venturi outlet provides a negative pressure during expiration. Position of stopcock regulates amount of negative pressure. Ventilator may be attached to provide positive pressure during inspiration.	Keuskamp DHG: Automatic ventilation in paediatric anaesthesia using a modified Ayre's T-piece with negative pressure during expiratory phase. Anaesthesia 18:46-56, 1963.

B

BACKGROUND NOISE: Any nonspecific unwanted random sound or electric activity.

BACKGROUND RADIATION: The radiation due to radioisotopes in soil, bombardment of cosmic rays, and trace radioactive gases in the atmosphere. This must be taken into account when quantitating total radiation dose. See Electromagnetic spectrum.

BAINBRIDGE REFLEX: A phenomenon demonstrated best in laboratory animals and seen inconstantly in humans. It occurs when a rapid infusion of intravenous fluids raises a low resting heart rate.

BALANCED ANESTHESIA (COMBINED ANESTHESIA): A term introduced in 1926 which refers to the induction of anesthesia using a combination of agents, each for its specific effect, rather than using a single agent with multiple effects. Diethyl ether inhaled with room air is the prototypic single-agent anesthetic. A combination of muscle relaxants, intravenous barbiturates, narcotics, and N_2O/O_2 is an example of balanced anesthesia, which is characterized by relaxation and unconsciousness, but not necessarily areflexia. Balanced anesthesia has been disparagingly referred to as "garbage anesthesia" because of the ease with which the drug combinations may change depending on which drugs are readily available in a particular operating room on a particular day.

BALLAST: See Fluorescent lamp.

BALLISTOCARDIOGRAPH: A device used to record the movement of the entire body caused by the movement of the heart during contraction. Laboratory techniques exist to convert these body movements into a direct readout of cardiac output.

BALLOON PUMPING: See Intra-aortic balloon pump.

BANDWIDTH: The range within a band of wavelengths, frequencies, or energies. See Frequency.

BARALYME: A trade name for barium hydroxide lime. See Carbon dioxide absorption, Carbon dioxide absorption canister, Soda lime.

BARBITAL: See Barbiturate.

BARBITONE: The British term for barbital. See Barbiturate.

Barbiturate: Structure of barbituric acid
and classification of common barbiturates.

Generic Name (Trade Name)	Substituents in Position 5	Duration of Action
Thiopental* (Pentothal)	Ethyl, 1-methylbutyl	Ultrashort
Thiamylal* (Surital)	Allyl, 1-methylbutyl	(intravenous
Hexobarbital** (Evipal)	Methyl, cyclohexenyl	anesthetics)
Secobarbital (Seconal)	Allyl, 1-methylbutyl	Short
Pentobarbital (Nembutal)	Ethyl, 1-methylbutyl	
Butabarbital (Butisol)	Ethyl, sec-butyl	Intermediate
Amobarbital (Amytal)	Ethyl, isoamyl	
Vinbarbital (Delvinal)	Ethyl, 1-methyl-1-butenyl	
Phenobarbital (Luminal)	Ethyl, phenyl	Long
Mephobarbital** (Mebaral)	Ethyl, phenyl	
Barbital (Veronal)	Ethyl, ethyl	

 * Thiobarbiturate.
** A CH_3 group is attached to the nitrogen atom.

BARBITURATE: A class of drugs, derived from barbituric acid, which act as generalized depressants of cellular function. The first barbiturate, barbital, was introduced into clinical practice in 1903, and since then many other derivatives have
been prepared by substitutions of the side chains on the basic molecule. Clinically,
onset, duration of action, and, to a lesser extent, speed of degradation are the determining factors in the use of a particular barbiturate. All barbiturates have been
classified as ultrashort acting, short to intermediate acting, and long acting. However, a large dose of an ultrashort acting barbiturate will have an effect indistinguishable from a moderate dose of a long-acting barbiturate. See Fig.

BARBITURIC ACID: See Barbiturate.

BARBOTAGE: The repeated withdrawal and injection of cerebrospinal fluid mixed
with a local anesthetic to ensure the maximal distribution of the anesthetic.

BARIUM HYDROXIDE LIME (BARALYME): See Carbon dioxide absorption, Carbon
dioxide absorption canister, Soda lime.

BARIUM SULFATE ($BaSO_4$): A bulky, fine powder which is odorless and tasteless
and is used as a contrast medium in radiology of the digestive tract. A contrast medium, by filling a hollow space, outlines and differentiates specific areas. Other
barium salts including bromide, carbonate, and chloride were previously used in
medicine for the treatment of various diseases. These practices have been dis-
carded. See Fig.

BAROMETER: An instrument used to measure atmospheric pressure.

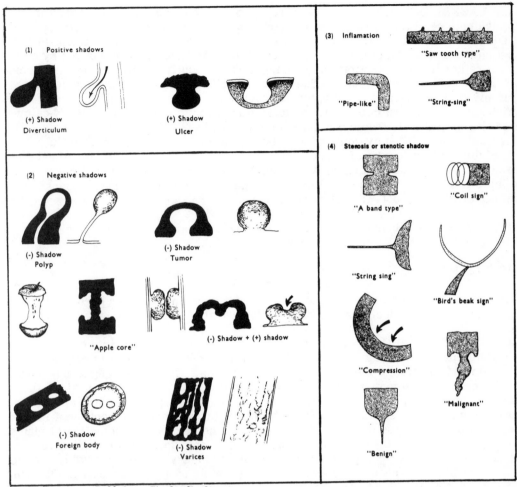

(1) Positive shadows

(+) Shadow
Diverticulum

(+) Shadow
Ulcer

(2) Negative shadows

(-) Shadow
Polyp

(-) Shadow
Tumor

"Apple core"

(-) Shadow + (+) shadow

(-) Shadow
Foreign body

(-) Shadow
Varices

(3) Inflamation

"Saw tooth type"

"Pipe-like"

"String-sing"

(4) Stenosis or stenotic shadow

"A band type"

"Coil sign"

"String sing"

"Bird's beak sign"

"Compression"

"Malignant"

"Benign"

Barium Sulfate: Study findings.

BARORECEPTOR (PRESSURE RECEPTOR): A stretch receptor in the walls of the heart and all large arteries. These receptors are stimulated by distention of the structures in which they are located; they discharge at an increased rate as the pressure rises in these structures. Their afferent nerve fibers pass via the glossopharyngeal and vagus nerves to the vasomotor center and the cardioinhibitory center. Baroreceptor impulses inhibit vasoconstrictor nerves and excite the cardioinhibitory center, eliciting vasodilatation, decrease in blood pressure, bradycardia, and a decreased cardiac output.

BASAL ANESTHESIA: The technique of giving preoperative medication beyond the point where consciousness is lost. It is an older method of anesthesia which has fallen into disuse because of its dangerous consequences. It was originally advocated for children, who were more likely to be frightened by the surgical suite.

BASE: A substance which acts to bind hydrogen ions (H^+) when in solution. Strong bases bind H^+ much more readily than weak bases. It may be positively charged, negatively charged, or neutral. See Acid, Acid-base balance.

BASE DEFICIT: See Base excess.

BASE EXCESS (BE): The base concentration of whole blood. It is measured in milliequivalents per liter by titration of blood to a pH of 7.4 with a strong acid at a PCO_2 of 40 torr at 37 degrees Celsius. Negative BE values (blood deficient in base) must be titrated with a strong base. The BE or deficit can also be derived by calculation (rather than by titration) or by using a nomogram if the pH, PCO_2, and hemoglobin concentration are known. The BE or deficit is used clinically to determine appropriate corrections for metabolic acid-base derangements. In the case of base deficit (by far the most common), the total correction is calculated as BE X calculated extracellular fluid compartment volume (usually 25-33% of total body weight) to arrive at the milliequivalents of bicarbonate needed. Usually one-third to one-half of this amount is administered, and then acid-base status is redetermined after the body has had time to equilibrate. Complete restoration of a normal (zero) base deficit should not be attempted with a single large dose of bicarbonate because of the danger of overshoot. See Bernard rules.

BASIC: An easy-to-learn computer language which is an acronym for Beginner's All-purpose Symbolic Instruction Code.

BASIC LIFE SUPPORT: See Cardiopulmonary resuscitation.

BATTERY: The unlawful beating of or use of force against another person without his or her consent, which may be grounds for a malpractice suit.

BATTERY, ELECTRIC: A device which in its simplest form consists of two dissimilar plates placed in an electrolyte bath. Electricity (current flow) is produced by the chemical reaction of the electrolyte on the plates. Current strength and duration depend on plate composition and size. A primary battery is one in which the electric current is produced without prior electric charging. A secondary battery has to be charged by sending a current through it in the reverse direction of its discharge, which reverses the chemical reaction of the electrolyte on the metal plates. Consequently, a primary cell can deliver current immediately but cannot revert to its original state after complete discharge; the secondary cell is reversible and can be recharged and discharged repeatedly. An example of a primary cell is the standard carbon-zinc flashlight battery; an example of a secondary cell is the rechargeable nickel-cadmium battery.

BAUD: A unit of signaling data or transmission speed; in the binary system 1 baud is equal to 1 bit/sec. See Binary code; binary number system. See Bit.

BECKMAN ANALYZER: See Oxygen analyzer.

BECLOMETHASONE (VANCERIL INHALER): A potent steroid, related to prednisolone, usually given to asthmatics in a dose-metering aerosol unit. This drug can be given to patients who are unsuitable for treatment with systemic steroids because of potential adverse reactions.

BEL: A logarithmic unit of measurement comparing the ratio of two amounts of power. The most commonly used unit is the decibel (one-tenth of a bel), which measures sound intensity. A 3-decibel change upward doubles and a 3-decibel change downward halves signal strength.

BELLADONNA (BELLADONNA ALKALOIDS): See Atropine.

BENDS: See Caisson disease.

BENZEDRINE: See Amphetamine.

BENZOCAINE: An ester-type local anesthetic. It is often combined with other agents, such as tetracaine, and is useful as a topical preparation in a gel, liquid, or ointment form. See Local anesthetic.

BENZODIAZEPINE: A class of sedative, hypnotic, antianxiety drugs. The derivative diazepam (Valium) is one of the most frequently prescribed drugs. Other examples of benzodiazepines include oxazepam (Serax), chlordiazepoxide hydrochloride (Librium), flurazepam hydrochloride (Dalmane), nitrazepam (Mogadon), and lorazepam (Ativan). The popularity of this drug class appears to stem from the fact that central nervous system depression and antianxiety action seem to occur at dosages much lower than those causing total body cellular depression. See Anxiety.

BENZOIC ACID: A naturally occurring acid used as a food preservative and antifungal agent.

BENZOQUINONIUM (MYTOLON): A neuromuscular blocking agent which combines some features of the nondepolarizing and depolarizing types. It currently has little clinical use.

BENZTROPINE MESYLATE (COGENTIN): An anti-Parkinson agent with atropine-like effects. It is also used in the treatment of the Parkinson-like syndrome induced by the phenothiazines.

BENZYL ALCOHOL: A compound formed by combining benzene and methyl alcohol. It has some local anesthetic effects and may be useful in patients who have demonstrated sensitivity to the more common local anesthetics.

BERNARD RULES: The three principles that govern the estimate of the appropriate change in serum bicarbonate levels when $PaCO_2$ changes. When the estimated appropriate bicarbonate level differs from the measured level, the contribution of metabolism to acid-base status can be determined. Rule 1 states that the increase in serum bicarbonate which accompanies an acute elevation in $PaCO_2$ is approximately 1 mEq/L of bicarbonate for each 10 torr rise in $PaCO_2$ over 40 torr. Rule 2 states that the decrease in serum bicarbonate which accompanies an acute decline in $PaCO_2$ is approximately 2 mEq/L of bicarbonate for each 10 torr fall in $PaCO_2$ below 40 torr. Rule 3 states that the increase in serum bicarbonate which accompanies a chronic increase in $PaCO_2$ is approximately 4 mEq/L of bicarbonate for each 10 torr increase in $PaCO_2$ above 40 torr.

BERNOULLI LAW: The relationship of velocity of fluid flow to cross-sectional diameter in a horizontal pipe. Stated simply, a fluid will gain speed as it passes from a wide to a narrow portion of the pipe. Conversely, the pressure is lowest where the velocity is highest and vice versa. If a horizontal pipe contains a constriction and then opens out to its original diameter slowly, the fluid slows down but regains its original pressure. This is a description of a Venturi tube. The Venturi tube generates a negative pressure at the constriction. The relationship between the negative pressure at the constriction and the positive pressure upstream can be related to flow. This pressure difference is used to measure gas flow in the water depression flowmeter.

BETA PARTICLE: A rapidly moving, energetic electron or positron emitted by some radioisotopes during decay. Each element capable of beta decay emits beta particles over a characteristic range of energies.

BETA-ENDORPHIN: See Endorphins.

BETAMETHASONE: A potent glucocorticoid, often encountered as a topical preparation.

BETHANECOL CHLORIDE (URECHOLINE): A parasympathomimetic drug (not destroyed by cholinesterase) which has a specific effect on the smooth muscles of the gastrointestinal tract and urinary bladder. It is used to treat postoperative abdominal distention (due to loss of muscle tone and impairment of persistalsis) and urinary retention (due to loss of muscle tone).

B FIBER: See Nerve fiber, anatomy and physiology of.

BIER BLOCK: See Nerve fiber, anatomy and physiology of.

Decimal Digit	Binary Code
0	0000
1	0001
2	0010
3	0011
4	0100
5	0101
6	0110
7	0111
8	1000
9	1001

Binary Code; Binary Number System: First 10 digits of the decimal system expressed in binary notation.

BINARY CODE; BINARY NUMBER SYSTEM: A notation system using two digits, usually 1 and 0, to represent all decimal numbers. In the binary coded decimal (bcd) system each number is indicated by a series of four binary digits (nibble). In an electronic circuit the presence or absence of an impulse is indicated by the bit 1 or 0 and the rate of flow is measured in bauds. The binary code is the universal method of transcribing data in computers. See Fig. See Baud, Bit.

BIOAVAILABILITY: A measure of the degree to which an administered substance becomes available to the target tissue.

BIOLOGIC DEATH: The cessation of life; the irreversible termination of cerebral function, spontaneous respiration, and spontaneous function of the circulatory system.

BIONICS: The science concerned with relating living systems to artificial devices and machinery. The goal of bionics is to simulate, duplicate, and enhance biologic functions.

BIOTRANSFORMATION: The alteration of an administered pharmacologic agent due to metabolic processes. See Elimination, drug.

BIRD CORPORATION: A company which manufactures and sells respirators such as the MARK 7 through the MARK 10 series. Later derivatives are the BABYbird, the IMVbird, and the MINIbird. Dr. Forrest M. Bird formed the organization in 1957. It is (as of January 1981) in the Medical Products Division of Minnesota Mining & Manufacturing Company (3M), and is referred to as Bird Products/3M. The Bird Corporation is located in Palm Springs, California.

BIT: An abbreviation of Binary digIT used in computer technology to signify either digit, the 1 or 0. See Binary code; binary number system.

BLACK BOX: An electronic device which performs its function so automatically it appears magical to its user. It may also denote the unobtainable, ideal solution to a difficult problem (i.e., "Let's black box the solution").

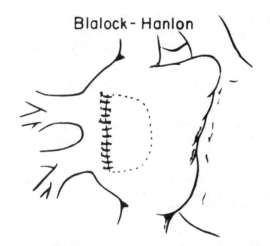

Blalock-Hanlon

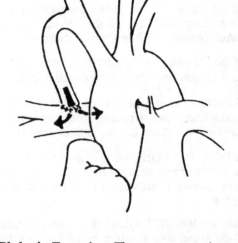

Blalock-Hanlon Procedure: In the Blalock-Hanlon procedure a surgical excision of part of the atrial septum is performed.

Blalock-Taussig: Three common types of procedures to increase pulmonary blood flow in congenital cardiac defects.

BLALOCK-HANLON PROCEDURE: A palliative surgical procedure for treating a congenital cardiac anomaly in which there is transposition of the great arteries. It consists of resecting the right lateral portion of the interarterial septum. A segment of the right and left atria and septum is clamped prior to the excision so there will be no interruption of blood flow. This procedure is performed only on those patients who are not good candidates for intracardiac repair. See Fig.

BLALOCK-TAUSSIG SHUNT: An end-to-side anastomosis of the subclavian artery with the pulmonary artery. This is a palliative procedure used in pediatric patients with defects reducing pulmonary blood flow, such as tetralogy of Fallot, pulmonary atresia with a ventricular septal defect, or transposition of the great vessels coupled with pulmonary stenosis. This shunt allows a controlled increase of pulmonary blood flow. See Fig.

BLEEDING DISORDER: A condition in which the normal clotting function of the blood is compromised either partially or completely. It can be either primary or secondary, congenital or acquired. Under certain circumstances (such as open heart surgery), it can be the result of pharmacologic management of the patient. See Anticoagulant, Blood coagulation, Blood storage, Disseminated intravascular coagulation, Hemophilia, Von Willebrand disease.

BLEEDING TIME: A screening test to determine coagulability. Typically, a puncture is made on the earlobe (Duke method) and the wound is blotted at 30-sec intervals until the bleeding is stopped. The total time elapsed from onset to cessation of bleeding is considered the bleeding time. The "normal values" are difficult to standardize because of probable variations in puncture technique by different individuals. The Ivy method of measuring bleeding time requires an incision to be made distal to an inflated blood pressure cuff on the forearm. The blood drops are absorbed at 30-sec intervals. The normal time for the cessation of bleeding is under 8 min.

BLEND: A setting on electrosurgical machines which combines the damped, sinusoidal wave pattern of the coagulation setting with the continuous undamped output of the cutting setting. This combination allows for some cutting and some coagulating simultaneously. See Coagulation current.

BLIND NASAL INTUBATION: The technique of introducing an endotracheal tube through the nose without visualizing the trachea.

BLOCK: The deposition of a local anesthetic near a nerve trunk to prevent nerve conduction. See Brachial plexus block, Caudal anesthesia, Digital block, Epidural anesthesia, Field block, Spinal anesthesia.

BLOCKADE MONITOR: A device which delivers various configurations of electric current across skin electrodes to evaluate neuromuscular blockade. These devices have open-circuit voltages of approximately 250 volts. See Peripheral nerve stimulator.

BLOOD-BRAIN BARRIER (BBB): A functional impediment to molecular diffusion which separates the brain and the cerebrospinal fluid from the blood. In the brain

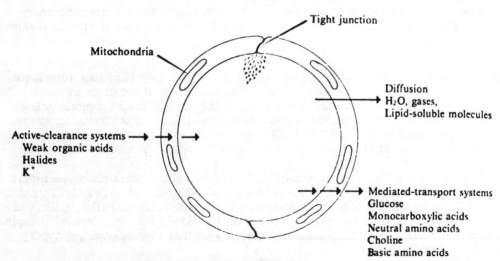

Blood-Brain Barrier: Transport processes across capillary endothelial cells in brain parenchyma. The tight junctions between endothelial cells preclude movement of large molecules.

the endothelial cells of the capillaries are joined by tight junctions. Lipid-soluble molecules easily penetrate the brain and equilibrate between the blood and the brain very rapidly. Lipid-insoluble molecules and proteins penetrate brain tissue extremely slowly. When the brain is damaged (irradiation, infection, tumor, or surgical retraction), this selective permeability of the blood-brain barrier breaks down. See Fig.

BLOOD COAGULATION: The process by which blood forms a fibrin clot. One of the most elegant and complex physiologic functions, coagulation depends on the interaction of multiple proteins. These proteins, either circulating in the blood or contained in platelets, are induced to form a multiple chemical cascade upon encountering an environment other than the interior of blood vessels. See Figs. See Blood storage.

BLOOD FLOW; BLOOD FLOW VELOCITY: The movement of blood by cardiac contraction determined by the change in pressure (delta P) along a given vessel length

Blood Coagulation: (I) Clotting factors and some of their common names.

Factor	Synonym
I.	Fibrinogen
II.	Prothrombin, prethrombin
III.	Tissue factor, thromboplastin (platelet factor 3)
IV.	Calcium (Ca^{++})
V.	Labile factor, proaccelertin, plasma accelerator globulin (ac-G)
VI.	No factor assigned to this numeral
VII.	Stable factor, proconvertin, autoprothrombin I, serum prothrombin conversion acceleration (SPCA)
VIII.	Antihemophilic globulin (AHG) Antihemophilic factor A (AHF) Thromboplastinogen, platelet cofactor I, antihemophilia factor A
IX.	Plasma thromboplastin component (PTC), Christmas factor, autoprothrombin II, antihemophilia factor B, platelet cofactor II
X.	Stuart-Prower factor, autoprothrombin C (or III)
XI.	Plasma thromboplastin antecedent (PTA), Rosenthal syndrome, antihemophilia factor C
XII.	Hageman factor, glass factor
XIII.	Fibrin-stabilizing factor (FSF), Laki-Lorand factor, fibrinase serum factor, urea-insolubility factor

78

Blood Coagulation: (II) Generally accepted scheme of the coagulation cascade modified to emphasize the sites of platelet and heparin activity. Substances enclosed in boxes represent platelet or platelet derivative activity. Underlined factors identify sites of heparin activity. The right portion of the final common pathway illustrates the theoretic interaction of heparin with PF−4. Heparin in combination with circulating anti-Xa/IIa inactivates Xa and IIa. PF-4 antagonizes this heparin activity.

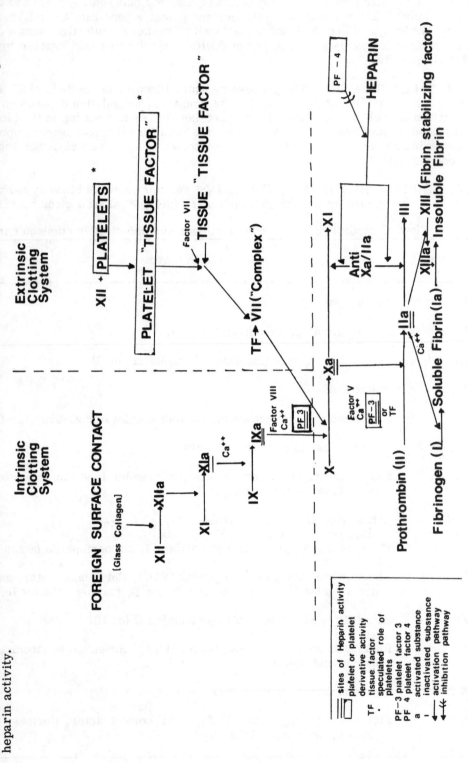

divided by the resistance to flow (R). The velocity of blood flow in each segment of the arterial circulation is inversely proportional to its area in cross-section. See Blood flow, methods for measuring.

BLOOD FLOW, METHODS FOR MEASURING: The various techniques used to measure blood flow. (1) The rotameter (experimental use only) is a device inserted into a cut vessel enabling the previously anticoagulated blood to flow through. The rotameter float reading is directly calibrated to blood flow. (2) The electromagnetic flowmeter (clinically useful) operates on the principle that an electric conductor, such as blood, moving in a magnetic field generates a weak electric current within itself. This current can be measured between two electrodes placed on the vessel wall and is proportional to the blood flow velocity. (3) The ultrasonic flowmeter is a crystal transmitter/receiver combination which is placed around a vessel. The transmitter alternates sending sound waves up and down the vessel length. The sound waves are altered in frequency by the Doppler shift in an amount proportional to the blood velocity. (4) The plethysmograph is an instrument for estimating volume change of a limb, organ, or part. When used to estimate blood flow, a limb, e.g., forearm, is inserted into an airtight chamber and a blood pressure cuff is then placed on the arm and inflated to less than 40 mmHg; this prevents venous return but not arterial inflow. The rate of forearm swelling is proportional to the rate of blood flow into the forearm.

BLOOD GAS FACTOR: The percentage of error exhibited by an O_2 electrode calibrated by a known gas mixture which then measures PO_2 in a known blood sample. It is expressed as PO_2 gas - PO_2 equilibrated blood/PO_2 gas X 100. (This error can be as large as 10-20%.)

BLOOD GAS MACHINE: A device for determining PO_2, PCO_2, and pH of a blood sample using specific electrodes. See Fig.

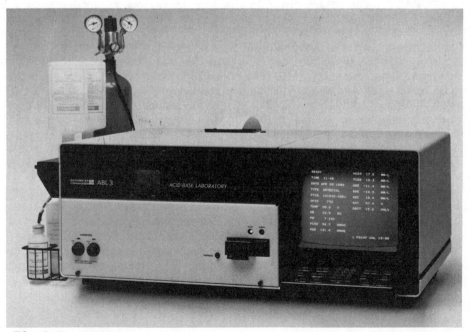

Blood-Gas Machine.

BLOOD LOSS, ESTIMATE OF: An attempt to determine as accurately as possible the amount of blood lost from the patient during surgery. The most accurate and practical technique involves weighing all the sponges and pads as they are used during the procedure and keeping a running total (1 ml blood weighs about 1 mg). Blood which is removed (suctioned) from the incision site is placed in a calibrated chamber and its volume is then determined (subtracting the volume of wash and irrigation solutions used). More elaborate situations involve operating tables which continually weigh the patient with various corrections for drapes and instruments and washing machines which wash all the drapes, pads, etc. after the procedure, with the hemoglobin content of the rinse water being determined.

BLOOD PATCH: See Epidural patch.

BLOOD PRESSURE: See Arterial blood pressure, Arterial pressure determination by palpation, Central venous pressure, Mean arterial pressure, Photoelectric determination of blood pressure.

BLOOD PRESSURE CUFF SIZE SELECTION: The choice of cuff size as it relates to accurate blood pressure measurement. The sizing of the blood pressure cuff is a common source of error in auscultatory methods of blood pressure determination. If the cuff is too narrow in relation to the arm, it must be blown up to a falsely high pressure in order to produce the proper tissue pressure on the artery. An inappropriately wide cuff in contradistinction will give relatively low readings. Loose wrapping of the cuff gives the same effect as a narrow cuff. The air bladder should occupy at least one-half of the arm circumference. In general, the minimum width of the cuff should be approximately 20% greater than the diameter of the arm. This usually works out to be anywhere from one-half to two-thirds the length of the upper arm. Cuff size which is incorrectly selected also affects in a similar way all indirect methods for determining blood pressure.

BLOOD STORAGE: The saving of whole blood or its various components for use in transfusions. Whole blood is stored on a unit basis. One unit contains approximately 450 ml of whole blood to which 50 ml of an anticoagulant, acid-citrate-dextrose (ACD) or citrate-phosphate-dextrose (CPD), are added. Anticoagulants only protect the red blood cells in whole blood and are therefore not added when storing components of blood. Until recently, ACD was added most frequently. When compared with whole blood, ACD-stored blood has a much lower pH, a much higher PCO_2, a very low 2,3-diphosphoglycerate (2,3-DPG) level, a decrease of factors V and VIII, and a serum potassium in excess of 15 mEq/L. Stored at 4 degrees Celsius, it has a shelf life of approximately 21 days. CPD-stored blood, at 4 degrees Celsius, has at least a 7-day longer shelf life. It is less acidic, has lower potassium levels, and its 2,3-DPG levels are not as depressed as in acid-stored blood. Neither ACD- nor CPD-stored blood contains viable platelets. In component therapy, only the specific blood fraction needed is administered, e.g., concentrated factor VIII is given to patients with classic hemophilia. Other commonly used fractions include fresh frozen plasma (FFP), which is used to restore clotting factors; platelet concentrates (stored at room temperature), which are useful in treating thrombocytopenia; albumin, the major blood protein, which is used to expand volume; and red cell concentrates (stored at 4 degrees Celsius), which replace lost hemoglobin and thereby increase O_2-carrying capacity. Red cells may also be suspended in glycerin and deep-frozen for an indefinite period. Once thawed, they must be used within 24 hr. See Blood coagulation.

Blood Group	Antigen(s) on RBC	Antibodies in Serum
A	A	Anti-B
B	B	Anti-A
AB	A and B	Neither anti-A nor anti-B
O	Neither A nor B	Both anti-A and anti-B

I

	Approximate Frequency (%)	
Phenotype	Whites	Blacks
O	44	49
A	45	27
B	8	20
AB	3	4

II

Blood Types: (I) The relationship between major ABO red cell antigens and reciprocal serum antibodies. (II) Frequency of occurrence of ABO blood types.

BLOOD TYPES (BLOOD GROUPS): The characterization of the blood by type of antigen on the red cell surface and type of antibody found in the serum. These antigen-antibody combinations are genetically determined. A major blood type system is the ABO, which depends on the presence or absence of the two antigenic factors A and B. (O signifies that neither A nor B is present.) Agglutinogens are the antigens located on the membranes of human red cells; antibodies against these agglutinogens are called agglutinins. Individuals with type A blood have agglutinogen A on their red cells and anti-B agglutinins in their serum. Therefore, if their plasma is mixed with type B cells, clumping and destruction of the blood will occur. The reverse is true for people with type B blood. Individuals with type O blood have circulating anti-A and anti-B agglutinins whereas those with type AB blood have no circulating agglutinins. Another major blood-typing system is concerned with the Rh factor. This system is composed of many antigens, the most important being D. (Alternate terminology for the Rh factor is blood group D.) The Rh+ (positive) person has agglutinogen D on the red cells and the Rh- (negative) person has no D antigen. Transfusion reactions occur when a patient is given incompatible blood resulting in hemolysis. This leads to hemolytic anemia. Clinically, in the awake patient, signs and symptoms may include hives, chills, chest pain, shortness of breath, headache, and skin flushing. (Reactions vary in severity depending on such factors as the degree of incompatibility and the amount of blood transfused.) During general anesthesia many of the symptoms may be masked. In both the awake and anesthetized patient, coagulation disorders, cardiovascular collapse, and hemoglobinuria may be seen. Researchers have identified a plethora of tissue and blood antigen-antibody systems, but 90% of all transfusion reactions occur as a result of incompatibility within the ABO and Rh systems. In most hospitals, three levels of preparation for transfusion are maintained preoperatively. The "type and hold," in which a patient's blood type only is characterized, is the lowest level of preparedness. In the "type and screen," the blood is characterized and checked for ABO and Rh incompatabilities against a panel of standard antigens. In "type and crossmatch," all possible antigen-antibody reactions are determined between the recipient and all possible donors. Compatible units are then stored and used only for that particular patient. See Figs.

BLOOD VOLUME MEASUREMENT: An estimate of circulating blood volume. This measurement can be made by either of two radioactive tracer techniques: the radioiodine-tagged albumin technique or the chromium-tagged red cell technique. Both methods measure dilution of radioactive material by the blood pool of nontagged albumin in one test and of red cells in the other. Both are subject to errors due to an unequal dilution of the radioactive material. Clinically, relative blood volume is determined by measuring the filling pressure of the right and left ventricles, the cardiac output, and the total peripheral resistance. In addition, when a baseline series of these pressures and outputs is known, blood volume trends can be monitored.

BLUE BLOATER: See Pink puffer.

BODY FLUID COMPARTMENT: A model for body fluid distribution which assumes that water is present in two compartments, intracellular (within cells) and extracellular (outside cells). The extracellular compartment is further subdivided into interstitial (between cells) and intravascular (within the blood vessels). Fluid transfer between compartments is determined by electrolyte gradients which in turn are controlled by cellular membranes, at times with energy expenditure. See Fig.

BODY PLETHYSMOGRAPH: An apparatus for ascertaining changes in body volume. It is useful in measuring the functional residual capacity of the lung, i.e., the volume of gas in the lung after a normal expiration. The patient sits in a large airtight chamber and is asked to force ventilation at the end of expiration against a closed mouthpiece. The gas in the lungs is compressed and lung volume decreases. The gas volume in the box increases as the box pressure decreases. According to Boyle law, at a given temperature, pressure times volume is constant. Therefore, if the initial pressure in the airway and in the box, the initial volume, and the new pressure in the box are known, the functional residual capacity of the lungs can be calculated. The body plethysmograph measures the total volume of gas in the lungs, including gas trapped behind closed airways.

BOHR EFFECT: A phenomenon exhibiting the increased affinity of O_2 for hemoglobin at low concentrations of CO_2 and the decreased affinity of O_2 for combining with hemoglobin at high levels of CO_2. The Bohr effect aids O_2 transport by favoring O_2 loading onto hemoglobin in the lungs (decreased PCO_2) and by favoring unloading from hemoglobin in the peripheral tissues (increased PCO_2). See Haldane effect.

BOHR EQUATION: A method for determining physiologic dead space. The equation states that the dead space volume divided by the tidal volume equals the $PACO_2$ minus the expiratory gas $PACO_2$, divided by the $PACO_2$. In normal subjects, the physiologic dead space approximates that of the anatomic dead space. See Anatomic dead space, Physiologic dead space.

BOILING POINT: The temperature at which a vaporizing liquid has a vapor pressure equal to atmospheric pressure. As a consequence bubbles of gas form throughout the volume of liquid.

BOND ENERGY: The energy required to break a chemical bond between two atoms in a molecule. The amount of energy is dependent on the type of atom and the nature of the molecule.

BOUNCING BALL: See Oscilloscope.

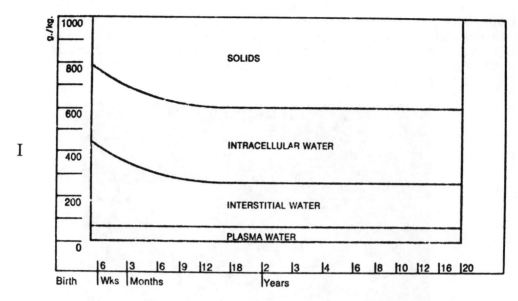

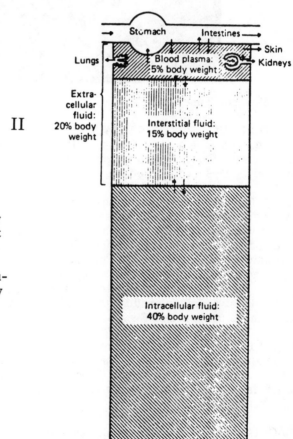

Body Fluid Compartment: (I) Body
content and distribution of water at
various ages. (II) Adult body fluid
compartments. The arrows show
fluid movement. Transcellular fluids, a very small part of total body
fluid, are not shown.

BOUNDARY LAYER: The fluid layer most proximal to the solid boundaries restraining that fluid, e.g., the layer of blood immediately adjacent to the inner wall of a blood vessel. Its thickness is determined by the viscosity of the blood, the friction between the blood and the vessel wall, and the speed at which the blood is moving. See Reynolds number.

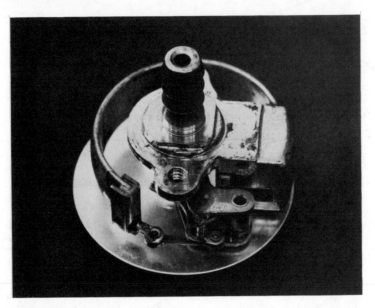

Bourdon Tube.

BOURDON TUBE PRESSURE GAUGE: A device measuring cylinder gas pressure which incorporates a curved tube. Elevation of internal tube pressure tends to straighten the tube. This straightening in turn may be mechanically linked to move a pointer across a dial. See Fig.

BOYLE BOTTLE: An older vaporizer which can be classified as a variable-bypass, flow-over, and/or bubble-through vaporizer. The amount of gas which is allowed into the vaporizer is controlled by the position of the on-off lever. The path of the gas through the vaporizing chamber depends on the height of the plunger which redirects flow across or under the surface of the liquid in the vaporizer. The Boyle bottle has no temperature compensation and may be used with multiple anesthetic agents. Anesthestic concentration is basically regulated by monitoring the clinical signs. This vaporizer produces unpredictable results due to the many variables involved in its usage. See Fig.

BOYLE LAW: A principle stating that if a given mass of gas is compressed at a constant temperature (T), but the pressure (P) is increased or decreased, the volume (V) of gas varies inversely to pressure. (At constant T, $PV = P'V'$.) Although the law is only an approximation for real gases, it is accurate enough for most clinical circumstances.

BRACHIAL PLEXUS BLOCK: A regional nerve block used for surgical procedures of the hand, forearm, and upper arm, in which a local anesthetic is injected unilaterally near the brachial plexus. There are essentially three approaches to brachial plexus block: supraclavicular, interscalene (a variation of the supraclavicular), and axillary. Phrenic nerve paralysis, Horner syndrome, and hematoma are po-

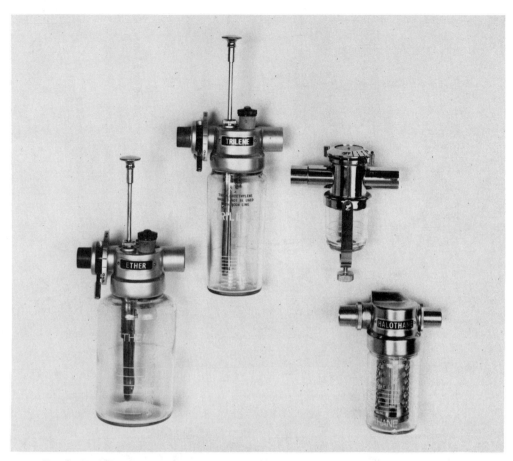

Boyle Bottle.

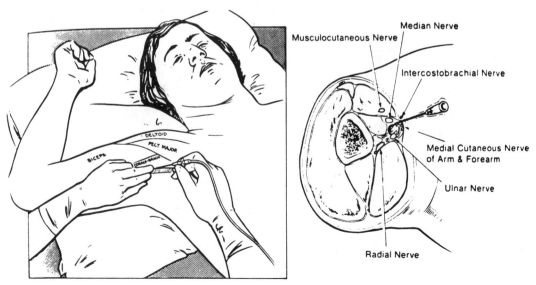

Brachial Plexus Block: (I) Axillary technique.

86

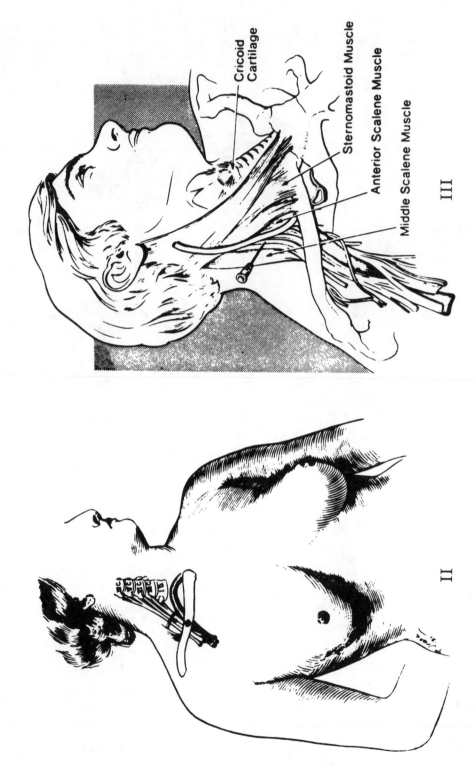

Cricoid
Cartilage

Sternomastoid Muscle

Anterior Scalene Muscle

Middle Scalene Muscle

III

II

Brachial Plexus Block: (II) Supraclavicular technique. (III) Interscalene technique.

tential complications of the supraclavicular and interscalene approaches. Pneumothorax occurs in 1-3% of cases with the supraclavicular approach. Intravascular injection and nerve injury are potential complications of the axillary approach. See Figs.

BRADYKININ: A polypeptide found in precursor form in plasma and therefore also known as plasma kinin. It is bound to the α_2-globulin fraction of the plasma, but the action of the proteolytic enzyme kallikrein enables the bradykinin to be released. Bradykinin causes profound relaxation of vascular smooth muscle and an increase in capillary permeability. It is assumed to play a role in inflammatory processes and anaphylatic shock syndromes. See Allergic response.

BRAIN (ENCEPHALON): The large mass of nerve tissue located within the cranium. The brain consists of five parts. (1) The cerebrum, the largest part of the brain, consists of a right and left hemisphere, each of which is composed of five lobes (temporal, parietal, occipital, frontal, and insula). One hemisphere is functionally dominant. Various functions such as behavior, memory, intelligence, spatial relations, hearing, taste, smell, and sight are regulated within the cerebrum. (2) The cerebellum functions in muscle coordination and equilibrium. (3) The medulla oblongata is the portion of the brain stem which helps regulate heartbeat, blood pressure, and respiration and influences the autonomic reflexes for swallowing, coughing, sneezing, and vomiting. (4) The pons varolii is the segment of the brain stem in which the trigeminal, abducens, facial, and vestibulcochlear nerves originate. (5) The midbrain is the portion of the brain stem which contains the nerve centers for the oculomotor and trochlear nerves. All parts of the brain stem control and transmit impulses between the brain and spinal cord.

BRAIN DEATH: The currently accepted criterion for biologic death. Two electroencephalograms taken 24 hr apart must demonstrate no electric activity. There must be no influence from temperature, ventilation, or drugs. The concept of brain death supplants the concept of the cessation of spontaneous ventilation, which may be supported by appropriate mechanical and pharmacologic intervention for long periods of time.

BRASS: An alloy containing copper and zinc in which the zinc content ranges up to 40%.

BREAKDOWN, ELECTRIC: A sudden, disruptive electric discharge through an insulator. It proceeds from a state of little or no current flow to a state of massive current flow. The insulation around wires used to conduct electric current is often rated by breakdown voltage. The higher the breakdown voltage, the better the quality of the insulation.

BREATHING BAG (RESERVOIR BAG): A device which is used to store and conveniently pressurize (by hand squeeze) a volume of gas which will be used to ventilate the lung. There are two types of breathing bags. (1) The self-inflating bag is designed with an internal spring or sponge to return it to its normal volume and configuration after the release of external pressure. It is usually used in combination with a one-way valve which directs exhaled gas to the atmosphere and prevents the negative pressure generated by the expanding spring from affecting the patient's airway. (2) The non-self-inflating bag, also called the rebreathing or anesthesia bag, is simply a rubber sack which is squeezed and then reinflated by fresh gas inflow, and the patient's exhaled volume. The non-self-inflating bag is usually used in combination with an overflow device (pop-off valve) to prevent overinflation. Rebreath-

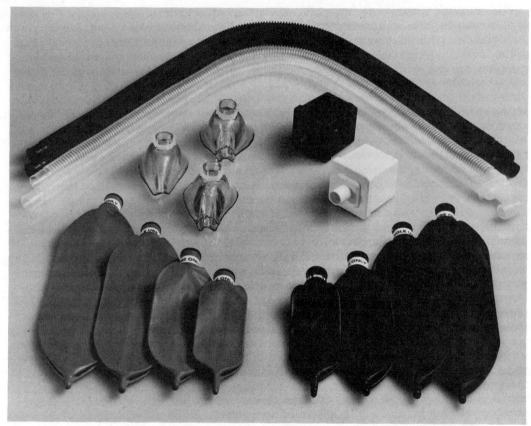

Breathing Bag: Breathing bags with other disposable breathing circuit parts.

ing of expired CO_2 is prevented by the valve in the self-inflating bag and by proper control of fresh gas flow and CO_2 absorption (when on an anesthesia machine) in the self-inflating bag. The self-inflating bag can be used to administer at most 40-60% O_2 as the bag reexpands too fast for normal O_2 supplies (10-20 L/min) to fill the bag. (The remaining volume comes from the atmosphere.) The non-self-inflating bag can administer 90-100% O_2 as fresh O_2 flow is augmented by the O_2 returning from the patient. (A patient breathing 40% O_2 will exhale approximately 36% O_2.) The Ambu resuscitator is a type of self-inflating bag. See Fig.

BREMSSTRAHLUNG (BRAKING RADIATION): The electromagnetic radiation produced when a fast-moving charged particle, usually an electron, decelerates as it approaches an atomic nucleus.

BRETYLIUM (BRETYLOL): A drug originally marketed as an oral antihypertensive agent and now accepted for use as an antiarrhythmic agent. It is approved for intravenous or intramuscular administration in patients with life-threatening ventricular arrhythmias which have failed to respond to lidocaine, procainamide, or dilantin. It tends to decrease the blood pressure.

BREVITAL: See Barbiturate.

BROMETHOL (AVERTIN, TRIBROMETHANOL): See Rectal anesthesia.

BROMIDE: The ionic form of the element bromine. It was given in the last century in the form of potassium bromide for the treatment of epilepsy and other seizure disorders. With an extremely long half-life, it tends to accumulate in the body if taken daily. This is of concern since it is found in many over-the-counter drugs and preparations. Chronic use may cause depression, confusion, and lethargy. In addition, since bromide is released as a degradation product of halothane, it may be one of the causes of prolonged sedation after extended administration of halothane.

BRONCHIAL INTUBATION: See Endobronchial intubation.

BRONCHIOLE: A distinct part of the respiratory tree containing occasional alveoli and connecting the terminal bronchioles (without alveoli) to the alveolar ducts (which are completely lined with alveoli).

BRONCHOGRAPHY: A procedure which allows radiographic visualization of the bronchial tree following instillation of a radiopaque material. The procedure can cause bronchial irritation and has a well-recognized morbidity rate.

BRONCHOMOTOR TONE: The continuous state of contraction of the bronchial musculature during respiration. It is apparently affected by vagal impulses as well as by circulating catecholamines.

BRONCHOPLEURAL FISTULA: An abnormal communication between the air passageways of the lung and pleural cavity. It is most likely to occur after lung surgery, rupture of a lung abscess, or the spread of an empyema. It can lead to pneumothorax and severe impairment of respiratory function.

BRONCHOSCOPE, FLEXIBLE: An instrument which allows direct visualization of the bronchi and their distal segments. (It is based on the fiberoptic principle by which an image is transmitted along flexible bundles of coated glass or plastic fibers having optical properties.) This device can be guided to specific locations directly or under fluoroscopy. The patient is usually mildly sedated and topical anesthetics, e.g., lidocaine, are administered through the bronchoscope. Brush catheters (for obtaining cytologic specimens) and small biopsy forceps are inserted through the scope to sample the lesion(s) visualized. See Fig.

BRONCHOSCOPE, RIGID: A firm, hollow stainless steel tube which is used to directly visualize the interior of the trachea and the mainstem bronchi. General anesthesia is often required during insertion of the scope. With the aid of lenses and a light source within the bronchoscope, the surgeon can readily observe anatomic abnormalities and pathologic conditions. In addition, secretions can be aspirated, foreign bodies removed, and suspicious lesions biopsied through the bronchoscope.

BRONCHOSPASM: The sudden, forceful, and involuntary contraction of the bronchial portion of the respiratory tree. Usually it is a reflex response secondary to the introduction of irritants, including inhalation anesthetics. If mild, bronchospasm can be treated by the prompt removal of the irritant; if severe (during anesthesia), it can be treated by (1) providing positive pressure ventilation, (2) deepening anesthesia, and (3) administering a bronchodilating drug. It is a well-observed paradox in the administration of anesthesia that low doses of some inhalation anesthetics, if introduced too quickly, will cause bronchoconstriction, whereas high doses, when they are administered slowly, will cause bronchodilation.

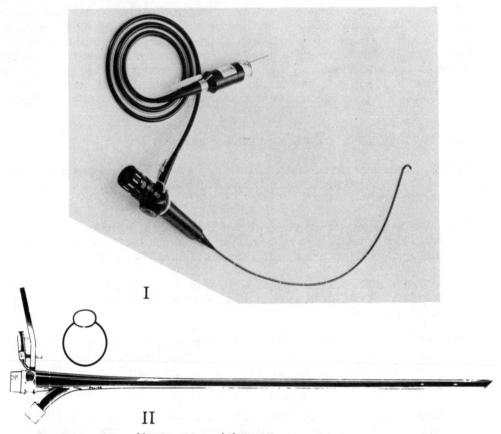

I

II

Bronchoscope: (I) Flexible. (II) Rigid.

BRONCHOSPIROMETRY: The determination of the O_2 intake, vital capacity, and CO_2 excretion of a single lung, usually using a double-lumen tube. A differential bronchospirometer can measure the function of each lung separately.

BRONCHUS: One of two main (primary) branches from the trachea which form the major passageways to the lungs. The right main bronchus is more vertical than the left and foreign objects entering the air passages are more likely to become lodged in it. The primary bronchi are composed of incomplete rings of cartilage and are lined by ciliated columnar epithelium. See Conducting airways.

BRONZE: A copper alloy in which the main alloying metal is usually tin.

BROWNIAN MOVEMENT: The random, continuous, irregular motion of small particles when suspended in a liquid. This is a visible demonstration that the molecules of the liquid are constantly bombarding the small particles.

BRUSH CELL: See Alveolar cell types.

BRUSH, ELECTRIC: A specialized electric conductor, usually made of carbon, which serves to maintain contact with a rotating communication.

BRYCE-SMITH TUBE: See Double-lumen tube.

BUBBLE OXYGENATOR: A device used with heart-lung machines in which exchange of gases takes place during cardiopulmonary bypass procedures. It breaks up a stream of supplied O_2 into continually forming bubbles which diffuse through a column of blood on the bypass machine. Gas exchange occurs on the surface of the bubbles. Rapidity of O_2 transfer to the blood depends on bubble size (surface area) and length of bubble path through the blood. Small bubbles produce a large surface area and thus good oxygenation, but are difficult to eliminate before the blood is returned to the patient. Some large bubbles are required for adequate elimination of CO_2. See Cardiopulmonary bypass.

BUBBLE JAR: An apparatus used for increasing the humidity of fresh gas supplied to a patient by bubbling the gas through a jar of water. Efficiency is contingent on the size of the bubbles, water pathway length, the temperature of the jar, and the rate of bubble production.

BUFFER: A substance which tends to preserve the original hydrogen ion concentration in solution, thereby maintaining the pH despite the addition of quantities of acid or base usually made up of a combination of a weak acid and its salt. The major body buffer systems are bicarbonate, phosphate, nondefined serum proteins, and hemoglobin. Currently, bicarbonate is the only directly measurable buffer system of the body. It is a mixture of carbonic acid and sodium (or magnesium, potassium, or calcium) bicarbonate. See Acid-base balance, Acidosis, Alkalosis.

BUFFER BASE: A clinical measurement used to evaluate acid-base balance. It indicates the sum of buffer anions in whole blood. This total is divided (approximately) equally between bicarbonate ions and hemoglobin ions. It has become obsolete because its determination varies depending on the pH of the blood specimen at the time of measurement. See Base excess.

BUG: A flaw in a set of instructions to a computer or in the computer circuitry which causes it to provide inappropriate results. (Debugging is the process by which errors in computer programming or wiring are eliminated.)

BUNSEN SOLUBILITY COEFFICIENT: See Ostwald solubility coefficient.

BUOYANCY: See Archimedes principle.

BUPIVACAINE: See Local anesthetic.

BUS: A pathway for transmitting information from one location to another. For example, in an electronic typewriter, the impulses generated by the key strokes are carried to the microprocessor by a bus.

BUS BAR: A conductor which can carry heavy current or connect many points in an electric system.

BUSHING: A type of adaptor used in altering the internal diameter of a system component.

BUTABARBITAL: See Barbiturate.

BUTISOL: See Barbiturate.

BUTYLPARABEN: See Preservative.

BUTYROCHOLINESTERASE: An enzyme which is found in plasma, liver, and many organs. It is the correct name for nonspecific cholinesterase or pseudocholinesterase. Its physiologic function is unknown. See Pseudocholinesterase.

BUTYROPHENONE: See Antipsychotic agent.

BYPASS: See Cardiopulmonary bypass.

BYPASS CAPACITOR: A device for providing an alternate path of relatively low impedance, i.e., the total opposition afforded to a flow of alternating current at a specific frequency, for alternating current around a circuit. It effectively prevents alternating current from entering inappropriate parts of a circuit.

C_m: See Minimum blocking concentration.

C_{MAX}: The maximum plasma concentration of a drug achieved following its administration.

CAFFEINE: A white powder alkaloid with the general formula $C_8H_{10}N_4O_2$. It is soluble in alcohol and water and has been used medically as a nonspecific stimulator of the central nervous system.

CAFFEINE TEST: A laboratory test to determine a patient's predisposition to malignant hyperthermia (MH). A muscle biopsy is performed, and the tissue is suspended in a bath into which O_2 and CO_2 are bubbled. Caffeine is added to the bath causing the muscle to contract. When halothane is added to the bath, no further increase in muscle tension is noted in normal muscle, whereas contraction continues in the muscle from a patient susceptible to MH.

CAISSON DISEASE (BENDS, DECOMPRESSION SICKNESS, DIVER PARALYSIS, DYSBARISM): A disorder which may occur following rapid decrease of air pressure in persons who have been breathing compressed air in hyperbaric chambers or caissons (pressurized underwater chambers). (Divers may be subject to this condition on ascent.) Under pressure, gases (N_2 in particular) are forced into tissues in direct proportion to the pressure. When this pressure is relieved, as when a diver surfaces, N_2 starts to leave the tissues very rapidly. Gas bubbles form in cells and small vessels just as they do in a carbonated beverage which is opened to the atmosphere. These bubbles act as occluding plugs, causing ischemia, severe pain, and, in acute cases, rapid elevation of total peripheral resistance and death. The only treatment for caisson disease is repeat exposure to higher pressures with gradual return to normal pressure.

CALCIUM: An element vital to multiple body processes. It is a major bivalent cation of the extracellar fluid and is essential for blood clotting (calcium is factor IV). By binding calcium with citrate, as in citrate-phosphate-dextrose (CPD) blood storage, clotting is prevented. Over 90% of body calcium is stored in bone as phosphate or carbonate. Calcium also plays an essential role in muscle contraction and is important in neuromuscular transmission.

CALCIUM CHANNEL BLOCKER: A class of drugs which interferes with cross-membrane transfer of calcium ions. The calcium channel blockers temper the role of calcium in the development of the cardiac action potential and in the coupling of electric excitation to contraction. The first available intravenous calcium-blocking agent, verapamil, is effective for paroxysmal supraventricular tachycardia. Verapamil and nifedipine (an oral calcium blocker) appear to be effective in treating angina, hypertrophic cardiomyopathy, and chronic atrial fibrillation.

CALCIUM CHLORIDE: An inorganic salt, normally administered intravenously, used for its direct inotropic effects on the heart. Extremely irritating to tissues and veins and capable of causing tissue necrosis, calcium chloride contains approximately three times more calcium than two of the major organic salts, calcium gluconate and calcium gluceptate (also used as inotropes). Therefore only one-third to one-half the amount of calcium chloride is necessary when used instead of these other salts. The calcium ion will cause the entire blood pathway to clot if it is erroneously injected into the same intravenous line as transfused blood which contains citrate.

CALCIUM GLUCEPTATE: See Calcium chloride.

CALCIUM GLUCONATE: See Calcium chloride.

CALCIUM TUNGSTATE: See Intensifying screen.

CALIBRATION: The process of comparing a measuring device to a known standard to determine its accuracy or to devise a new scale. For example, in the calibration of an invasive electronic blood pressure monitoring device, a transducer connected to the monitor is opened to room air. This is selected as a zero point and the electronics are set to zero. The transducer is closed and a mercury column sphygmomanometer in parallel with the transducer applies a set pressure (usually 200 torr). The invasive electronic monitoring device is then adjusted to agree with that pressure. See Accuracy.

CALIBRATION SIGNAL: See Self-test capability.

CALOMEL ELECTRODE: A reference electrode, at times employed in pH determinations, consisting of mercury in contact with a solution of potassium chloride saturated with calomel (mercurous chloride). See Fig.

CALORIE: A unit of heat measurement. The large calorie (kilocalorie or Cal) is the unit used in metabolic studies and is equal to the amount of heat necessary to raise the temperature of 1 kg H_2O 1 degree Celsius at a pressure of 1 atmosphere. The small calorie (gram calorie or cal) is 1/1000 of a Cal.

CANDELA: The standard international unit of light intensity.

CANNON WAVE: See Central venous pressure.

CANNULA: A tube introduced into a duct or body cavity often with the aid of a trocar. The trocar makes the initial puncture into the space the cannula is to occupy. It is then withdrawn, clearing the lumen of the cannula. The term cannula is often used interchangeably with the term catheter. See Catheter.

CANNULIZATION, ARTERIAL; ARTERIAL LINE: See Allen test, Arterial blood pressure, Cardiac catheterization.

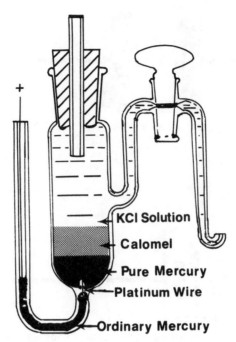

Calomel Electrode.

CAPACITANCE, ELECTRONIC: The buildup (storage) of electrons on one conductor balanced by the buildup of positive charges on a second conductor separated from the first by an insulator. If the insulator breaks down, current will flow to balance and neutralize the charged states. See Capacitor.

CAPACITANCE, FLUIDIC: The relative ability of a vessel or container to increase linearly in volume without a linear increase in pressure.

CAPACITANCE VESSELS: See Resistance vessels.

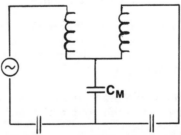

Capacitive Coupling. C_M represents the capacitance seen between the two parallel circuit elements and exists because these two conductors lie in close proximity to each other separated by an air gap which functions as the dielectric in a conventional capacitor.

CAPACITIVE COUPLING: The process of linking together two portions of a circuit so that energy is transferred from one to the other by means of mutual capacitance. Any two conductors separated by an insulator (even an air gap) can function as a capacitor. Capacitive coupling is one of the ways stray signals may leak between channels. See Fig. See Capacitor.

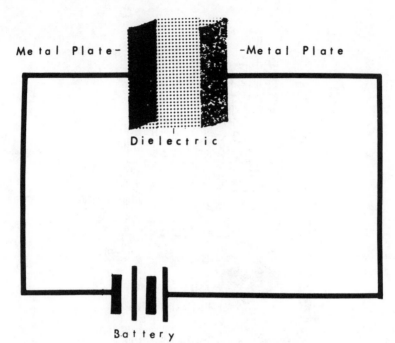

Metal Plate-

-Metal Plate

Dielectric

Battery

Capacitor: Three elements of a capacitor. They include two conductors separated by an electric insulator called the dielectric. The ability of the capacitor to store charges is related to the area of the two conductors and the relative electric impermeability of the dielectric.

CAPACITOR: An electronic device composed of two conducting plates separated by an insulator. It holds and stores electric energy, blocks the flow of direct current (blocking capacitor), and allows the flow of alternating current proportional to frequency and capacitance. (Capacitance is measured in farads and is determined by plates and insulation material, surface area, and distance between the plates.) Cardiac defibrillators, for example, use large capacitors to store electrons. See Fig.

CAPILLARY BLOOD FLOW: See Microcirculation.

CAPNOGRAPH: An alternate name for an infrared CO_2 analyzer.

CAPSTAN: A rotating shaft, found in the drive mechanism of a tape recorder, which controls the speed of tape movement.

CARBACHOL: An analog of acetylcholine which is used in the treatment of glaucoma. Solutions of carbachol applied to the conjunctiva decrease intraocular pressure and produce miosis.

CARBAMAZEPINE (TEGRETOL): A drug which treats epilepsy, trigeminal neuralgia, and related central nervous system disorders. Its toxic side effects involve the skin, liver, and bone marrow. It also has been implicated in teratogenic effects. See Trigeminal neuralgia.

CARBAMINOHEMOGLOBIN: A chemical combination of hemoglobin and CO_2. It is one of the principal forms in which CO_2 exists in the blood. The lower the O_2 saturation of hemoglobin, the greater the amount of carbaminohemoglobin that can be found in the blood.

CARBIDE: A compound made up of carbon with one other element, e.g., tungsten, silicon. Silicon carbide is one of the hardest manufactured materials and is frequently used as an abrasive.

CARBOCAINE: A trade name for mepivacaine. See Local anesthetic.

CARBON BLACK: An amorphous powdered form of elemental carbon, usually made from the incomplete combustion of a gas. It is mixed with rubber in a controlled manner (so the carbon chain connections are not broken) to make it conductive.

CARBON DIOXIDE (CO_2): A colorless, odorless, noncombustible gas with a molecular weight of 44. CO_2 and the carbonates aid in maintaining the neutrality of the blood and tissues. Low concentrations (approximately 5%) of CO_2, which alter the pH of the blood, stimulate respiration, whereas high concentrations of CO_2 depress it. In solid form (Dry Ice) CO_2 is used in cryocautery to destroy abnormal tissue. See Carbon dioxide absorption, Carbon dioxide combining power, Carbon dioxide response, Carbon dioxide total in blood, Carbon dioxide transport in blood, Carbonic anhydrase.

CARBON DIOXIDE ABSORPTION: The elimination of CO_2 from rebreathing systems. This is usually accomplished by allowing exhaled gases to flow through an absorber, normally soda lime or Baralyme, which selectively reacts with the CO_2 from the gas mix. The stages of this reaction for soda lime are as follows: CO_2 combines with H_2O at the surface of the granules to form carbonic acid; carbonic acid combines with sodium and potassium hydroxides to yield sodium and potassium carbonates plus H_2O; and the sodium and potassium carbonates combine with the calcium hydroxide to produce calcium carbonate plus sodium and potassium hydroxides. The chemical reaction of CO_2 with a strong base is exothermic and equals 13,500 cal for each gram-molecular weight of CO_2. Two indicators of absorption ability are effective absorption ability (expressed as the volume of CO_2 absorbed/ 100 g of absorbent) and effective absorption efficiency (the percent of CO_2 absorbed out of the volume entering a canister). See Carbon dioxide absorption canister, Soda lime, To-and-fro carbon dioxide absorption.

CARBON DIOXIDE ABSORPTION CANISTER: A device within the breathing circuit of the patient which removes CO_2 from the recirculating gases. It contains either soda lime or Baralyme as the absorber. The standard canister, uniformly and properly packed with the appropriate absorbent, has a minimal capacity of 8 hr of continuous service in the anesthesia circuit. It should hold approximately 1 kg of absorbent granules. See Carbon dioxide absorption, Soda lime.

CARBON DIOXIDE COMBINING POWER: An in vitro analysis which measures arterial blood gases to determine the contribution of PCO_2 in pH changes. It is derived by measuring (in millimoles per liter) the total CO_2 (free plus bound) in a plasma sample equilibrated with CO_2 at a pressure of 40 mmHg at room temperature. (If a sample starts with an elevated CO_2 content, its combining power is less.) This kind of analysis is no longer in general use because it is too dependent on sampling technique.

CARBON DIOXIDE DISSOCIATION CURVE: The plot which shows the relationship between total CO_2 and PCO_2 in the blood. The curve shifts according to the PO_2. See Haldane effect.

CARBON DIOXIDE ELECTRODE: The element of a blood gas machine which detects

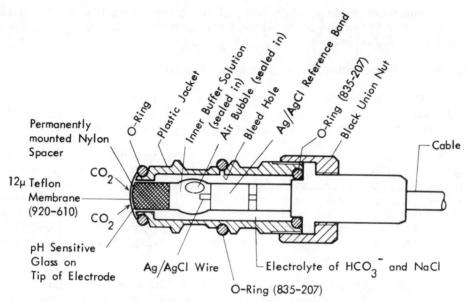

Carbon Dioxide Electrode: Standard CO_2 electrode.

and determines CO_2 concentration in a blood sample. It is a modified pH electrode with a semipermeable plastic membrane on one end which comes in contact with the sample. Carbon dioxide diffuses through this membrane and raises the hydrogen ion concentration of the buffer solution contained behind the membrane. The hydrogen ions diffuse through a glass membrane in the electrode and register on a detector as a variation in ion current. The strength of the ion current is related via appropriate electronics to reflect the CO_2 concentration in the sample. See Fig. See Oxygen electrode, pH electrode.

CARBON DIOXIDE METHOD FOR DETERMINING ALVEOLAR VOLUME: A technique based on the fact that gas exchange does not occur in the anatomic dead space. If exhaled volume is measured and CO_2 concentration in the exhaled volume is also measured along with alveolar CO_2 concentration [approximated very well in the healthy individual by arterial partial pressure of carbon dioxide (PaCO$_2$)], then a relationship can be drawn to determine alveolar volumes. See Anatomic dead space.

CARBON DIOXIDE RESPONSE: The reaction by the patient to changes in CO_2 concentration. If CO_2 is increased in inspired air, the normal patient will increase minute ventilation. Initially depth is augmented followed by the rate. The tension of CO_2 in the arterial blood is one of the most sensitive variables in the body. Normal CO_2 tension in arterial blood is 38-42 torr and venous blood averages 6-7 torr higher. Elevated CO_2 in the arterial blood causes an immediate increase in cerebral blood flow which is almost linear to the increase in CO_2 tension. A decrease in arterial CO_2 causes a proportional decrease in cerebral blood flow. Increased metabolism in the tissues leads to a buildup of CO_2 eliciting local peripheral dilatation. However, this may be counteracted by a centrally regulated effect. See Cerebral blood flow, Intracranial pressure.

CARBON DIOXIDE TOTAL IN BLOOD: The amount of CO_2 in blood or plasma which is liberated upon acidification of the sample. It is measured in millimoles per liter. A more clinically useful derivative of total CO_2 is actual bicarbonate, which is the total CO_2 minus CO_2 found as carbonic acid and physically dissolved CO_2. Actual bicarbonate can be determined from the Henderson-Hasselbalch equation if pH and PCO_2 are determined by multiplying the PCO_2 by 0.03 (a factor representing the solubility of CO_2 in blood) and subtracting the value from total CO_2.

CARBON DIOXIDE TRANSPORT IN BLOOD: The movement of CO_2 in the blood. This is accomplished by three different routes. In the first route, CO_2 dissolves in the fluid portion of the blood. At a partial pressure of 45 torr, 2.7 ml CO_2 dissolves in 100 ml blood (while at 40 torr, the amount is 2.4 ml/100 ml blood). Approximately 7% of the CO_2 exhaled per minute is transported to the lungs via this route. In the second route, CO_2 is transported in the blood as bicarbonate ions. The reaction is $CO_2 + H_2O \rightarrow H_2CO_3$, which yields $H^+ + HCO_3^-$ (catalyzed by carbonic anhydrase contained in red cells). The bicarbonate ions leave the red cells to be carried in the fluid portion of the blood. These ions are replaced in the red cells by chloride ions; therefore, the chloride content of venous red blood cells is higher than that of arterial red blood cells. This phenomenon is called the chloride shift. This route accounts for the transport of 70% of CO_2 exhaled. In the third route, CO_2 is transported via a loose bonding to hemoglobin as carbaminohemoglobin. A small quantity is also transported joined to other plasma proteins. This route accounts for approximately 20% of CO_2 exhaled. By all three methods the concentration of CO_2 in tissue or blood at a PCO_2 of 45 torr is 52 vol %. The concentration falls to 48 vol % when blood is arterialized in the lungs.

CARBONIC ANHYDRASE: An enzyme found in red blood cells, gastrointestinal mucosa, kidney tubules, and glandular epithelial cells. (Zinc is an integral component of carbonic anhydrase.) The principal function of the enzyme is to catalyze, in both directions, the reversible reaction of CO_2 and H_2O forming carbonic acid. Normally, the reaction requires several seconds, but carbonic anhydrase allows the reaction to proceed 5000 times faster. Its presence in red blood cells allows huge amounts of CO_2 to be transported in blood as bicarbonate, a product of carbonic acid dissociation. In the kidney, the presence of carbonic anhydrase facilitates resorption of bicarbonate. When a carbonic acid inhibitor such as acetazolamide (Diamox, a mild diuretic) is administered, bicarbonate reabsorption is prevented and some acidosis occurs in the body as a whole.

CARBON MONOXIDE (CO): A gas generated by the incomplete oxidation of carbon. Carbon monoxide reacts with hemoglobin (Hb) to form carboxyhemoglobin (COHb), which is highly toxic because it cannot carry O_2. Hemoglobin has 210 times more affinity for CO than it does for O_2. Carbon monoxide, in very low concentrations, is used to test the diffusion capacity of the lung. See Diffusion capacity of the lung.

CARBON TETRACHLORIDE: A compound first prepared in 1845 and used initially as an anesthetic. Due to its extreme toxicity, however, its use was discontinued. While it can be decidedly toxic to the heart, causing arrhythmias and marked hypotension, its more deadly effects are on the liver and renal tubular cells.

CARBONYL CHLORIDE: See Phosgene.

CARCINOID SYNDROME: The complex of signs and symptoms associated with slowly growing malignancies of the enterochromaffin (argentaffin) cell type (found in the gastrointestinal tract, especially the ileum and small intestine, bronchus, and ovary). The tumor cells secrete serotonin (5-HT), bradykinin, and histamine. These vasoactive substances are responsible for the signs and symptoms associated with carcinoid, including cutaneous flushing, diarrhea, telangiectasia, valvular heart disease, bronchial constriction, and asthma. Anesthetic complications arise from surgical manipulation of the tumor which releases the vasoactive agents.

CARD: In computer technology, a card is a stiff piece of paper used to record either information or instructions for a computer. The information is recorded on the card by holes punched in it at a particular X-Y location; each card has the same number and spacing of sites for holes. The presence or absence of a hole corresponds to the binary code, 1 or 0 notation. A card punch or keypunch machine actually makes the holes, and a card-reading machine reads the location and function of the holes accordingly.

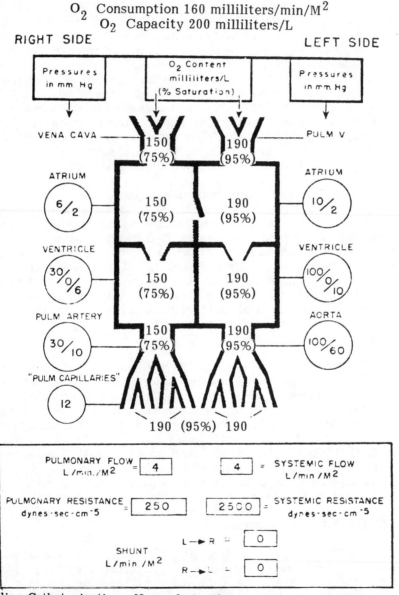

Cardiac Catheterization: Normal circulatory dynamics with O_2 contents, expected pressures, and percent saturations encountered during cardiac catheterization in adults.

CARDIAC CATHETERIZATION: A diagnostic technique in which a catheter is passed along veins or arteries into the heart to examine the structure of the heart. The catheter also measures pressures and blood gas values in the heart and visualizes the flow characteristics of the coronary circulation. A radiopaque dye is injected through the catheter for angiography. See Fig. See Swan-Ganz catheter.

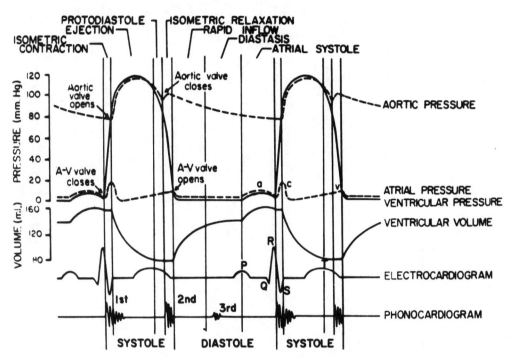

Cardiac Cycle: Events of the cardiac cycle, showing the changes in left atrial pressure, left ventricular pressure, aortic pressure, ventricular volume, the electrocardiogram, and the phonocardiogram.

CARDIAC CYCLE: The electric and mechanical sequences which begin with the heart at rest, continue through contraction and relaxation of the heart chambers, and return to the heart at rest. See Fig. See Electrocardiogram.

CARDIAC GLYCOSIDES: A group of drugs, derived from the Digitalis or Strophanthus plants, which have a powerful and specific action on the myocardium and circulation. The term digitalis is often used to designate all the cardiac glycosides, but generic names of the more commonly used ones are digoxin, digitoxin, ouabain, and deslanoside. Since the basic effect of all the cardiac glycosides is the same, their use in anesthesia is more often determined by rapidity of onset, i.e., the faster the onset, the shorter the duration of action. (The fastest is ouabain with an onset of 3-10 min. The slowest is digitoxin with an onset of 25 min or more.) The cardiac glycosides have a profound positive inotropic effect, i.e., they stimulate the force of myocardial contractions without increasing demand. The action of the cardiac glycosides on a molecular level is not understood but is known to involve facilitation of calcium ion transport. Cardiac glycoside toxicity is enhanced by hypokalemia and hypercalcemia. The cardiac glycosides are most often used in treating congestive heart failure, atrial fibrillation, atrial flutter, and paroxysmal tachycardia. See Fig.

Cardiac Glycosides.

Generic Name (Trade Name)	Onset	Half-Life	Peak Effect	Comments
Digitalis Leaf (Digifortis) (Major active component is digitoxin)	2-6 hr PO	4-6 days	12-24 hr	Digitalis leaf is available in a powdered form for oral administration though it has largely been replaced by the purified glycosides. It is only moderately absorbed from the GI tract (20-40%). As with all the digitalis glycosides, its therapeutic indications are for congestive heart failure and various arrhythmias, especially atrial flutter and fibrillation. Side effects mark the onset of toxicity and include GI disturbances (e. g., anorexia, nausea, diarrhea, and pain) and neurologic disturbances (e. g., blurred vision, paresthesias, fatigue, weakness in the extremities, and toxic psychosis). Toxic levels of digitalis also can lead to arrhythmia and increasing heart failure which is worsened by hypokalemia and hypomagnesemia.
Digoxin (Lanoxin)	15-30 min IV	36 hr	1-5 hr	Digoxin is becoming the most widely used of the cardiac glycosides due to its intermediate duration of action. GI absorption is fairly good (60-80%) but is affected in patients with malabsorption syndromes and by antacids, kaolin, and pectins. It is eliminated from the body via the kidneys.

Digitoxin (Crystodigin)	0.5-2 hr IV	4-6 days	4-12 hr	Digitoxin is well absorbed from the GI tract (90-100%). It should be used cautiously in patients with liver disease as it is excreted primarily via the hepatic route. It is slowly metabolized in the body.
Deslanoside (Cedilanid-D)	10-30 min IV	33 hr	1-2 hr	Deslanoside is used for rapid digitalization. It is eliminated from the body via the kidneys.
Ouabain (G Strophanthin)	5-10 min IV	21 hr	0.5-2 hr	Ouabain is used for rapid digitalization. It has the most rapid onset and shortest duration of action. It is eliminated from the body via the kidneys.

CARDIAC INDEX (CI): The relationship of the cardiac output to body surface area measured as cardiac output per square meter of surface area. A normal CI for a 70-kg man is between 2.5 and 3.5 L/min/m^2. See Cardiac output.

CARDIAC OUTPUT (CO): The volume of blood pumped in 1 min by either the right or left side of the heart. Since the two ventricles pump in series, their output must be the same in a given time period. In the healthy individual, CO is considered to be the stroke volume (60-90 ml/beat in the 70-kg male) X the heart rate/min. There are three principal methods for assessing CO.In the thermal dilution method, which is the most common, a known volume of cold solution is introduced into the circulation in a given time period. The extent and duration of the temperature change in the blood is measured by a thermistor distal to the injection point. If a curve is traced in which the Y axis is equal to the temperature difference and the X axis is equal to time, the area under the curve is related to the CO. The thermal dilution method usually employs a Swan-Ganz catheter. In the dye dilution technique, an indicator dye, such as Cardio-Green (indocyanine green), is injected in precise quantity into the central venous circulation. Arterial sampling is done by passing the arterial blood through a dye detector. (Here the Y axis equals dye concentration and the X axis equals time.) The dye detector then traces out a curve,the area of which is related to the CO. Aside from requiring samples (which the thermal dilution technique does not), the dye dilution method shows the phenomenon of recirculation (dye which has been returned to the heart and pumped out again). The third method

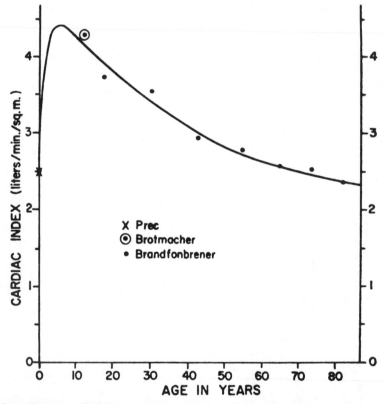

Cardiac Output: Cardiac index is the cardiac output divided by the surface area of the patient in square meters. Note the rise in cardiac index through the age of 10 and then its gradual dropoff to old age.

is based on the Fick principle which states that the CO is equal to the uptake of O_2 per minute in milliliters per minute divided by the arteriovenous O_2 difference in milliliters per milliliter of blood. To be performed properly, it requires the collection of expired gases and right heart catheterization to obtain mixed venous blood. See Fig. See Swan-Ganz catheter.

CARDIAC RISK IN ANESTHESIA: A score (first described in 1977) assigned to each preoperative patient (for noncardiac surgery) based on the measurement of nine possible variables. These factors include age greater than 70 years, myocardial infarction (MI) in the previous 6 months, an S3 gallop or jugular venous distention, significant valvular aortic stenosis, electrocardiogram rhythm disturbances, major acid-base disturbances or serum electrolyte abnormalities, site of operation, urgency of the operation, and more than five premature ventricular contractions/min at any time. As an example of the two major risk factors, an MI in the preceding 6 months is worth 10 points whereas an S3 gallop or jugular venous distention is worth 11 points. A total of 26 points or greater (out of a possible 53) places the patient in a high-risk category.

CARDIAC TAMPONADE: The compression of the heart due to fluid accumulation in the pericardial sac, causing a decrease in cardiac output and potential circulatory failure. Acute cardiac tamponade is a true medical emergency. Its critical state may be reached with as little as 250 ml blood or fluid. When it is chronic, it may take over 1000 ml of effusion to compromise the heart. Trauma is a prime cause of tamponade; however, tuberculosis, infection, and local tumor growth are also associated with fluid accumulation in the pericardial sac. Signs of cardiac tamponade include tachycardia, decline in blood pressure and pulse pressure, distention of the jugular veins, rapid enlargement of the liver and equalization of right- and left-sided cardiac pressure. Jugular vein distention is increased during inspiration (Kussmaul sign) or when pressure is applied over the liver (hepatojugular reflux), due to the inability of the right side of the heart to accommodate the increased inflow of blood.

CARD INHALER: A vaporizer for oral administration of a volatile anesthetic, most frequently used with trichloroethylene or methoxyflurane. It has a fixed upper limit of anesthetic concentration which, theoretically, makes it safe for self-administration.

CARDIOGENIC SHOCK: See Shock.

CARDIO-GREEN: See Indocyanine green.

CARDIOPULMONARY BYPASS (EXTRACORPOREAL CIRCULATION): The technique of replacing the circulatory and respiratory functions of a patient in order to rest the heart during cardiac surgery. The anticoagulant heparin must be administered to the patient prior to cardiopulmonary bypass. The bypass requires withdrawal of the blood returning to the heart with large-bore cannulas. The blood is then oxygenated and CO_2 removed via an oxygenator. The blood is then pumped back to the root of the aorta (via another cannula) where it enters the arterial side of the circulation. The blood can also be heated and cooled by a heat exchanger in line with the heart-lung machine. (The heart-lung machine is operated by a highly trained perfusionist.) The heart is deliberately fibrillated while on bypass, usually through the use of cryocardioplegia solution (an iced potassium electrolyte mixture). The heart-lung machine may have at least three and as many as six separate pumps. It is capable of maintaining cardiac output in liters per minute at least equal to the output of the patient's heart at rest. It can pump to the coronary arteries (separately if nec-

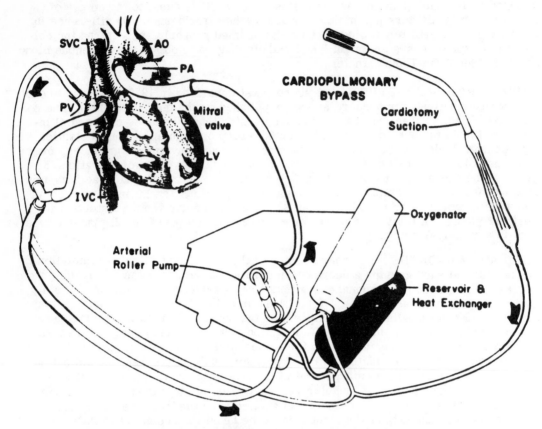

Cardiopulmonary Bypass: Blood drains by gravity from the patient to the oxygenator where gas exchange occurs. A roller pump returns blood to the patient and is the driving force for the systemic circulation.

essary), pump the cryocardioplegia solution, and drain the left ventricle of the blood which flows into it from the thebesian veins. Total bypass eliminates the heart and lungs from the circulation. Partial bypass (in which blood is removed from the femoral vein and returned to the femoral artery) can be used for short periods of time to assist the failing heart prior to more definitive treatment. See Fig. See Activated clotting time, Bubble oxygenator, Heparin, Membrane oxygenator, Rotating disc oxygenator, Screen oxygenator.

CARDIOPULMONARY RESUSCITATION (CPR): The technique for providing respiration and cardiac output for a patient. There have been recent efforts to encourage the general population to learn the basic techniques of CPR. (These techniques, termed either the basic rescue level or basic life support are mouth-to-mouth respiration and closed-chest massage.) Advanced life support techniques usually require specially trained personnel and include such methods as pharmacologic intervention, electric countershock, and cardiac pacing. Encouragement for basic CPR stems from a recognition that mouth-to-mouth resuscitation can supply all the O_2 necessary for life. (Exhaled breath contains only 14-18% O_2 and external cardiac massage can generate only one-third the normal cardiac output.) See Fig.

CARDIOVERSION (ELECTROCONVERSION): A method which uses electricity to re-

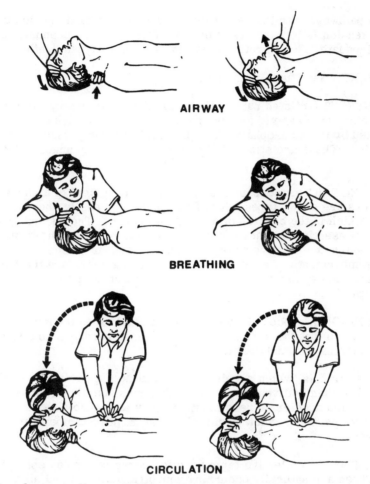

AIRWAY

BREATHING

CIRCULATION

Cardiopulmonary Resuscitation: Fundamentals of adult cardiopulmonary resuscitation.

store normal cardiac rhythm. A shock is given to the heart through the use of external paddles placed against the chest. Commonly, the term cardioversion is interpreted narrowly to mean a technique used to treat any of a number of atrial, junctional, and some ventricular dysrhythmias. The currents used are much less than for ventricular defibrillation. Intravenous administration of barbiturates or diazepam is useful to counteract the pain caused by this procedure. Internal cardioversion is the placing of paddles through the open chest at the end of open heart surgery to reestablish a normal rhythm when the heart is fibrillating. See Defibrillation, Synchronization mode.

CARDIOVERSION SYNCHRONIZATION: See Synchronization mode.

CARLENS TUBE: See Double-lumen tube.

CAROTID BODY: A small mass of cells located between the origins of the external and internal carotid arteries. The carotid bodies lie adjacent to the carotid sinus but are different in both function and structure. Their blood supply comes directly from the carotid artery and their basic function is to monitor arterial O_2 tension.

Connected by pathways with the respiratory center of the brain (which they stimulate when O_2 tension falls), they have been implicated in the phenomenon known as paradoxical O_2 death. See Carotid sinus, Paradoxical oxygen death.

CAROTID SHUNT: See Stump pressure.

CAROTID SINUS: The dilated part of the internal carotid artery located above the division of the common carotid artery and its two major branches. The carotid sinus, innervated by the glossopharyngeal (IX cranial) nerve, contains baroreceptors within its walls. These are stimulated by blood pressure changes. See Carotid body.

CARRIER, ELECTRIC: A concept used to explain movement of a charge through a solid. Carriers are of two types. The first (and more easily understood) type is the electron, which is the carrier of a negative charge. The second type of carrier is the hole, representing the lack of an electron where one normally would be found. This hole is assigned a positive charge which migrates from one side of a solid to another. The movements of electrons and holes as carriers are the foundation of solid state electronics, in which charges are moved under precise control through semiconductors.

CASE HARDENING: A process by which carbon is added to the surface of low-carbon steel or iron so that the surface has an increased hardness compared with the core, which remains soft and ductile.

CATALYST: A material which accelerates or initiates a chemical reaction without entering into that chemical reaction itself. Enzymes, catalysts found in living cells, not only initiate and accelerate reactions, but they also enable certain reactions to occur at body temperature which would otherwise require temperatures of many hundreds of degrees.

CATECHOLAMINE: A collective term used for norepinephrine, epinephrine, and dopamine. These are naturally occurring neurotransmitters and all are catechols (i.e., their major molecular structure is that of an orthodihydroxybenzene; they contain an amino group on a side chain). See Fig. See Autonomic nervous system.

CATGUT (GUT): A stringlike material made from the intestines of sheep which is used for suturing. The sheep intestines are soaked and cleaned in an alkali solution, then drawn through holes in a plate, sterilized, and graded according to size. Since this material is degradable by various enzyme systems in living tissue, catgut sutures are not permanent. Absorption of the suture can be delayed by adding various minerals which retard degradation, such as chrome (chromic catgut).

CATHETER: A tube used to introduce or remove fluids from a body, channel, or hollow organ. It is made of rubber, plastic, or metal and is usually slender and flexible. The most frequently used is the intravenous catheter. The term catheter is often used interchangeably with the term cannula. See Cannula.

CATHODE: The negative electrode or source of electrons, i.e., negative charges, in a battery or vacuum tube.

CATHODE-RAY TUBE (CRT): An evacuated glass cylinder, one end of which is coated on the inside surface with a phosphor. (The characteristic of this phosphor

Catecholamines: Molecular formulas for the naturally occurring catecholamines, their precursor tyrosine, the intermediate compound dopa, and the artificial analog isoproterenol.

109

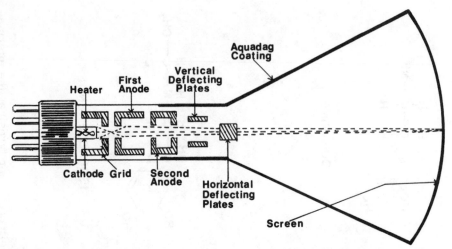

Cathode Ray Tube: Common elements of the cathode ray tube. The heater provides the electron emission, the first and second anodes concentrate the electron beam, the vertical and horizontal deflecting plates sweep the beam across the screen, and the Aquadag coating returns the electrons to ground.

is such that it will emit light when struck by a stream of electrons.) The other end of the glass cylinder contains a source of electrons, usually a heated wire. The electrons emitted by the heated wire are shaped and directed into a thin beam by either electric or magnetic fields applied from the outside of the tube. This beam strikes the phosphor setting it aglow and can be deflected to draw either pictures, letters, or combinations. CRTs are used in both oscilloscopes and televisions. See Fig.

CATION: A positively charged ion. The principal cations in the body are sodium (Na^+), calcium (Ca^{2+}), potassium (K^+), and magnesium (Mg^{2+}).

CAUDA EQUINA SYNDROME: A lesion of the tail of the spinal cord characterized by urinary retention, loss of sensation in the perineum, and loss of sexual function. It has been reported as a consequence of inadvertent injection of toxic or contaminated drugs during spinal anesthesia.

CAUDAL ANESTHESIA: A type of regional anesthesia produced by injecting local anesthetic agents through the sacral area at the base of the spinal column. Caudal anesthesia is functionally a kind of epidural anesthesia, since the local anesthetic is deposited outside of the dura covering the spinal cord. It is a popular technique for rectal and obstetric procedures. See Fig.

CAUSALGIA (CAUSALGIC STATES; REFLEX SYMPATHETIC DYSTROPHY): A term now applied to a group of disease states, e.g., shoulder-hand syndrome, posttraumatic pain syndrome, Sudeck atrophy, and postfrostbite syndrome, which exhibit a similar symptomatology, including hyperesthesia, motor disturbances, and skin changes (dryness). The patient suffering from severe causalgia goes to extremes to prevent the affected area from being touched or moved. Causalgia as a single entity was first described after the American Civil War in soldiers who had received injuries to the extremities from projectiles. Causalgia is a controversial entity. It is believed to be either peripheral dysfunction or hyperactivity of the sympathetic nervous system. Sympathetic blockade(s) can cause dramatic reversal of the condition,

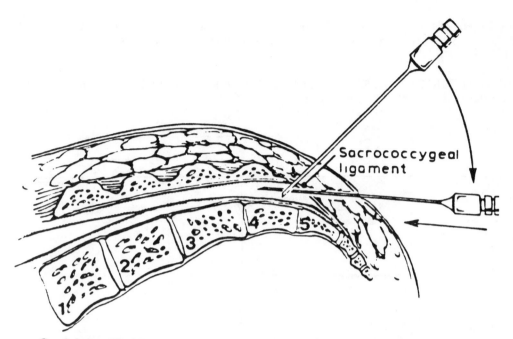

Caudal Anesthesia: Approach to the caudal part of the epidural canal through the sacrococcygeal ligament. The needle is initially placed at nearly right angles to the skin. Once the ligament is pierced the needle is moved to form an angle of 20 degrees with the skin and then advanced 1-2 cm.

although blockade will be less effective if the condition has continued for a year or more.

CAUSALITY: The legal principle which states that every effect is the consequence of an earlier cause(s). Causality can be true even if the antecedent causes are too numerous, too complicated, or too obscure for analysis.

CAUTERIZATION: The process of burning tissue with a caustic drug or heat. An electrocautery, often used in this process, is a metal instrument which is electrically heated and used to burn, cut, or coagulate tissue. It is different from an electrosurgery instrument, which uses radiofrequency current for the same purpose, but does not necessarily become heated in the process.

CELIAC PLEXUS BLOCK: A regional anesthetic technique in which a local anesthetic is injected into the retroperitoneal area beyond the first lumbar vertebra while the patient is in a prone or lateral position. A 12-cm needle is used. Celiac block is indicated for patients with intractable pain due to acute or chronic pancreatitis or advanced carcinoma of the pancreas, liver, or bladder.

CELLULOSE: A polysaccharide in which the basic building block is $C_6H_{10}O_5$ repeated in strands and cross-linkages as many as 2000 times. It is the main constituent of plant cell walls. In medicine, cellulose is often used as a hemostatic agent and as a volume expander for intravenous use.

CELSIUS SCALE: A temperature scale with the ice point of water at 0 degrees and the boiling point of water at 100 degrees. The Celsius scale (since 1948) is the official term of the centigrade temperature scale. One degree Celsius (C) is 1/100th of the temperature differential and is equal in magnitude to the Kelvin (K) scale (1 K = 1 degree C).

CENTIMETER-OF-WATER TO MILLIMETER-OF-MERCURY CONVERSION: An equation stating that 1.36 cm water equals 1.0 mmHg.

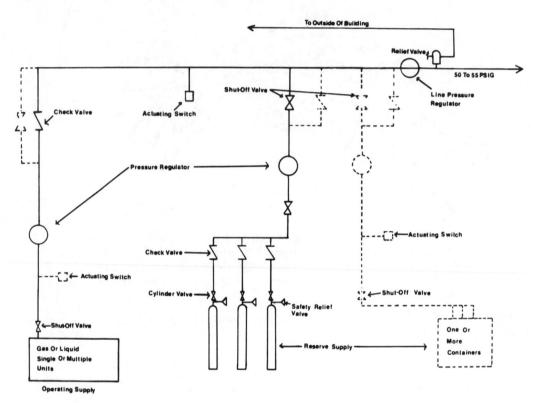

Central Gas Supply: Typical hospital bulk supply system. Dotted lines indicate a reserve supply. Reprinted with permission from NFPA 56F-1977, Standard for Nonflammable Medical Gas Systems, Copyright © 1977, National Fire Protection Association, Quincy, MA 02269. This reprinted material is not the complete and official position of the NFPA on the referenced subject, which is represented only by the standard in its entirety.

CENTRAL GAS SUPPLY: A system for supplying gas throughout hospital, clinic, or office where the cylinders or tanks are at a remote location from the site at which the gas is being used. The central supply usually consists of a facility for storage of gas, controls to deliver the gas through an in-the-wall piping system (at the appropriate working pressure), and an alarm system which indicates abnormal gas pressure changes. See Fig.

CENTRAL NERVOUS SYSTEM: The part of the nervous system made up of the brain and the spinal cord. See Fig. See Amygdala, Brain, Cerebrospinal fluid, Cranial nerves.

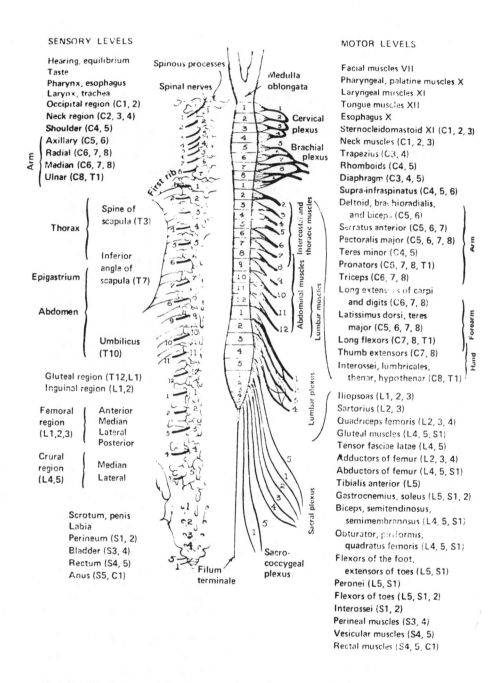

SENSORY LEVELS

Hearing, equilibrium
Taste
Pharynx, esophagus
Larynx, trachea
Occipital region (C1, 2)
Neck region (C2, 3, 4)
Shoulder (C4, 5)
Axillary (C5, 6)
Radial (C6, 7, 8)
Median (C6, 7, 8)
Ulnar (C8, T1)

Spinous processes
Spinal nerves
Medulla oblongata

First rib

Spine of scapula (T3)
Thorax

Inferior angle of scapula (T7)
Epigastrium

Abdomen

Umbilicus (T10)

Gluteal region (T12, L1)
Inguinal region (L1, 2)

Femoral region (L1, 2, 3)
Anterior
Median
Lateral
Posterior

Crural region (L4, 5)
Median
Lateral

Scrotum, penis
Labia
Perineum (S1, 2)
Bladder (S3, 4)
Rectum (S4, 5)
Anus (S5, C1)

Filum terminale

MOTOR LEVELS

Facial muscles VII
Pharyngeal, palatine muscles X
Laryngeal muscles XI
Tongue muscles XII
Esophagus X
Sternocleidomastoid XI (C1, 2, 3)
Neck muscles (C1, 2, 3)
Trapezius (C3, 4)
Rhomboids (C4, 5)
Diaphragm (C3, 4, 5)
Supra-infraspinatus (C4, 5, 6)
Deltoid, brachioradialis, and biceps (C5, 6)
Serratus anterior (C5, 6, 7)
Pectoralis major (C5, 6, 7, 8)
Teres minor (C4, 5)
Pronators (C6, 7, 8, T1)
Triceps (C6, 7, 8)
Long extensors of carpi and digits (C6, 7, 8)
Latissimus dorsi, teres major (C5, 6, 7, 8)
Long flexors (C7, 8, T1)
Thumb extensors (C7, 8)
Interossei, lumbricales, thenar, hypothenar (C8, T1)

Iliopsoas (L1, 2, 3)
Sartorius (L2, 3)
Quadriceps femoris (L2, 3, 4)
Gluteal muscles (L4, 5, S1)
Tensor fasciae latae (L4, 5)
Adductors of femur (L2, 3, 4)
Abductors of femur (L4, 5, S1)
Tibialis anterior (L5)
Gastrocnemius, soleus (L5, S1, 2)
Biceps, semitendinosus, semimembranosus (L4, 5, S1)
Obturator, piriformis, quadratus femoris (L4, 5, S1)
Flexors of the foot, extensors of toes (L5, S1)
Peronei (L5, S1)
Flexors of toes (L5, S1, 2)
Interossei (S1, 2)
Perineal muscles (S3, 4)
Vesicular muscles (S4, 5)
Rectal muscles (S4, 5, C1)

Cervical plexus
Brachial plexus
Intercostal and thoracic muscles
Abdominal muscles
Lumbar muscles
Lumbar plexus
Sacral plexus
Sacro-coccygeal plexus

Arm
Forearm
Hand

Central Nervous System: The motor and sensory levels of the central nervous system.

CENTRAL PAIN: The pain occurring as a result of a central nervous system lesion.

CENTRAL PROCESSING UNIT (CPU): The functional center of any computer which actually performs the mathematic operations necessary to alter input information.

Data-processing buffers and temporary storage devices are often used to hold the various batches of information so that the CPU can operate on them individually. See Computer, Data-processing buffer.

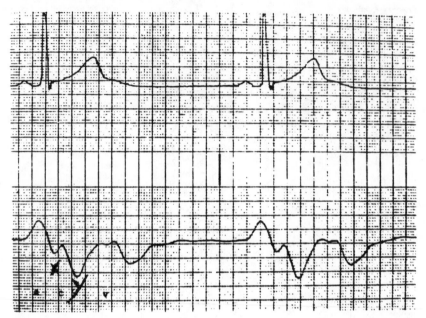

Central Venous Pressure: Tracing of the central venous pressure showing the five waveforms.

CENTRAL VENOUS PRESSURE (CVP): The pressure measured in the great veins of the thorax. This pressure is considered to be the filling pressure of the right side of the heart and is an indication of both the adequacy of blood return to the heart and the performance of the right ventricle. The normal CVP tracing has five separate wave patterns: a, c, x, v, and y. (The wave patterns labeled a, c, and v are positively directed and the wave patterns x and y are negatively directed.) The a wave is caused by right atrial contraction; the c wave is caused by the pushing of the tricuspid valve into the right atrium as the right ventricle contracts. These two waves are followed by the x wave, which results from further atrial relaxation and the downward displacement of the ventricle during contraction. The v wave is formed by the filling of the right atrium against the closed tricuspid valve. The y wave is caused by the opening of the tricuspid valve as blood begins to flow from the right atrium into the right ventricle. The wave of particular importance is the a wave, as it is absent in patients with atrial fibrillation. Enlarged a waves occur during conditions of increased resistance to right atrial emptying, such as right ventricular hypertrophy, pulmonary stenosis, tricuspid stenosis, or pulmonary hypertension. A huge a wave may be seen when the right atrium contracts with the tricuspid valve closed. This can be seen in nodal rhythms of the heart and results in a "cannon wave." See Fig.

CENTRIFUGE: A machine in which samples of solutions, suspensions, or mixtures may be spun rapidly to separate out the lighter portions (due to centrifugal force).

CEPHALOSPORINS: A group of antibiotics structurally similar to the penicillins. The antibacterial spectrum of the cephalosporins resembles the broad-spectrum

Cephalosporins.

Generic Name (Trade Name)	Spectrum of Activity	Comments
Cephalothin (Keflin) IM IV	Active against both G+ and G− microbes (especially Escherichia coli, Proteus mirabilis) including penicillinase-producing Staphylococcus.	Cephalothin, like other cephalosporins, is the primary agent against Klebsiella pneumoniae infections. Side effects include rash, fever, increased SGOT, blood dyscrasias, anaphylactoid reactions, and serum sickness. Severe pain can occur after IM injection and repeated injections can lead to phlebitis.
Cephaloridine (Loridine) IM	Similar to cephalothin plus Mycobacterium fortuitum. E. coli and Clostridium perfringens are more sensitive to cephaloridine than to cephalothin.	Cephaloridine shows higher and more sustained blood levels and is better tolerated than cephalothin. Side effects include rash, eosinophilia, and nephrotoxicity, especially at higher doses.
Cephalexin (Duricef) Monohydrate PO	Similar to cephalothin.	Cephalexin monohydrate is excreted unchanged in urine and is useful in urinary tract infections caused by E. coli, Pr. mirabilis, and some Klebsiella.
Cefazolin Sodium (Ancef) IM IV (Kefzol)	Similar to cephalothin though it is more active against E. coli, Klebsiella, some Enterobacter, indole-positive Proteus, and Hemophilus influenzae.	Cefazolin sodium is recommended for the treatment of urinary tract, skin, respiratory, and soft tissue infections. There is less pain after IM injection than with cephalothin. Side effects include rash (uncommon), increased SGOT, and increased alkaline phosphatase.
Cephradine (Anspor) IM IV (Velosef)	Similar to cephalexin though it may be less effective against E. coli and Pr. mirabilis. It is active against Enterococci.	Cephradine shows excellent absorption after oral administration.

Generic Name (Trade Name)	Spectrum of Activity	Comments
Cephapirin (Cefadyl) IM	Similar to cephalothin though it is more active against Streptococcus pyogenes and Pneumococcus.	Cephapirin is not well tolerated IM. Nausea is quite common after adminis-tration.
Cefamandole (Mandol) Nafate IM IV	Wider spectrum than cephalothin. Increased activity against Entero-bacter, indole-positive Proteus, and H. influenzae.	Cefamandole is not well tolerated IM. More active than cephalothin against G^- microorganisms. Pseudomonas is resistant.
Cefoxitin (Mefoxin) IM IV	Less active than cefamandole against most G^+ and G^- organisms. Increased activity against indole-positive spe-cies of Serratia, Proteus, and Bacillus fragilis.	Highly resistant to beta-lactamases produced by G^- bacilli.

penicillins. A cross-sensitivity reaction between cephalosporins and penicillins exists in some individuals. See Fig.

CEPHALOTHIN: A cephalosporin. See Antibiotic.

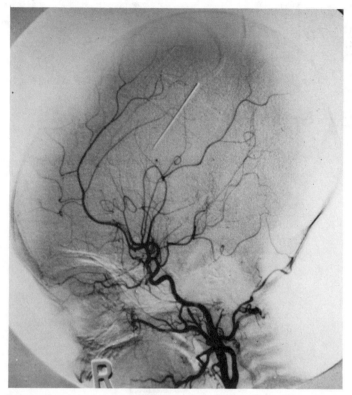

Cerebral Angiography: An angiogram outlining the vasculature of the right side of the brain in a child.

CEREBRAL ANGIOGRAPHY: A radiographic examination of the vascular system of the brain after injection of dye into the carotid artery. Previously the primary technique for the study of neuropathology, it is a relatively safe procedure that has a small but known morbidity and mortality. This procedure is now being replaced or supplemented by computerized axial tomography (CAT) scanning and similar techniques. See Fig.

CEREBRAL BLOOD FLOW: The amount of arterial blood perfusing the brain each minute. In the normal adult this equals 700 ml/min, and in the brain as a whole approximately 46-54 ml/100 g/min. Regional cerebral blood flow is individualized by the structure and function of the brain; it is highest in the gray matter (up to 140 ml/min in the superior colliculus with the eyes open) and lowest in the white matter (down to 20-25 ml/min in the corpus callosum). In the past, cerebral blood flow was determined by the Fick principle using N_2O uptake; more recently it has been measured by radioisotope tracer techniques. See Fig.

CEREBRAL DEHYDRATION: A condition brought about by the intravenous injection of drugs, such as mannitol or urea, to increase the osmolarity of the blood. This removes water from all cellular structures, particularly the brain, causing the neu-

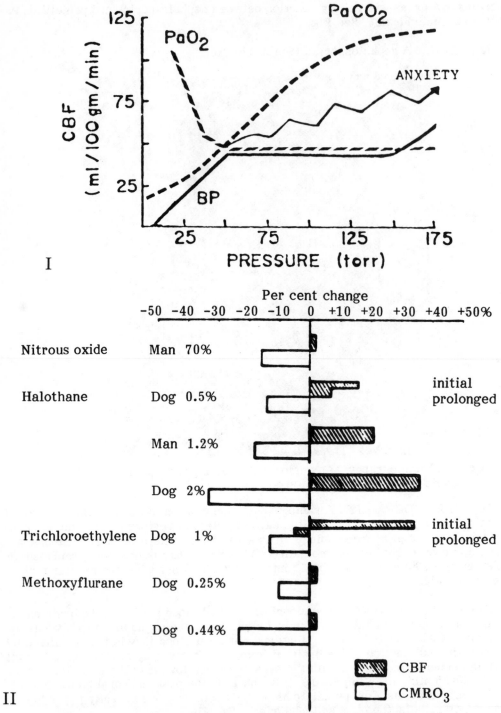

Cerebral Blood Flow: (I) Changes in cerebral blood flow brought about by changes in PaO_2, $PaCO_2$, and blood pressure, and by the variable effect of anxiety. (II) Effects of the gaseous and intravenous anesthetic drugs on cerebral blood flow and cerebral metabolic rate.

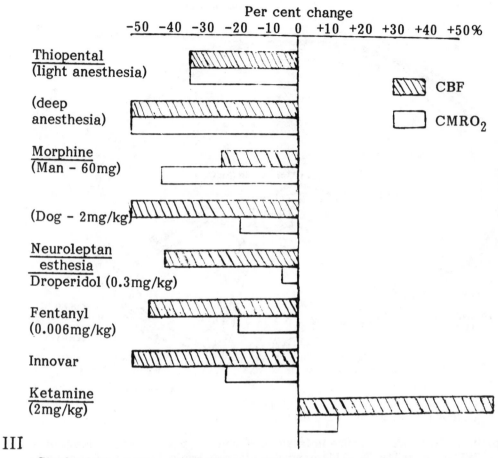

III

Cerebral Blood Flow: (III) Effects of the gaseous and intravenous anesthetic drugs on cerebral blood flow and cerebral metabolic rate.

rons to shrink in volume. It is usually employed as a technique for neurosurgery to "relax the brain" and to allow better access without having to enlarge the incision.

CEREBRAL FUNCTION MONITOR: One of the first clinically available devices for monitoring the electroencephalogram (EEG) intraoperatively. It uses a single pair of electrodes to measure the amplitude of the EEG signal. It also monitors the impedance between those electrodes to show any changes in the contact between the scalp and the electrodes. The device has not been well accepted in anesthesiology.

CEREBRAL METABOLIC RATE (CMR): The rate at which the brain uses O_2 (CMR_{O2}) and glucose (CMR_g).

CEREBRAL PERFUSION PRESSURE: The amount of difference between arterial blood pressure and intracranial pressure. In cases of severe trauma, the intracranial pressure can be higher than the systolic blood pressure, completely shutting off arterial blood flow to the brain. See Subarachnoid screw.

CEREBROSPINAL FLUID (CSF): The fluid which bathes and supports the brain. In the normal adult it totals about 140 ml. Measured by lumbar puncture (in the later-

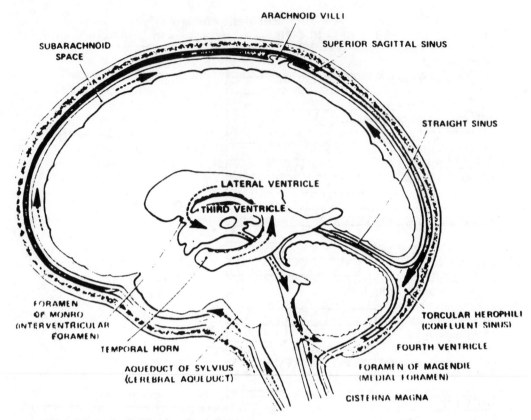

ARACHNOID VILLI

SUBARACHNOID SPACE

SUPERIOR SAGITTAL SINUS

STRAIGHT SINUS

LATERAL VENTRICLE

THIRD VENTRICLE

FORAMEN OF MONRO (INTERVENTRICULAR FORAMEN)

TORCULAR HEROPHILI (CONFLUENT SINUS)

TEMPORAL HORN

FOURTH VENTRICLE

AQUEDUCT OF SYLVIUS (CEREBRAL AQUEDUCT)

FORAMEN OF MAGENDIE (MEDIAL FORAMEN)

CISTERNA MAGNA

Cerebrospinal Fluid: Circulation.

al position), the CSF pressure is between 10 and 15 cm of water. The specific gravity of CSF is about 1.007. This normally clear and colorless fluid is produced by the choroid plexus, a specialized secretory tissue of the lateral third and fourth ventricles, at a rate of about 0.5 ml/min. The turnover of the entire CSF volume takes about 5 hr. The flow of the CSF is from the lateral ventricles to the third ventricle and then to the fourth ventricle via the cerebral aqueduct. From the fourth ventricle, the CSF enters the subarachnoid space where it ultimately bathes the brain and spinal cord. It is eventually absorbed by the arachnoid villi, which are specialized tissues projecting into the dural venous sinuses, thereby creating elevations known as arachnoid granulations. See Fig.

CERENKOV RADIATION: The light energy emitted by a particle when it passes into a transparent medium at a speed which is higher than the velocity of light in that medium. The light is the physical evidence of the instantaneous deceleration of the particle to the speed of light in that medium.

CESIUM-137: A radioactive element which emits gamma rays with a half-life of 33 years. The gamma radiation energy spectrum is less than cobalt-60. It has some medical applications as a radioactive tracer and a radiation treatment modality.

CETACAINE: A trade name for a liquid topical anesthetic containing a small amount of tetracaine with benzocaine. See Local anesthetic.

C FIBER: See Nerve fiber, anatomy and physiology of.

CGS SYSTEM OF UNITS: A system of measurements in which the centimeter is the unit of length, the gram is the unit of mass, and the second is the unit of time. The CGS system has been superseded by the SI system. See SI unit.

CHANNEL: A defined pathway for information signals. The most obvious example is the channel on a standard television set. Each channel number actually refers to the frequency range of the carrier signal over which the information (the television program) is sent.

CHARGE: A measurable property of certain elementary particles. The terms positive and negative are semantic inventions in the most simplified sense. They signify that a particle has either an excess of electrons (negatively charged) or a scarcity of electrons (positively charged).

CHARLES LAW: A physical law which governs the behavior of an ideal gas. It states that at a constant pressure and 0 degrees Celsius the volume of a fixed mass of gas increases by 1/273 for each degree Celsius rise in temperature. For example, if at constant pressure a gas occupies 1 L at 0 degrees Celsius, it will occupy a volume of 1 L plus 100/273 L (136.3L) at 100 degrees Celsius.

CHASSAIGNAC TUBERCLE: See Stellate ganglion block.

CHEMICAL SOLUTION: A liquid mixture in which a chemical reaction has occurred between the solvent and the solute, such that the solute is unrecoverable by physical processes.

CHEMILUMINESCENCE: The phenomenon in which bacteria or fireflies produce light without the production of heat. This is usually accomplished through the oxidation of a species-specific pigment called luciferin promoted by the enzyme luciferase. See Anesthesia, pressure reversal of.

CHEMTRON CORPORATION: A major manufacturer of anesthesia and medical equipment and a modern day descendant of the National Cylinder Gas Company. It is now part of the Allied Health Care Products, Inc., a division of Allegheny Ludlum Industries, Inc., Pittsburgh.

CHENG NEEDLE: See Epidural needle.

CHEST PHYSIOTHERAPY: A procedure referring to postural drainage in conjunction with chest percussion and vibration. See Postural drainage.

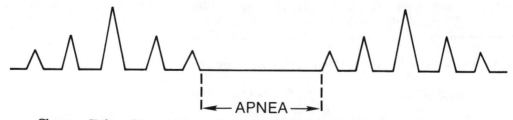
Cheyne-Stokes Respiration: Pattern of Cheyne-Stokes respiration.

CHEYNE-STOKES RESPIRATION: A state of periodic breathing and apnea seen in various disease states, especially those with damage to the central nervous system. This type of respiratory phenomenon is often demonstrated in patients with uremia and congestive heart failure. See Fig.

CHI-SQUARE TEST (X^2): A test used to compare frequency distribution and to determine statistical significance of the differences, i.e., a comparison of the observed frequency with the expected frequency. It is useful as an alternative to the Student t test on small samples.

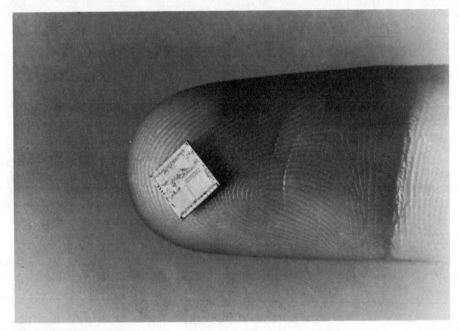

Chip: Typical integrated circuit.

CHIP: A slang term, originally from electronics, for an integrated circuit. See Fig. See Circuit, integrated.

CHLORAL HYDRATE: A sedative-hypnotic drug first used in the 1870s. Most of its effect is believed to be due to its rapid reduction to the active metabolite trichloroethanol. After having been supplanted by the barbiturates, chloral hydrate has again become relatively popular as a children's sedative or as a hypnotic the night before surgery. Combined with ethanol it forms the "Mickey Finn" cocktail. (The power of this cocktail to "knock out" its imbiber is somewhat overrated.)

CHLORAMPHENICOL: A broad-spectrum antibiotic first employed clinically in 1948 and used widely during the 1950s and early 1960s. Its documented tendency to cause serious and often fatal blood dyscrasias, however, has now limited use to the most serious of infections as the drug of last choice.

CHLORAZEPATE DIPOTASSIUM (TRANXENE): See Benzodiazepine.

CHLORDIAZEPOXIDE (LIBRIUM): See Benzodiazepine.

CHLORIDE: The principal extracellular anion in the body. Its normal plasma concentration is given variously as 95-105 mEq/L. Intracellularly, it has an extremely low concentration (2 mEq/L). Early technical breakthroughs allowed simple, accurate measurement of chloride in serum and urine before it was possible to measure any other ion (sodium, potassium) correctly. Hypochloremia may be indicative of alkalosis, which is a major consequence of persistent vomiting. Excess chloride appears to be easily excreted by the kidney.

CHLORIDE SHIFT: See Carbon dioxide transport in blood.

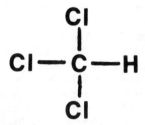

Chloroform.

CHLOROFORM: A general anesthetic first discovered soon after the initial demonstration of ether anesthesia in the 1840s. It has been quite popular in England and Europe for many decades. Chloroform (CHCl3) is a potent, nonexplosive anesthetic agent that has a fairly rapid induction and emergence time. Associated with severe liver damage and sudden fatal cardiac arrhythmias, it is seldom used in contemporary anesthetic practice. See Fig.

CHLOROPROCAINE (NESACAINE): A short-acting, ester-type local anesthetic which is a derivative of procaine. See Local anesthetic.

CHLORPHENIRAMINE MALEATE (CHLOR-TRIMETON): A commonly used antihistaminic agent, usually administered orally.

CHLORPROMAZINE (THORAZINE): See Phenothiazine.

CHOLINERGIC CRISIS: A medical emergency precipitated by an overdose of an anticholinesterase agent. The crisis shows muscarinic effects (such as sweating, miosis, salivation, lacrimation, and bowel hyperactivity) as well as nicotinic effects (such as muscle fasciculation and paralysis).

CHOLINERGIC NERVOUS SYSTEM: See Autonomic nervous system.

CHOLINERGIC RECEPTOR: A proteinaceous structure on the surface of a cell which specifically binds to the neurotransmitter acetylcholine and its congeners. Cholinergic receptors vary in makeup and density at different sites and can be divided into two types by their response to the natural alkaloids, muscarine and nicotine.

CHOLINESTERASE (PSEUDOCHOLINESTERASE): An enzyme that catalyzes the hydrolysis of choline esters. See Acetylcholinesterase, Dibucaine number.

CHORDOTOMY: A neurosurgical procedure which diminishes chronic intractable pain. In a chordotomy, the pain pathways on one side of the spinal cord are interrupted by a precise incision. This is in contrast to rhizotomy, in which only the nerve roots of the particularly painful area are sectioned.

CHRISTIAN SCIENCE: A system of religious teaching founded in 1866 in the United States. Christian Scientists deny the reality of the world and argue that illness and sin are illusions which can be overcome by the mind. They therefore refuse medical help for illness.

CHRISTMAS DISEASE: A bleeding disorder which is due to a factor IX deficiency. The disease is named after the family in which it was first diagnosed. See Hemophilia.

CHRONIC OBSTRUCTIVE PULMONARY DISEASE (COPD): A lung disorder seen almost exclusively in heavy smokers and characterized by irreversible airway obstruction associated with emphysema and chronic bronchitis. The emphysematous component results in destruction of the alveolar walls with subsequent abnormal enlargement of the air spaces distal to the terminal nonrespiratory bronchioles. This destruction of alveolar walls causes loss of support and some degree of collapse of the distal nonrespiratory bronchioles which, in turn, causes narrowing of their lumens, particularly on expiration. The chronic bronchitis component leads to hyperplasia of mucous glands, inflammation, mucosal edema, bronchospasm, along with impacted secretions. The single most consistent finding in COPD is the loss of the 1-sec forced expiratory volume (FEV_1). Practically, this means that the patient with COPD finds it increasingly difficult to expel a given volume of air in a finite period of time. The consequences of COPD are progressive respiratory embarrassment with elevated PCO_2 and decreased PO_2. Treatment of COPD is aimed at providing respiratory support during acute exacerbation and at fighting infection. Recently a genetic predisposition to emphysema has been discovered. Those individ-

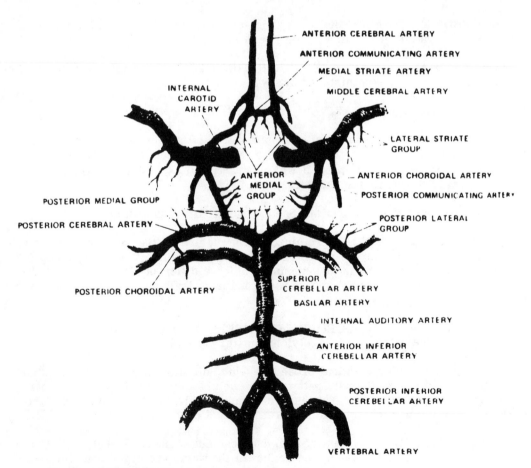

Circle of Willis (Circulus Arteriosus): Its origins and branches.

uals have a deficiency of alpha-1-antitrypsin on serum assay. They appear to be uniquely susceptible to autodigestion of pulmonary tissue by the naturally occurring proteases, since the antitrypsin molecule is not present to protect them. These cases may account for as much as 2-3% of all emphysema cases.

CHRONOTROPISM: The ability to influence the cardiac rate via the adrenergic sympathetic nerves. Positive chronotropic drugs increase the heart rate whereas negative ones decrease it, e.g., acetylcholine.

CINCHOCAINE (NUPERCAINE): The British term for dibucaine. See Dibucaine, Local anesthetic.

CIRCADIAN RHYTHM: The cyclic repetition of certain phenomena which occurs on a 24-hr basis. Physiologic functions which seem to follow this periodicity include body temperature, adrenal cortical function, electrolyte concentration, and urine volume. For example, in those people who sleep at night and are awake during the day, adrenal cortisol secretion is at peak levels upon awakening. Its level progressively falls throughout the rest of the day.

CIRCLE OF WILLIS: The circular formation of arteries at the base of the brain. It is the origin of the six large vessels supplying the cerebral cortex. Composed of the internal carotids and the anterior and posterior cerebral arteries, it is not unusual for the Circle of Willis to be incomplete. See Fig.

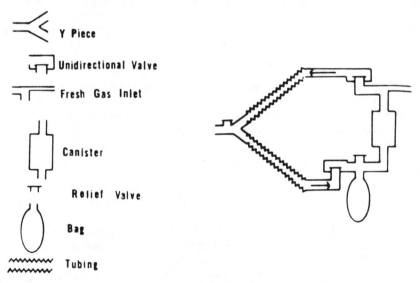

Circle System: One of the many configurations of valves, fresh gas inlet, CO_2 canister, relief valve, and breathing bag possible with a circle system.

CIRCLE SYSTEM: An assembly of hoses and valves which are unidirectional. Theoretically and (for the most part) practically, gas flows through the system in only one direction. The system is considered to be semiclosed or partially rebreathing in type, i.e., part of the gas expired by the patient goes through a CO_2 absorber and forms part of the fresh gas supply of the succeeding inspiration. See Fig.

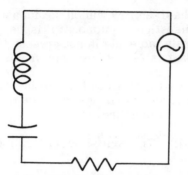

Circuit: Simple circuit showing the symbols for a power source (circle with a sinusoid waveform); resistance (jagged line); capacitance (two lines perpendicular to the current path separated by an air space); and inductance (series of loops).

CIRCUIT: A system of active and passive electric components which carry or act on an electric current. The term usually refers to the smallest combination of two or more electric components which perform a specific function on a current (amplification, rectification, etc.). For example, two diodes can be used to form a current which will change alternating to direct current. See Fig.

CIRCUIT BREAKER (OVERCURRENT PROTECTOR): A device used to protect an electric circuit. It interrupts the current flow when the flow exceeds a predetermined limit. A fuse performs the same function; however, it usually can be used only once as it is destroyed by an overcurrent condition and its destruction interrupts that condition. Circuit breakers are usually mechanical spring-loaded devices which can be reset rather than replaced.

CIRCUIT, INTEGRATED (IC): A single unit of semiconductive material which contains thousands of electrically active elements. Integrated circuits are usually made by photoetchings from photomicrographs. The desired circuit is initially drawn full size and then photographed. The negative is then markedly reduced in size. This negative is used to control a laser which, in turn, cuts a layered piece of semiconductive material of the proper electric characteristics. The end result of this entire process is the IC. Miniaturization is becoming so advanced that limits are being approached which approximate the physical size of electrons. Circuit element densities can be routinely made greater than 5 million elements/in^3.

CIRCUIT, SOLID STATE: A set of electric components which operate on a current in such a way that the current always flows through solid materials. This is in contrast to vacuum tube circuitry in which current partially flows through the evacuated glass envelopes of the vacuum tubes. Solid state circuits (in contrast to vacuum tube circuits) are characterized by small size, low heat generation, and ruggedness.

CIRCULATOR, REVELL: A device which uses an external source of power (gas pressure or suction) to move the anesthetic gases continuously around the anesthesia machine breathing circle. This reduces the dead space under the mask by providing fresh gas to this volume even during pauses in ventilation. The circulator, by operating at a flow rate which just "floats the valves," decreases the resistance of these valves, thereby reducing the work needed for spontaneous ventilation. Certain disadvantages have prevented the circulator from gaining wide acceptance. These include the need for a power source and the tendency to gas leakage due to the slight increase in pressure during operation.

CLADDING: A process in which one metal is bonded to the surface of another to prevent corrosion of the protected metal. For example, zinc and nickel are often used to clad iron.

CLARK ELECTRODE: See Oxygen electrode.

CLEARANCE: The elimination of a biologically active substance from an organism. For example, total body clearance (usually abbreviated as Qb) is a measure of the rate of removal of a given drug from the body.

CLOCK, ELECTRONIC: A device which is used to precisely time and, therefore, synchronize the various functions of a multipurpose circuit.

CLOSED ANESTHESIA SYSTEM: See Anesthesia system, closed.

CLOSED CIRCUIT TELEVISION (CCTV): A system usually used in the surveillance or security of limited-access areas, e.g., an operating room. All parts of the system, including the cameras, the control mechanisms, and the TV receiver, are physically linked by cables, eliminating the need to transmit by aerials.

CLOSING CAPACITY: The lung volume at which small airways narrow and close during continuous exhalation. In health, this point should exist at the far end of the expiratory reserve volume but increasing age, smoking, and obesity move it toward the tidal volume (airways close earlier and earlier during exhalation). In general, any reduction of the functional residual capacity will shift the closure of a significant number of small airways from a point in the expiratory reserve volume to a point in the tidal volume. See Fig. See Absorption atelectasis, Lung volumes and capacities.

CLOSTRIDIUM BOTULINUM TOXIN: A systemic poison elaborated by the bacillus Clostridium botulinum which causes botulism. It prevents the release of acetylcholine by cholinergic nerve fibers and gives rise to neurologic symptoms. This toxin is the most potent organic poison ever discovered.

COAGULATION CURRENT: A type of output available from an electrosurgical instrument which allows maximal coagulability with a minimal incision. The waveform is a damped, intermittent sine wave. See Fig.

COARCTATION OF THE AORTA (COARC): A condition in which there is a stricture or contraction, usually localized, of the aorta. Often seen as a congenital anomaly, it can cause severe cardiac decompensation due to the elevated resistance to left ventricular output. Hyperperfusion occurs above the "coarc" and hypoperfusion below the "coarc." From an anesthetic viewpoint, excessive bleeding may become a problem during the surgical procedure due to the hypertension in the vessels proximal to the stricture.

COAXIAL CABLE: A conductor used for the transmission of high-frequency signals. It consists of a central wire surrounded by an insulator with an outer coaxial conducting cylinder. Coaxial cables are more expensive than the usual twin lead cables, but do not produce nor are they affected by external electric fields. Therefore, they are used when low noise conditions are required.

COAXIAL SCAVENGER: A device fitted to the tail of the reservoir bag of the standard Jackson-Rees modification of an Ayre T-piece for pediatric anesthesia. Basically, the device removes undesirable gases via a reservoir which is fitted around the tailpiece of the bag.

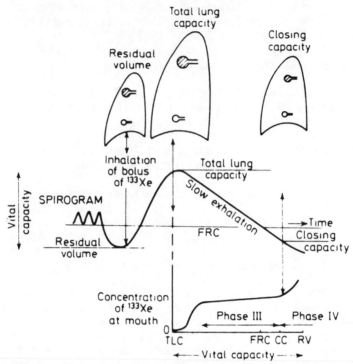

Closing Capacity: Measurement of closing capacity using a radioactive gas as a tracer. The bolus of tracer is inhaled near residual volume and due to airway closure is distributed only to those alveoli with air passages still open (shaded area). During expiration, concentration of the tracer gas becomes constant after the dead space is washed out. This plateau (phase III) gives way to a rising concentration of tracer gas (phase IV) when there is closure of airways leading to alveoli which did not receive the tracer gas.

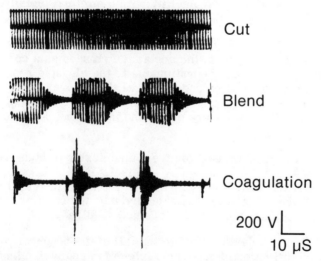

Coagulation Current: Oscillographic picture of cutting, blend, and coagulation currents.

COBALT (Co): A metallic element with the atomic weight of 59. Its radioisotope, cobalt-60, has a half-life of 5.3 years and emits highly penetrating gamma rays in the range of 1.1-1.3 million electron volts. Nonradioactive Co is alloyed with chrome to make a number of superhard materials (Vitallium and Tyconium) which are not attacked by body fluids. These are used as bone replacements and in making dentures. Depending on the ratios of Co to chrome, these materials can be made superhard with tensile strength in excess of 300,000 lb/in^2.

COBOL: An acronym for COmmon Business Oriented Language, computer terminology frequently used for commercial data application.

COCAINE: The first local anesthetic to be discovered and used. This complex molecule is unique in that it produces both anesthesia and local vasoconstriction. These effects are probably due to its ability to block the reuptake of norepinephrine at nerve terminals, thereby prolonging its own action. It is a drug much abused by inhalation of the powdered form. See Local anesthetic.

CODE BLUE: In common hospital parlance, the announcement that cardiopulmonary resuscitation is required at a given location.

CODEINE: The weakest of the available narcotics. See Narcotic.

CODMAN, ERNEST AMORY: See Anesthesia chart.

COEFFICIENT OF EXPANSION: A physical characteristic of all materials that represents the percentage of change in a given measurement per degree Celsius.

COEFFICIENT OF VARIABILITY: A value indicating the ratio of the standard deviation (SD) to the mean. It is determined by dividing the SD by the arithmetic mean and multiplying by 100. This calculation for two or more data sets allows for direct comparison of their frequency distribution without concern for different units of measurement. The data set with the smaller coefficient of variation (read as a percent) has the smaller frequency distribution. For example, if the SD of blood pressure is 15 with a mean of 100, then the coefficient of variation is 15%. If the SD of serum sodium is 5 with a mean of 140, the coefficient of variation is 3.5%.

COGENTIN: See Benztropine mesylate.

COLD SALINE INJECTION: A treatment modality in which large quantities of iced saline are injected under the dura. It is used for relief of intractable pain. It is usually performed during general anesthesia as the side effects are extremely unpleasant for the patient. This is not a widely used technique.

COLLATERAL RESPIRATION: A phenomenon seen when lung segments distal to an obstructed small bronchus are inflated via the surrounding tissues. Collateral respiration does not occur if a main bronchus is occluded.

COLLODION (COLLODIUM): A highly flammable, colorless, thick solution of gun cotton in ether and alcohol, used as a protective dressing for cuts and surgical wounds. [Gun cotton (nitrocellulose or pyroxylin) is produced by reacting cotton with nitric and sulfuric acids.] Collodion is extremely flammable.

COLLOID THEORY OF ANESTHESIA: An old hypothesis of anesthetic behavior which states that anesthetic agents cause a reversible change in the protoplasm of neurons. This reversible condition interferes with protein function and resembles the physical state known as a colloidal suspension. Currently, this theory is unacceptable since no physical evidence for this effect exists. (Refer to the major journals for the next few years to see if it makes a comeback.)

COLLOIDAL OSMOTIC PRESSURE: See Oncotic pressure.

COLORIMETRY: A chemical quantitation method which uses the intensity of color (produced as the result of a test reaction or test sequence) to determine the concentration of a sought-after variable. For example, hemoglobin concentration can be determined by aiming a light source of a frequency known to be absorbed by hemoglobin through an unknown solution at a photocell. The amount of light absorbed by the unknown solution is directly proportional to the amount of hemoglobin present.

COLTON, GARDNER QUINCY: See Morton, William T. G.

COMA (COMATOSE): A condition in which a patient is unaware of his or her surroundings and is unarousable by powerful stimulation. These terms are used relatively indiscriminately and subcategories such as presence or absence of spontaneous ventilation should be stressed. A method for evaluating the comatose state is the Comascore, which can be used to show patient trends in the intensive care unit. See Figs.

COMBINED ANESTHESIA: See Balanced anesthesia.

COMBUSTION: The rapid and vigorous oxidation of fuel molecules leading to the emission of heat and light. Flames are visible evidence of combustion.

COMPARATOR: An electronic or mechanical device which compares two signal inputs. The output of the device depends on some preprogrammed or predetermined relationship between the two inputs. For example, the alarm mechanisms on most physiologic monitors use comparators to relate the pulse rate to some internal standard. If the alarm is set to sound at a pulse of 180, the patient's pulse (usually the interval detected between successive R waves) is compared with the alarm time interval (0.33 sec). If the patient's pulse is higher, the comparator actuates an alarm. See Fig.

COMPENSATORY DAMAGES: See Punitive damages.

COMPETITIVE ANTAGONISM (REVERSIBLE INHIBITION): A pharmacologic phenomenon seen between two drugs which have affinity for the same tissue receptor site. The number of receptor sites the drugs occupy depends on their concentration. Thus, a relative overabundance of one drug will displace the other. Narcotics and narcotic antagonists share a competitive antagonistic relationship. The narcotic effect can be terminated with the displacement of the narcotic by an antagonist at its tissue receptor sites. See Noncompetitive antagonism.

COMPETITIVE INHIBITION: See Neuromuscular blocking agent.

COMPLIANCE: A calculation of the elasticity or expandability of the lungs measured when the flow of air into the lungs has ceased, e.g., while holding one's breath. This is best demonstrated in the paralyzed, anesthetized patient. It is the volume change (in liters) divided by the pressure change caused by the expansion to that vol-

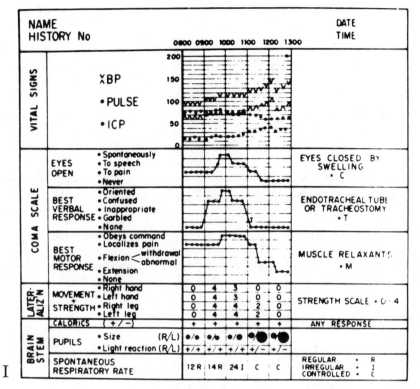

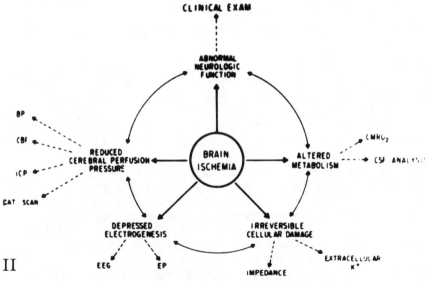

Coma: (I) Example of a neurologic status record. It consists of a vital sign chart, a coma scale, and estimation of lateralization and brain stem function. The patient being followed was initially comatose, emerged from the coma, and then relapsed. (II) Summary of the pathophysiologic consequences of cerebral ischemia and the specialized monitoring involved in detecting them. The outer circle represents the physiologic disorders caused by cerebral ischemia. The dashed arrows indicate the monitoring methods needed to determine these derangements.

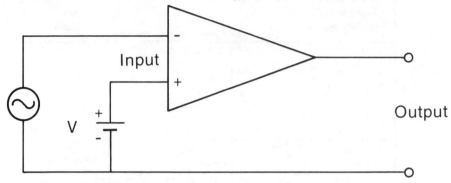

Comparator: Operational amplifier comparator.

ume. In the normal individual, the compliance of the lungs and thoracic wall are measured together. It is approximately 100 ml/cm water pressure. For example, if the lungs are inflated to a volume of 1 L in a normal anesthetized patient, a pressure gauge connected to the airway should read about 10 cm water when air movement stops.

COMPONENT THERAPY: See Blood storage.

COMPRESSED SPECTRAL ARRAY: A display technique used in the interpretation of the electroencephalogram. See Fourier analysis.

COMPRESSION NERVE PALSY: The injury often arising during anesthesia due to poor or careless positioning of the patient, thereby affecting the main nerve trunks. The facial, radial, ulnar, and tibial nerves are susceptible to compression nerve palsies.

COMPRESSION VOLUME: The portion of the tidal volume delivered to a patient by a bag squeeze or ventilator which functions to distend the hoses leading to the patient. In general, most anesthesia equipment has a compression volume of 3 ml/cm water pressure. This means that if a ventilator delivers a peak pressure of 24 cm water during patient inspiration, 75 ml of the volume pushed by the ventilator does not reach the patient but distends the pliable parts of the ventilator circuit.

COMPUTER: An electronic device which processes information. Most computers, regardless of their complexity, have a number of common subdivisions which include input and output devices, an arithmetic or calculating section (the central processing unit, CPU), temporary and permanent storage facilities, communication units, and a control unit. Extremely large computers handle sophisticated tasks such as playing chess. The computer's move at any particular point in the game is based on mathematic calculations; it is designed to make the move which gives it the best mathematic chance for success. Some new computers have a fantastic ability to "number crunch." The Cray-1 series of computers can perform 100 million arithmetic computations/sec. See Analog computer, Central processing unit, Computer logic.

COMPUTERIZED AXIAL TOMOGRAPHY (CAT): A diagnostic radiology technique using advanced computer methods to form a visual image of a body plane with minimal doses of radiation. The older tomographic x-ray system moved the x-ray head and x-ray film simultaneously, pivoting around an imaginary point within the patient.

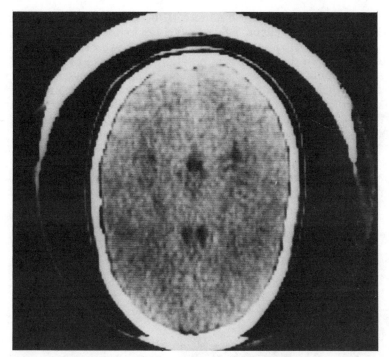

Computerized Axial Tomography: Typical CAT scan of a cross-section of the brain.

This point would be in focus while all points above and below it would become blurred. The CAT scanner moves stepwise around the body or segment to be visualized (usually 1 degree/step). The beam which emerges from the body is detected by a photomultiplier tube and is electronically assigned a value from white to gray to black, in proportion to its energy. (A beam blocked by bone would be greatly attenuated and appear white.) Each point in a plane would be crossed by an x-ray beam multiple times as the x-ray projector steps about the area being examined. The computer adds these densities together and draws a composite picture of the findings on a cathode ray tube. Accurate CAT scanning requires the patient to be immobile. A general anesthetic and a muscle relaxant may be administered to the uncooperative patient for an extended procedure. See Fig.

COMPUTER LOGIC: A reference to the five functions that any computer can perform: subtraction, addition, division, multiplication, and comparison of results. These processes encompass all necessary functions since the most complicated equation or process can be separated into these individual steps.

CONCENTRATION EFFECT: An explanation of the observation made during inhalation anesthetic induction that the higher the inspired concentration of an anesthetic, the faster the relative rise in alveolar concentration. (The alveolar concentration of an agent administered at a 20% concentration rises more than twice as fast as the same agent given at a 10% concentration.) The concentration effect is made up of two parts, the concentrating effect and the increased ventilation effect. In the latter, gas is drawn down the trachea to replace alveolar gas which has entered the blood. This tends to augment minute ventilation. For example, if a 70%N_2O/30%

O_2 source is connected to a patient, the mix will be pulled down the trachea to re-place any N_2O taken up in the blood. Since alveolar concentration of N_2O would be less than 70% (because of blood uptake), this would tend to restore it to the inspired level of concentration. In the concentrating effect the uptake by blood of an anesthetic changes the alveolar concentration of that agent to a lesser degree if it is in high concentration initially. For example, in an alveolus containing 50% agent and 50% O_2, uptake of half the agent (O_2 considered in equilibrium with no uptake) leaves more than 25% agent in the alveolus [i.e., old volume 50 parts N_2O + 50 parts O_2 = 100 parts (50% O_2); new volume 25 parts N_2O + 50 parts O_2 = 75 parts (33% N_2O + 67% O_2) . If we start with 25% agent, uptake of half agent and the new volume is 12.5 parts agent plus 75 parts O_2 = 14.2%. Note that the higher concentration decreased relatively less than the lower concentration. All calculations assure equilibrium of O_2, water vapor, CO_2, and N_2. See Diffusion hypoxia, Second gas effect.

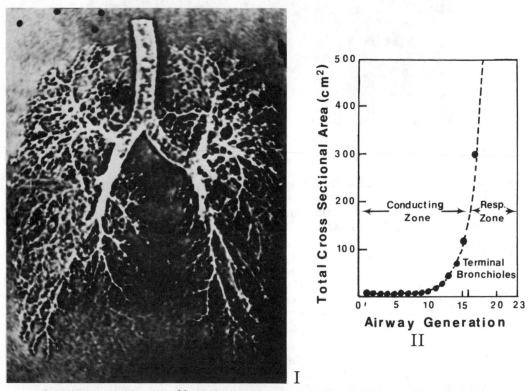

Conducting Airways: (I) Cast of human conducting airways with the alveoli trimmed away. The arborization of the airways from the trachea to the terminal bronchioles is shown. (II) Relationship of cross-sectional area, in square centimeters, to the number of divisions of the airways as they proceed from the trachea. The respiratory zone occurs at approximately the sixteenth division soon after the cross-sectional area begins to increase dramatically.

CONDUCTING AIRWAYS: The passages which start at the trachea, divide into the right and left mainstem bronchi, then into the lobar and segmental bronchi, continue to the terminal bronchioles, and end before the alveoli. There are 23 divisions from the trachea to the terminal bronchioles. These conducting areas contain no alveoli and therefore do not participate in gas exchange. They constitute the anatomic dead space. See Figs.

CONDUCTION: The transmission of some form of energy (heat, electric, or mechanical) from one point to another. It is also used to indicate the transmission of nerve impulses.

CONDUCTION ANESTHESIA: The interruption of nerve pathways, particularly sensory pathways, without loss of consciousness. Conduction anesthesia includes local infiltration, local nerve blocks, regional nerve blocks (epidural, caudal, and spinal anesthesia), and nerve blocks by direct pressure and refrigeration. A major conduction block usually refers to spinal, epidural, and regional blocks, whereas all other blocks are called minor conduction blocks.

CONDUCTIVE FLOORING: A floor which is deliberately rendered conductive to electricity. It is a requirement in enclosed areas, such as operating rooms, where the atmosphere may become flammable or explosive. By being conductive, the floors harmlessly dissipate stray electric charges which may build up as static electricity on personnel and objects in the room. In order for the flooring to perform its function, a conducting path must be maintained between the floor and the personnel and objects. This is usually accomplished with conductive shoes, conductive chains hanging from equipment, or by deliberate wiring of equipment to the floor.

CONDUCTOR: A material in which resistance to the passage of an electric current is negligible.

CONFIDENCE INTERVAL: See Confidence level.

CONFIDENCE LEVEL (STATISTICS): The concept that the mean of a group of observations lies within a specified distance of the mean of all possible observations. The choice of confidence level can be any number, but the usual choice is 95%. This means that 19 out of 20 times the mean of a sample of observations will fall within ±2 standard deviations (SD) of the true mean. The mean plus or minus the specified number of SDs is called the confidence level. The confidence level is bounded by the confidence limits.

CONGENER: Any discrete object closely related to another. For example, a congener of a drug has a similar structure and function to the parent drug.

CONGESTIVE HEART FAILURE (CHF): A clinical condition in which the heart fails to pump blood adequately resulting in a decreased blood flow to the tissues and congestion in the pulmonary and/or systemic circulation. Pulmonary and peripheral edema and hepatomegaly develop. Usually, CHF is a chronic condition and is associated with sodium and water retention by the kidneys. This is due to an alteration in renal plasma flow and glomerular filtration. Although the function of one side of the heart may be primarily impaired, the function of the other side is also affected since both sides ultimately must work together for optimal efficiency. Primary left-sided failure refers to signs and symptoms of increased pressure and congestion in the pulmonary veins and capillaries. Primary right-sided failure refers to signs and symptoms of increased pressure and congestion in the systemic veins and capillaries. The most common cause of right-sided failure is left-sided failure. See Fig. See Pulmonary edema.

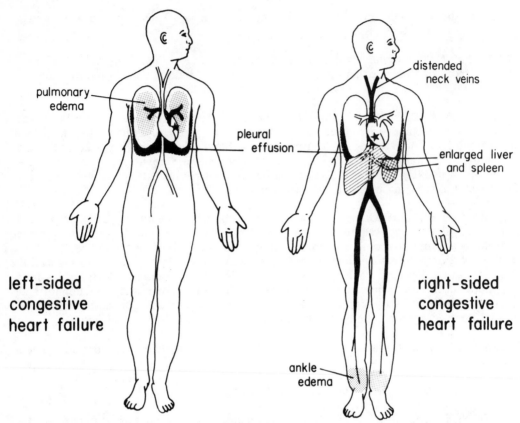

Congestive Heart Failure: Physical findings in left-sided and right-sided congestive heart failure.

CONJUGATE PAIR: An acid and the base it forms when it gives up a hydrogen ion. For example, carbonic acid (H_2CO_3) forms a conjugate pair when in solution with its conjugate base, the bicarbonate ion HCO_3^-.

CONNECTOR: A device or fitting that joins two or more components.

CONSCIOUS SEDATION: A technique of drug administration popular in outpatient dentistry. The goal of this technique is to produce a nonanxious, cooperative patient who can respond to commands. The patient's upper airway reflexes remain intact.

CONSENT FORM (PERMIT FORM): A legal document which is part of a patient's chart and medical record. By signing it, the patient agrees to undergo a specified medical and/or anesthetic procedure to be performed by specified personnel. While not completely unimpeachable, a signed consent form shows that an attempt was made to apprise the patient of needed treatment and possible complications before proceeding. See Fig. See Informed consent.

CONSERVATION OF MOMENTUM: A fundamental physical law which states that a body or particle in motion will continue to move unless acted upon by an outside force.

G-2d₂ **CONSENT FOR OPERATION OR PROCEDURE**

(See reverse for Monitored Telephone Call)

● File UNDER G-2a of same date ●

| DATE |
| HOSP NO |
| NAME |
| BIRTHDATE |
| ADDRESS |
| ☐ PVT ☐ CLP ☐ IND |
| IF NOT IMPRINTED, PLEASE PRINT HOSP NO., NAME AND LOCATION |

1. I authorize Dr. _____, or such associates as may

(Attending M.D., D.O., D.D.S.)

be selected by the doctor, to perform upon _____ the

(myself or name of patient)

following operation/procedure: _____

_____

(Technical name, followed by description in lay language)

_____

_____

2. In the event developments indicate that further operations/procedures may be necessary, I authorize the physicians to use their own judgment and do whatever they deem advisable during the operation/procedure for the patient's best interests, except the following: _____

_____

(List any exclusions. If none, write "none".)

3. I consent to the administration of such anesthetics as may be considered necessary or advisable by the anesthetist, with the exception of _____

_____

(List any exclusions. If none, write "none.")

4. The nature and purpose of the operation/procedure, possible alternative methods of treatment, the risks involved, the possible consequences, and the possibility of complications have been explained to me by Dr. _____. All of my questions concerning the operation/procedure and its possible outcome have been answered to my satisfaction.

5. I am aware that the practice of dentistry, medicine and surgery is not an exact science and acknowledge that no guarantees have been made to me by anyone concerning the results of the operation/procedure.

6. Any tissues surgically removed may be disposed of by the hospital in accordance with accustomed practice including use in research studies except as follows: _____

_____

(If none, write "none.")

Signature: _____

(Patient or person authorized to consent for patient)

Date: _____ Time: _____ A.M. / P.M.

Signature of Physician securing this consent:

_____

Continued On Reverse

6/80   **THE UNIVERSITY OF IOWA HOSPITALS AND CLINICS**

G 2d₂ — H — PATHOLOGY — I — DIAGNOSIS

Consent Form: Consent form used at The University of Iowa Hospitals and Clinics.

CONTINUOUS ANESTHESIA: The technique of introducing a catheter into a body space for the intermittent injection of local anesthetics over an extended period of time to maintain an anesthetic response. Continuous spinal, epidural, and caudal techniques have been used since the 1920s.

CONTINUOUS FLOW ANESTHESIA MACHINE: The complete name for the standard anesthesia delivery system. It is found in operating rooms worldwide. Flow from the machine continues regardless of changes caused by patient respiration. Gas issues from the common outlet, mixed according to the setting on flowmeters for each separate gas, and moves from the common outlet into the patient's circuit at all times, as long as the flowmeter is functioning. Gas leaves the common outlet at a

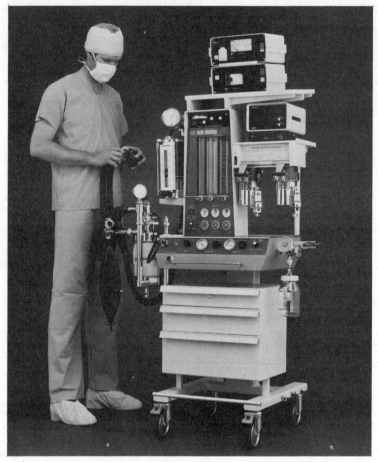

Continuous Flow Anesthesia Machine: Modern version.

pressure of 2-10 lb/in^2. Continuous flow machines are also currently available which use a single control for both O$_2$ and N$_2$O rather than two separate needle valves. See Fig.

CONTINUOUS MONITORING FOR POLLUTION: The constant use of a detector for trace anesthetic gases in an operating room. This can immediately determine leaks or faulty techniques.

CONTINUOUS POSITIVE AIRWAY PRESSURE (CPAP): A method of spontaneous or mechanical ventilation in which the pressure of the upper airways is not allowed to decrease to atmospheric pressure (zero). (CPAP is also referred to as continuous positive pressure breathing, CPPB.) It is particularly useful in patients whose distal airways would collapse if not kept continuously inflated by greater-than-atmospheric pressure. CPAP is frequently employed in the treatment of infants with respiratory distress syndrome. See Fig. See Infant respiratory distress syndrome.

CONTINUOUS POSITIVE PRESSURE BREATHING (CPPB): A synonym for continuous positive airway pressure (CPAP). See Continuous positive airway pressure.

CONTRACT: An agreement between two or more persons which sets up a binding

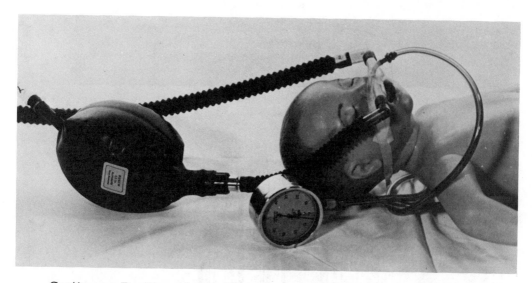

Continuous Positive Airway Pressure: Nasotracheal tube attached to a modified Jackson-Rees apparatus with a pressure gauge for the administration of continuous positive airway pressure as set up for an infant.

legal relationship. For an agreement to be a legal contract it must include the following elements. (1) The persons involved must be legally capable of making binding agreements. (2) They must be in some agreement as to the meaning of the contract. (3) The agreement must contain at least one promise and a consideration (something of value) which has to be either delivered, promised, or given. A contract exists when the promises and obligations are clear, well defined, and understood by all parties. Expressed contracts can be either verbal or written. An implied contract is not sharply delineated for the parties involved but flows from the circumstances of the individual case, e.g., a patient, by seeking out a physician for a physical examination, has implied a contract with that physician to pay for the service.

CONTRAST MEDIUM: See Barium sulfate.

CONTROLLED HYPOTENSION (INDUCED HYPOTENSION): The deliberate reduction of the blood pressure (particularly the mean arterial pressure) to some predetermined level and maintenance at that level to decrease bleeding during surgery.

COOL FLAME: A combustion process in which only partial oxidation occurs. The temperature of the cool flame is only a few hundred degrees Celsius. Cool flames are propagated by the most reactive fragments of fuel molecules. They are normally ignited by low-energy points of ignition and can occur only in fuel-rich mixtures. Cool flames can ignite a detonable mixture.

COPPER KETTLE: A device for the vaporization of a liquid anesthetic in a controlled and predictable manner. Invented by Dr. Lucian Morris at The University of Iowa in the early 1950s, the copper kettle is a "universal vaporizer." It will take any liquid anesthetic and vaporize it into a stream of O_2, the quantity of vapor being proportional to the vapor pressure at a given temperature. The underlying principle of the copper kettle is as follows: as finely divided bubbles of O_2 are allowed to rise through a standing volume of liquid, vapor penetrates them and reaches equilibrium. See Fig.

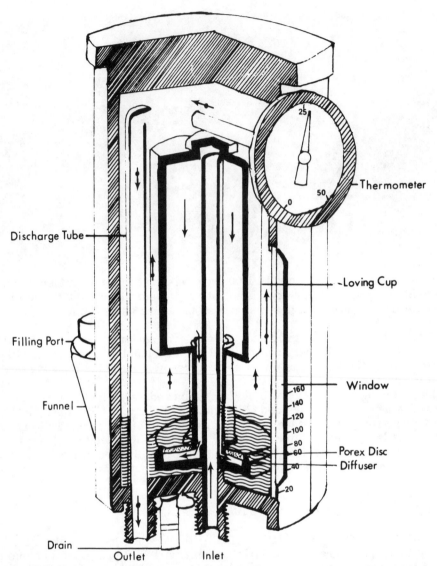

Copper Kettle: Cutaway drawing of a typical copper kettle showing the various functional parts.

CORE MEMORY: A type of information storage device often seen in large computers. Information is kept in binary form. In a magnetic core memory, microscopic metal areas become the storage media. Magnetized in one direction, they correspond to a 0; in the other direction they correspond to a 1.

CORE TEMPERATURE: The temperature of the blood measured at the level of the left atrium or, alternately, the temperature of the heart and brain.

CORNEAL ABRASION: An irritation, scratch, or wearing away of the external layer of the eye by a foreign body or object. Corneal abrasions are a potential hazard in the anesthetized or unconscious patient because the eyelid reflex which normally protects the cornea does not function in the anesthetized patient.

CORNEAL REFLEX (EYELID REFLEX; EYE BLINK): The automatic closing of the eyelids when the eyelashes or cornea are touched. This reflex is often tested to demonstrate the onset of general anesthesia. The reflex path involves the corneas, ophthalmic branch of the trigeminal nerve, synapse in the main sensory nucleus of the trigeminal nerve, medial longitudinal bundle, synapse in main motor nucleus of the facial nerve, then efferent impulses via the facial nerve to the orbicularis occuli. See Cranial nerves.

CORONARY ARTERIES: The arterial supply of the myocardium. The left coronary artery arises from the portion of the ascending aorta which protrudes between the main pulmonary artery and the left atrium. The left coronary artery runs under the left atrium and divides into the anterior descending (interventricular) and circumflex branches. The anterior descending artery supplies oxygenated blood to the ventricular walls whereas the circumflex artery supplies the walls of the left ventricle and left atrium. The right coronary artery arises from the two ostiums in the ascending aorta (in approximately 50% of patients) and runs into the right atrioventricular sulcus. It then divides into the posterior interventricular and marginal branches. The posterior interventricular artery supplies oxygenated blood to the walls of both ventricles whereas the marginal branch supplies the myocardium of the right ventricle and right atrium.

CORONARY CARE UNIT (CCU): A specialty care division for patients with recent or incipient myocardial infarctions. Increased monitoring and vigilance in the unit is aimed directly at reducing the incidence of myocardial electric instability (arrhythmia).

CORONARY OCCLUSION: The obstruction (acute or chronic) of blood flow in a coronary vessel which prevents an adequate flow to the portion of the myocardium supplied by that vessel. See Myocardial infarction.

CORONARY VEINS: The venous drainage system of the myocardium. There are three systems of coronary veins: thebesian, anterior cardiac, and coronary sinus and its branches. The thebesian veins (the smallest system) are located mostly in the septa of the right atrium and right ventricle. (They may be seen in the left side as well, but less commonly.) The anterior cardiac veins, which provide most of the venous drainage of the right ventricle, are formed over the anterior wall of the right ventricle. Their branches drain in the direction of the anterior right atrioventricular sulcus and empty into the right atrium. The coronary sinus and its branches are the largest system of coronary veins. They are responsible for the venous drainage of the left ventricle.

COR PULMONALE: A condition characterized by enlargement of the right ventricle secondary to malfunctioning lungs. Cor pulmonale is always associated with pulmonary hypertensive heart disease and is frequently associated with chronic obstructive pulmonary disease (bronchitis, emphysema). Severe pulmonary alveolar proteinosis may lead to cor pulmonale. See Pulmonary alveolar proteinosis.

CORTICOSTEROID: The general term for the steroids produced by the adrenal cortex and having 21 carbons. These are further classified as mineralocorticoids and glucocorticoids. The mineralocorticoids (aldosterone being the most significant one) are responsible for sodium retention (preventing excessive loss in the urine) and potassium excretion. Cortisol (hydrocortisone, compound F) is the most abundant and physiologically important glucocorticoid. (Corticosterone, compound B, is another glucocorticoid.) Glucocorticoids exert diverse effects on the body. (1)

Corticosteroids.

Steroid	Anti-Inflammatory Potency	Sodium Retention
Cortisone Acetate (Cortone)	0.8	0.8
Cortisol (Cortef)	1	1
Prednisone (Meticorten)	2.5	0.8
Prednisolone (Meticortelone)	3	0.8
Methylprednisolone (Medrol)	4	0
Triamcinolone (Aristocort)	5	0
Dexamethasone (Decadron)	20	0
Paramethasone (Haldrone)	6	0
Betamethasone (Celestone)	20	0
Desoxycorticosterone (DOC)	0	10-25
Fludrocortisone (Florinef)	12	100
Aldosterone	0.2	250

They stimulate gluconeogenesis (the biosynthesis of glucose from amino acid precursors), thereby influencing carbohydrate and protein metabolism. (2) They help store body fat. (3) They help the body resist and react to a range of stresses such as fright, temperature extremes, high altitude, bleeding, and infection. (4) They exert an anti-inflammatory effect. Therapeutically, the glucocorticoids are used for a myriad of disease conditions such as Addison disease, bronchial asthma, rheumatoid arthritis, adrenocortical insufficiency, systemic lupus erythematosus, sarcoidosis, allergic conjunctivitis, and acquired hemolytic anemia. Transient beneficial effects are seen when they are used to treat acute leukemia and multiple myeloma. It is important to recognize that these steroids do not provide a cure but only symptomatic relief to the patient. The administration of glucocorticoids represents replacement therapy only in the treatment of Addison disease and adrenocortical insufficiency. Small doses of glucocorticoids for a short period of time rarely cause adverse effects. However, chronic use (at a higher than physiologic level) may result in severe complications for the patient, relating to either the abrupt withdrawal of the steroid or prolonged use. (The dosage regimen must be reduced gradually to prevent acute adrenal insufficiency.) Common side effects include those characteristic of Cushing disease: "moon face," hirsutism, fatty deposits on the back, and amenorrhea. Other adverse effects are osteoporosis, hypokalemia, myopathy, aggravation of diabetes mellitus and peptic ulcer, psychotic disorders, and increased susceptibility to infections. Those patients whose bodies have been accustomed to high levels of circulating steroids are poor surgical risks and should be protected by corticosteroid supplementation prior to, during, and after surgery. See Fig.

CORTISOL: See Corticosteroid.

CORUNDUM: An extremely hard crystalline mineral found in nature. It is composed of aluminum oxide and is used as an abrasive. The ruby and sapphire are corundums colored with oxides.

COST-EFFECTIVENESS: A measurement of performance which analyzes the monetary cost of a device, process, or system in relation to the tangible benefits produced.

COULTER COUNTER: See Automated cell counter.

COUMARIN: See Anticoagulant.

COUNCIL ON ACCREDITATION OF EDUCATIONAL PROGRAMS OF NURSE ANESTHESIA: A group within the American Association of Nurse Anesthetists but whose members include both physicians and the lay public. They advise, formulate and/or adopt standards and guidelines, and accredit nurse anesthesia programs.

COUNTER: A device which detects and counts individual particles and photons. See Geiger counter, Photomultiplier.

COUPLING: The spatial or electric connection between two circuits which allows power or signals to be transferred from one to the other. See Capacitance, Inductance.

CPD BLOOD: See Blood storage.

CRANIAL NERVES: The twelve pairs of large nerves which directly exit from the brain. See Fig.

CRANIOSACRAL DIVISION: See Parasympathetic division.

CRANIOSACRAL OUTFLOW: See Parasympathetic division.

CRASH INDUCTION: See Induction.

CRAWFORD NEEDLE: See Epidural needle.

CREATINE PHOSPHOKINASE (CPK): A series of similar enzymes found in skeletal muscle, heart, gastrointestinal tract, and brain. CPK catalyzes the transfer of phosphate between different energy-storing molecules. The serum level of this enzyme rises in progressive muscular dystrophy and other primary diseases of skeletal muscle, cerebral infarcts, and following injuries to the heart or skeletal muscles. Serum samples of CPK are helpful in determining the presence of myocardial tissue necrosis. Elevated serum levels of CPK are found in patients with malignant hyperthermia. See Malignant hyperthermia.

CREATININE: A breakdown product of protein detectable in urine. High levels of creatinine may indicate kidney disease or malfunction.

CREMOPHOR EL: See Althesin.

CRICOTRACHEOTOMY: See Tracheostomy.

Cranial Nerves: Twelve cranial nerves and their components: (BM) brachial motor, (GSS) general somatic sensory, (SM) somatic motor, (SSS) special somatic sensory, (VM) visceral motor, and (VS) visceral sensory.

Nerve		Components	Primary Cell Body	Course	Peripheral Termination
I	Olfactory	SSS	Olfactory epithelium	Through roof of nasal cavity	Olfactory epithelium
II	Optic	SSS	Ganglionic layer of retina	Orbit → optic chiasm → optic tracts	Bipolar cells of retina rods and cones
III	Oculomotor	SM	Oculomotor nucleus	Orbit	Rectus superior, inferior, medial; obliquus inferior, levator palpebrae muscles
		VM	Edinger-Westphal nucleus	Ciliary ganglion → ciliary nerves	Constrictor pupillae and ciliary muscles of eyeball
IV	Trochlear	SM	Trochlear nucleus	Orbit	Obliquus superior muscle
V	Trigeminal	BM	Masticator nucleus	With mandibular	Muscles of mastication
		GSS	Semilunar ganglion	Ophthalmic, maxillary, mandibular branches	Face, nose, mouth
		GSS	Mesencephalic nucleus	With mandibular and maxillary branches	Proprioceptive to jaw muscles and tooth sockets
VI	Abducens	SM	Abducens nucleus	Under pons, into orbit	Rectus lateralis
VII	Facial	BM	Facial nucleus	Temporal bone, side of face	Muscles of expression, hyoid elevators
		VM	Superior salivatory nucleus	a) Greater superficial petrosal to spheno-palatine ganglion	a) Glands of nose, palate, lacrimal gland

No.	Nerve			b) Chorda tympani to submaxillary ganglion	b) Submaxillary and sub-lingual glands
VIII	Vestibular	VS	Geniculate ganglion	Chorda tympani	Anterior taste buds
		SSS	Vestibular ganglion	Internal acoustic meatus	Cristae of semicircular canals, maculae of utricle and saccule
	Cochlear	SSS	Spiral ganglion	Internal acoustic meatus	Organ of Corti
IX	Glosso-pharyngeal	BM	Nucleus ambiguus	Jugular foramen → side of pharynx	Superior constrictor, stylopharyngeus muscles
		VM	Inferior salivatory nucleus	Lesser superficial petrosal → otic ganglion → auriculotemporal nerve	Parotid gland
		VS	Petrous ganglion	Side of pharynx	Taste buds of vallate papillae
		GSS	Superior ganglion	Side of pharynx	Auditory tube
X	Vagus	BM	Nucleus ambiguus	Recurrent and external branch of superior laryngeal nerve	Pharyngeal and laryngeal muscles
		VM	Dorsal motor nucleus	Along carotid artery, esophagus, stomach	Viscera of thorax and abdomen
		VS	Nodose ganglion	With motor	Viscera of thorax and abdomen
		GSS	Jugular ganglion	Auricular branch	Pinna of ear
XI	Accessory	BM	Accessory nucleus	Side of neck	Sternocleidomastoid
XII	Hypoglossal	SM	Hypoglossal nucleus	Side of tongue	Muscles of tongue

145

CRITICAL FLICKER FREQUENCY (CFF): The threshold used to evaluate the effects of acute oral doses of psychotropic drugs. Stimulants tend to increase CFF whereas hypnotics decrease it. The patient reports his or her perception of a change in the flicker of a light source with constant intensity but varying frequency.

CRITICAL OPENING PRESSURE: The pressure which must be exceeded in a system, such as a collapsed arteriole, before any flow can begin. See Pulmonary perfusion, zones of.

CRITICAL PATH METHOD (CRITICAL PATH ANALYSIS): A method of temporal analysis based on the relationships between parts of a complex process. The critical path is the longest process in a multiprocess task. The entire complex task cannot take less time than the critical path task. For example, during the orthopedic replacement of a joint, the critical path is the length of time it takes bone cement to adhere and harden. Anesthesia induction, patient preparation, completion of the surgery, and emergence from anesthesia are all variable; the cement setting time is a physical constant which is difficult to change.

CRITICAL PRESSURE: The minimum pressure necessary to liquefy a gas at its critical temperature or, conversely, the saturated vapor pressure of a liquid when it is at its critical temperature.

CRITICAL TEMPERATURE: The temperature above which a gas cannot be liquefied by increase of pressure. The critical temperature of N_2O is 36.5 degrees Celsius.

CRITICAL VELOCITY: The velocity at which the motion of a fluid changes from laminar (parallel) to turbulent (erratic) flow. See Laminar flow, Turbulent flow.

CROSS-FILLING: See Transfilling.

CROSS-INFECTION: An infection in one patient which can be identified as having come from another patient.

CROSSOVER NETWORK: A type of filter circuit which is designed to pass high frequencies through one path and low frequencies through another. (The frequency at which these two pathways divide is known as the crossover frequency.) This particular type of network is often used in multispeaker systems for high-fidelity reproduction of sounds.

CROSS-TALK: A term first used in regard to telephone circuits and now expanded to relate to circuits in general. It indicates undesirable signals (caused by direct or indirect coupling) which degrade a normal circuit signal.

CRYOCARDIOPLEGIA: See Cardiopulmonary bypass.

CRYOGENICS: The science of the production and effects of very low temperatures.

CRYSTAL-CONTROLLED CLOCK (CRYSTAL-CONTROLLED OSCILLATOR): An electric circuit which oscillates at a precise frequency and is controlled by the piezoeffect of a quartz crystal. See Crystal, piezoelectric; Piezoelectric effect.

CRYSTAL, PIEZOELECTRIC: A piece of natural quartz or other crystal which vibrates at a desired frequency when placed in an appropriate electric circuit. It is used as an electromechanical transducer. See Crystal-controlled clock. Piezoelectric effect.

CUIRASS VENTILATOR: An obsolete, shell-like, airtight device which fits onto the thorax and abdomen and aids in respiration. Suction is applied under the cuirass to lift up the ribs and abdomen and cause inspiration. An advance over the "iron lung," it allows some degree of mobility, but is extremely uncomfortable and quite heavy.

CURARE: See Muscle relaxant, Neuromuscular blocking agent, Tubocurarine chloride.

CURIE (Ci): The unit used to measure the number of disintegrations per second of a radioactive substance. One curie is equivalent to 3.7×10^{10} disintegrations/sec.

CURRENT DENSITY: The ratio of the current or electron flow to the cross-sectional area of the conductor.

CURVE FITTING: A mathematic technique used to formulate an equation which describes a line drawn through plotted data points. The equation may then be used to predict new data points.

CUSHING, HARVEY: See Anesthesia chart.

CUSHING SYNDROME: See Corticosteroid.

CUSHING TRIAD (CUSHING RESPONSE): The consequences of raised intracranial pressure (ICP) named for the great neurosurgeon, Harvey Cushing. The Cushing response or reflex is elevation of arterial pressure accompanied by bradycardia as pressure on the brain increases. The triad adds respiratory irregularity to these first two. Other signs and symptoms associated with raised intracranial pressure (but not part of the triad) are headache, vomiting, and papilledema. See Intracranial pressure.

CUTDOWN: A surgical technique for gaining entry into a large vessel of a patient when percutaneous puncture has failed or is impossible.

CUTOFF FREQUENCY: The frequency at which the attenuation of a signal rapidly changes from a small value to a much higher one. For example, the input amplifiers of an electroencephalograph (EEG) usually have cutoff frequencies well below 60 cycles/sec, the frequency of line current which must never intrude on the EEG signal.

CUTTING CURRENT (PURE CUT): A selected output of an electrosurgery machine designed to maximize incision-making ability and minimize coagulation. The waveform of this modality is of constant amplitude with a fundamental frequency between 1 and 3 MHz. See Coagulation current.

CYANOSIS: A bluish discoloration, usually of the skin and the mucous membrane, indicative of a high concentration of reduced (deoxygenated) hemoglobin in the blood. Blueness of the skin is a subjective evaluation dependent on the observer, the patient's complexion, the lighting intensity, etc. It is generally thought to be seen consistently when at least 5 g/100 ml reduced hemoglobin exist in the patient's blood.

CYBERNETICS: The study of human, animal, and mechanical control and communication systems and their capabilities for handling, processing, and routing information. (The central nervous system can be compared to a mechanical-electric control system).

CYCLOPROPANE: A simple cyclic hydrocarbon (C_3H_6) which is a colorless, sweet-smelling, flammable, and explosive gas. It was introduced as a general anesthetic in 1933 by Waters and co-workers. Cyclopropane was the anesthetic agent of choice in certain circumstances because of its effects. These include rapid induction of anesthesia, wide safety margin between the anesthetic and lethal dose, and support of cardiovascular stability (maintains blood pressure and increases cardiac output). Cyclopropane is excreted almost entirely by the lungs and approximately half is removed from the body within 10 min of discontinuing its use. Frequently arrhythmias occur during induction. Cyclopropane shock is a term used to explain the sudden hypotension sometimes observed during emergence from deep cyclopropane anesthesia. The hypotension and collapse were thought to be due to the sudden withdrawal of the sympathetic actions of cyclopropane. Cyclopropane was widely used until the 1960s.

CYCLOPROPANE SHOCK: See Cyclopropane.

CYLINDER CONNECTIONS: See American standard compressed gas cylinder valve outlet connections.

Cylinder, Gas: Common medical gases and their color code.

Gas	Formula	United States	International	70% Service Pressure (psig)	State in Cylinder	Filling Density
Oxygen	O_2	Green	White	1800-2400*	Gas	
Carbon Dioxide	CO_2	Gray	Gray	838	Liquid 88°	68%
Nitrous Oxide	N_2O	Blue	Blue	745	Liquid 98°	68%
Cyclopropane	C_3H_6	Orange	Orange	75	Liquid	55%
Ethylene	C_2H_4	Red	Violet	1200	Liquid 50°	31-35%
Helium	He	Brown	Brown	1600-2000*	Gas	
Nitrogen	N_2	Black	Black	1800-2200*	Gas	
Air		Yellow ††	White & Black	1800	Gas	

*Depending on type of cylinder.

†† Air, including mixtures of oxygen with nitrogen containing 19.5%-23.5% oxygen, is color coded yellow. Mixtures of nitrogen and oxygen other than those containing 19.5%-23.5% oxygen are color coded black and green.

CYLINDER, GAS: A container for compressed gas. Medical gas cylinders are usually constructed of steel, with walls between 5/64 and 1/4 in thick; they must meet the standards of the Interstate Commerce Commission to be transported across state lines. The size of the tank is commonly letter-coded; contents are color-coded. See Fig.

CYLINDER PRESSURE GAUGE: A gauge which records and displays the pressure remaining in a gas cylinder.

CYLINDER VALVE: A device which allows controlled access to the contents of a gas cylinder. Each valve consists of (1) the body (the basic structure), (2) the port (the exit point for the gas), (3) the stem or shaft (when open allows the gas to flow to the port), (4) the handle or handwheel (turns the valve stem), (5) the safety relief device (allows discharge of cylinder contents) for preventing cylinder explosion if internal pressure goes above a preset maximum, (6) the conical depression (on small cylinder valves, receives the retaining screw of the yoke), and (7) the noninterchangeable safety systems (prevent attachment of an incorrect cylinder to the yoke or regulator). The most common safety system is the Pin-Index Safety System. Two types of cylinder valve designs exist, the packed type (also called the direct-acting valve), in which the stem is sealed by a resilient, compressible packing material such as Teflon, and the diaphragm type, which acts indirectly so that turning the stem raises or lowers a metal diaphragm. The latter valve operates better under low-temperature conditions and does not cause a great deal of wear to the valve seat.

CYSTIC FIBROSIS (FIBROCYSTIC DISEASE OF THE PANCREAS): A congenital disease of the exocrine glands (especially those which secrete mucus) which affects many organ systems. It is transmitted as a recessive trait. Among the important clinical manifestations are (1) pancreatic insufficiency, (2) dysfunction of the mucous glands of the entire gastrointestinal tract, and (3) susceptibility to heat, in which excessive sweating may result in loss of fluids and electrolytes, leading to hypochloremia, hyponatremia, and dehydration. The most disabling pathologic changes affect the lung. The patient may suffer from chronic bronchitis and emphysema and is quite susceptible to bronchial pneumonia. Patients usually succumb to progressive respiratory failure as the bronchi become obstructed by viscid mucous secretions. Diagnosis is usually made by a "sweat test" which measures the sodium and chloride concentrations in sweat. Appropriate respiratory care enables patients with moderate cases to live longer. These patients, however, should always be considered to have a compromised respiratory tract and manipulation of the respiratory tract should only be done with extreme care and precautions taken against infection.

CYTOCHROME P-450: See Enzyme induction.

CYTOPATHOLOGY: The study of cells in disease states. It is a recognized subspecialty of pathology, and its practitioners often rely on the expertise of trained cytotechnologists. Working together, these individuals are capable of diagnosing benign, atypical, premalignant, and malignant processes in cellular samples obtained from different body sites. Becoming increasingly more sophisticated and widespread, the technique of fine-needle aspiration biopsy allows cytopathologists and cytotechnologists to render a diagnosis on very limited samples. The aspirates may be performed: (1) preoperatively (in some cases eliminating the need for surgery and in others, altering the extent of the surgery, depending on the diagnosis), (2) intraoperatively (to diagnose a possible metastatic nodule not visualized by other techniques beforehand), or (3) postoperatively (as a follow-up). Frequently, the cytotechnologists will be in attendance during the actual aspiration to prepare and fix the slides, and then return to the laboratory to stain and microscopically examine the cellular material. Using a quick-stain technique, it is possible to arrive at a diagnosis within a few minutes. This is the cytopathologic equivalent of a frozen section. If the sample is inadequate, the procedure can be repeated in most cases. Cellular samples obtained by other methods, such as exfoliation, direct scraping, endoscopic brushing, or centesis, are examined by cytopathology personnel as well.

CYTOPLASM: The protoplasm of the cell which is not contained within the nucleus. It consists of a viscous, semitransparent fluid which contains the cellular organelles. It is the site where most of the chemical activities of the cell take place.

D

DALMANE: See Flurazepam.

DALTON LAW OF PARTIAL PRESSURE: The principle that the total pressure of a mixture of gases is the sum of the partial pressures of the separate components.

DAMAGES: The monetary compensation paid to an individual for loss or injury, usually as a result of a legal determination of negligence. See Punitive damages.

DAMPING: The progressive reduction of mechanical or electric oscillations due to the expenditure of energy by viscosity, resistance, friction, or other work. When the damping is such that the oscillations stop rather than continue, the oscillations are "critically damped." In "overdamped systems," the oscillations are attenuated very rapidly (more than is necessary for critical damping). In "underdamped systems," damping never reaches critical proportions; the oscillations continue although they may undergo shape changes. A water manometer connected to a central venous pressure line is an example of damping. The viscosity of the water in the column and the subsequent friction against the inside glass surface damp rapid oscillations in the central venous pressure but allow trends to be discerned.

Dantrolene.

DANTROLENE (DANTRIUM): A hydantoin derivative that appears to act on skeletal muscle beyond the neuromuscular junction. Although primarily used in athetosis and dystonia, it is also considered to be the only specific clinical treatment for malignant hyperthermia. See Fig.

DARVON: See Propoxyphene.

DATA, ANALOG: See Analog.

DATA BASE (DATA BASE MANAGEMENT): The compilation, management, and use of the fundamental facts or parameters of a particular case or class of individuals. For example, a patient's laboratory results represent a data base. The way this information is stored, retrieved, and disseminated constitutes data base management.

DATA-PROCESSING BUFFER: A device used in electronics or computer engineering to alter, prevent, or temper the interaction of two other devices. For example, a user may insert information into a small computer at a faster rate than it can be processed. The overflow insertions are stored in a buffer (often called a buffer register) which then feeds them to the processor at a slower rate. On large computers, buffers may be used to temporarily store an intermediate result which can then be reinserted into the processor as required. See Central processing unit.

DEAD SPACE: See Alveolar dead space, Anatomic dead space, Physiologic dead space.

DEAD SPACE EQUATION: See Bohr equation.

DEAD SPACE VENTILATION PER MINUTE: The volume of gas in each tidal volume which fills the respiratory passageways (but not the alveoli where changes in gas composition take place) times the number of breaths per minute. See Anatomic dead space, Single breath test, Ventilation/perfusion abnormality.

DEAFFERENTATION: The interruption or elimination of afferent nerve impulses by destruction of nerve pathways.

DEATH: See Biologic death.

DEBUG: See Bug.

DECADRON: See Dexamethasone.

DECAMETHONIUM (DRUG C-10): A depolarizing neuromuscular blocking agent used in brief anesthetic procedures. Phase II block is reported to be relatively frequent with large doses. Succinylcholine is frequently used instead of decamethonium bromide. See Neuromuscular blockade, assessment of; Neuromuscular blocking agent; Phase II block.

DECOMPRESSION SICKNESS: See Caisson disease.

DEFAMATION: The dissemination of false or objectionable information about an individual.

DEFIBRILLATION: The termination of ventricular fibrillation and the restoration of a normal cardiac rhythm by means of an externally applied large direct current (DC). (It is also referred to as external defibrillation.) Defibrillators are the devices which deliver the DC current. Most defibrillators are portable and battery-powered to allow easier access to the patient. In simplified form, a battery supplies power to an electronic circuit which boosts the battery voltage dramatically and uses this voltage to accumulate electrons on a very large capacitor. This charge is then fired across the patient's chest between two paddles (very large electrodes). The paddles are usually covered with a gel to break down resistance between the paddles and the skin. In modern designs, discharge occurs when the individual holding the paddles simultaneously presses a button on each paddle. Modern defibrillators can deliver energy in the range of 510 joules over a few thousandths of a second. This

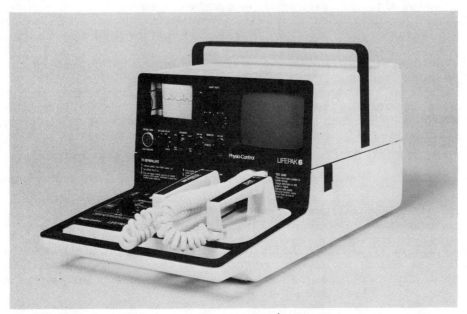

Defibrillation: Modern, portable monitor/defibrillator with paper-charting capacity.

is the equivalent of at least 2/3 hp. This large current or flow of electrons should, in theory, completely depolarize all polarizable membranes in the heart which will allow those areas which repolarize quickly, i.e., the normal specialized tissue which maintains the cardiac rate, to begin discharging in a normal fashion. See Fig.

DEFLAGRATION: The combustion of a fuel/air or fuel/O_2 mixture which is accompanied by a self-propagating flame. Once ignited, the flame will continue to burn any new fuel even if the original source of ignition is removed.

DEGAUSSING: The magnetic neutralization by current-conducting coils to prevent stray magnetic fields from interfering with electric phenomena, such as the display on a cathode ray tube.

DEHYDRATION: The loss of body fluids to the point that signs of fluid deprivation occur. Dehydration is termed isonatremic when the serum sodium levels remain normal (130-150 mEq/L), hyponatremic when serum sodium levels are less than 130 mEq/L, and hypernatremic when serum sodium levels are above 150 mEq/L. In infants and young children, the percent weight loss is evaluated to determine the degree of dehydration: 5% weight loss is mild, 10% is moderate, and 15% is severe. See Fig.

DELAY LINE: A transmission line or circuit element which introduces a known delay in signal transmission.

DELIRIUM: A mental disturbance characterized by illusions, confusion, hallucinations, disordered speech, restlessness, and incoherence.

DELIRIUM TREMENS: A mental disturbance related to alcohol withdrawal in the alcoholic. It is characterized by profound confusion, hallucinations, delusions, mus-

MAGNITUDE OF DEHYDRATION

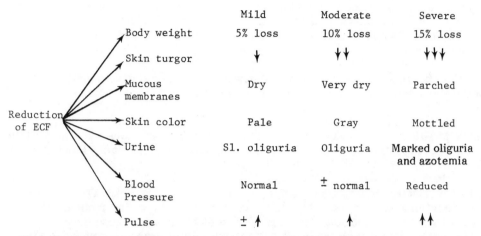

	Mild	Moderate	Severe
Body weight	5% loss	10% loss	15% loss
Skin turgor	↓	↓↓	↓↓↓
Mucous membranes	Dry	Very dry	Parched
Skin color	Pale	Gray	Mottled
Urine	Sl. oliguria	Oliguria	Marked oliguria and azotemia
Blood Pressure	Normal	± normal	Reduced
Pulse	± ↑	↑	↑↑

Dehydration: Correlation between the intensity of clinical findings with the magnitude of dehydration. It is specifically applicable to isotonic dehydration in an infant. Age and hypertonic or hypotonic dehydration may cause some variations.

cle tremors, anxiety, agitation, and gastrointestinal symptoms. It is usually accompanied by increased activity of the autonomic nervous system exemplified by tachycardia, hypertension, and profuse perspiration. Delirium tremens can be fatal in approximately 15% of patients due to cardiovascular collapse or hyperthermia. Treatment involves correction of fluid, electrolyte, and metabolic abnormalities, appropriate sedation, and cardiovascular and respiratory support.

DELTA Δ: A Greek alphabet letter usually written as a triangle. It stands for "change in" or "deviation from" some resting or standard condition.

DELTA-CORTEF: See Corticosteroid, Prednisolone.

DELTASONE: See Corticosteroid, Prednisone.

DEMAND FLOW MACHINE: See Continuous flow anesthesia machine.

DEMEROL: See Meperidine, Narcotic.

DENDRITE: A nerve cell process which carries an impulse toward the cell body. See Axon.

DENERVATION: The removal of nervous control of a structure, particularly muscle; alternately, the destruction of the neurons or neuron tract which supply a structure.

DENERVATION SUPERSENSITIVITY: A condition in which denervated muscle fibers become responsive to externally applied acetylcholine shortly after denervation. Prior to denervation, only the muscle motor end-plate region is sensitive to acetylcholine. It is thought that new acetylcholine receptors develop as a consequence of denervation.

DENITROGENATION: The elimination of N_2 from the body by breathing a gas mixture free of N_2, allowing no rebreathing of exhaled gas. This is often done deliberately when beginning inhalation anesthesia to saturate the body with 100% O_2 to gain as large a margin of safety as possible in case of decreased ventilation, e.g., airway obstruction or airway instrumentation. With normal lungs and normal alveolar ventilation, lung O_2 concentration reaches inspired O_2 concentration (100%) in approximately 3 min.

DENSITY: The mass per unit volume of substance. The relative density, i.e., the density of the substance divided by the density of water, is known as the specific gravity.

DENSITY MODULATED SPECTRAL ARRAY: A display technique used in the interpretation of the electroencephalogram. See Electroencephalogram, Fourier analysis.

DEPOLARIZATION: The neutralization or elimination by redistribution of electric charges found in a state of polarity. Depolarization is one of the most fundamental processes in nerve conduction. The membrane of the resting nerve is polarized, i.e., the inside is positively charged and the outside is negatively charged (70-90 mV). When the nerve conducts an impulse, the nerve membrane becomes depolarized, and the difference in electric charge effectively goes from -70 to 0 mV. In fact, it is transiently repolarized in the opposite direction to approximately 40 mV. The membrane returns to the resting state with the accumulation of negative charges inside and negative charges outside the membrane. See Action potential, Polarization.

DEPTH OF ANESTHESIA: An inexact term referring to the progressive attenuation of the patient's response to painful stimuli as increasing quantities of anesthetics are administered. See General anesthesia, Stages and planes of anesthesia.

DEPTH OF FIELD: The zone in which an image is acceptably sharp when observed through a camera lens.

DERMATOME: A skin segment in which innervation is supplied by afferent nerve fibers from a single spinal cord level. It is also an instrument for cutting thin layers of skin for grafting procedures. See Fig.

DERMATOMYOSITIS: An inflammation of the skin, subcutaneous tissues, and underlying muscles with necrosis of muscle fibers. The etiology of the disease is obscure but it appears to be associated with an autoimmune reaction. When this disease is confined to the musculature it is known as polymyositis. Patients with dermatomyositis or polymyositis may be particularly sensitive to muscle relaxants, and approximately half the adult patients have an underlying malignancy.

DESENSITIZATION BLOCK: See Phase II block.

DESICCATION: The process of drying up. Electrodesiccation (a technique of electrosurgery) involves the destructive drying of cells and tissues by short, high-frequency electric sparks which evaporate the intracellular water.

DESOXYCORTICOSTERONE: A naturally occurring mineralocorticoid. It is useful in treating electrolyte abnormalities in adrenal insufficiency. See Corticosteroid.

DETERGENT: A substance which decreases the surface tension of a liquid and al-

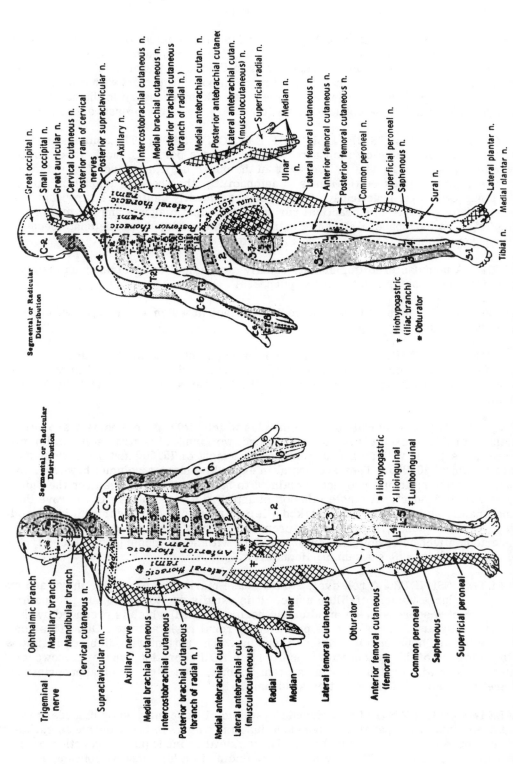

Dermatome: Distribution of the various dermatome levels on the anterior and posterior surfaces of the body.

lows it to spread further. Detergents are used in respiratory therapy aerosols to break down fixed secretions. See Surface tension.

DETERMINANTS OF FLUID FLOW: The physical parameters which modify flow in a conduit. Doubling the diameter of an infusion line or a needle increases the flow rate of a fluid 16 times (since the rate varies to the fourth power of the radius of a tube). Because of this relationship, it is more important to start with a large intravenous line if rapid flow is required, rather than adding pressure to the administration system or raising the bottle (or bag) to achieve a greater pressure gradient.

DETONABILITY, LIMITS OF (LIMITS OF EXPLOSIVENESS): The combinations of fuel and O_2 above and below the ratios which produce a powerful shock wave. In the lower limit, not enough heat is liberated; in the upper limit, too much fuel exists for the O_2 available. Between the limits of detonability, the speed of detonation varies over a narrow range; practically, detonations are equally destructive throughout the range of detonability. For practical purposes, anesthetic agents and air mixtures (ether/air, cyclopropane/air), while extremely flammable, do not detonate because of the physical characteristics of the flame front generated.

DEVICE: A manufactured implement, usually mechanical or electric in nature, used for a single purpose or related set of purposes.

DEW POINT: The highest temperature of a surface at which water vapor will condense from a humid atmosphere.

DEXAMETHASONE (DECADRON): An extremely potent glucocorticoid and often the drug of choice for steroid therapy in acute situations. It has been used to treat acute and chronic aspiration pneumonia, increased intracranial pressure, and shocklike states.

DEXTRAN: Any of numerous polysaccharides which yield glucose upon hydrolysis. Partial hydrolysis and cleavage have produced two forms of dextran solution for intravenous use: one with an average molecular weight of 75,000 and one with an average weight of 40,000. They are useful in expanding plasma volume; however, the newer, smaller molecule product is claimed to have some advantage over the older, higher weight product. A single infusion in appropriate quantities can improve the hemodynamic status for 24 hr. Marked allergic reactions can occur with both products. At higher doses, some dextran preparations have been noted either to have a deleterious effect on coagulation or to interfere with some techniques of blood typing and crossmatching. See Albumin, Hetastarch.

DIABETES INSIPIDUS: A relatively rare disease marked by excessive thirst and excretion of a large volume of dilute urine. It is usually due to inadequate production or release of vasopressin, an antidiuretic hormone (ADH) which is produced by the posterior pituitary. It can also be produced by renal resistance to ADH. This condition is termed nephrogenic diabetes insipidus. The patient with diabetes insipidus is the converse of the patient with inappropriate ADH secretion syndrome; however, both can occur with central nervous system trauma. See Fig. See Inappropriate antidiuretic hormone (ADH) secretion syndrome.

DIABETES MELLITUS (DM): A chronic systemic disease marked by disorders in the metabolism of the pancreatic hormone insulin, which, in turn, deranges carbohydrate, protein, and fat metabolism. There is either inadequate production or inadequate use of insulin. The key laboratory finding is a high fasting concentration

Diabetes Insipidus: Differences between pituitary diabetes insipidus and nephrogenic diabetes insipidus.

Pituitary Diabetes Insipidus	Nephrogenic Diabetes Insipidus
Idiopathic	Congenital
Familial	Familial
Brain tumor	Acquired
	Amyloidosis
Head trauma	Chronic renal failure
	Hyperthyroidism
Postneurosurgical	Multiple myeloma
	Nephrocalcinosis-hypercalcemia
Infection disorder (e. g. , encephalitis)	Obstructive uropathy
	Potassium deficiency
Vascular disorder (e. g. , postpartum	Sickle cell anemia
necrosis)	Sjögren's syndrome
	Drugs
Systemic disorder (e. g. , Hand-Schüller-	Demeclocycline
Christian disease, sarcoidosis, tumor	Lithium carbonate
metastasis)	

of glucose in the blood. The diagnosis, however, is only firm if this value can be repeated in the absence of factors which might influence this measurement, such as drugs, exercise, or diet. For the DM patient about to be anesthetized, the appropriate timing of exogenous insulin administration in conjunction with the patient's last nourishment before surgery is important. Insulin injection, in particular, can lead to severe hypoglycemia which, in the acute situation, has a much higher morbidity than the hyperglycemia which may result from withholding insulin.

DIACETYLMORPHINE: See Heroin, Narcotic.

DIALYSIS: See Hemodialysis.

DIAMETER INDEX SAFETY SYSTEM (DISS): A system which provides removable, noninterchangeable connections for low-pressure gas lines. These act as a safeguard against the incorrect coupling of gas supplies with the anesthetic equipment. Each type of gas has a specific sized receptacle and attached nipple for its gas line.

DIAPHORESIS (SWEATING): The exudation of fluid onto the surface of the skin in response to elevated heat production. The evaporation of sweat from the skin's surface cools the body. The sweat glands are innervated by cholinergic fibers of sympathetic origin. Sweating in the anesthetized patient is considered to be a sign that anesthesia is too light. By contrast, sweating in a patient being resuscitated indicates that effective circulation is taking place and resuscitative effort should therefore continue. See Autonomic nervous system, Insensible water loss.

DIAPHRAGM: The large, thin membranous muscle which separates the abdominal and thoracic cavities and is chiefly responsible for respiration (approximately 70% of inspired respiratory volume). The diaphragm is supplied by the left and right phrenic nerves which arise from the cervical plexus at C2, C3, and C4 levels. The downward contraction of the diaphragm creates a slight negative pressure in the thorax. This is aided by the contraction of the intercostal muscles which expands the rib cage. This negative pressure causes inspiration as air moves down the upper airway along the pressure gradient from atmospheric to subatmospheric areas.

DIAPHRAGMATIC HERNIA: A disorder in which the intestines, and often the stomach and spleen, protrude into the thoracic cavity through the diaphragm wall (on the left side in 90% of the cases). It may be either congenital or acquired. It is a surgical emergency in newborns. The lung on the affected side is often hypoplastic. Because the abdominal viscera occupy the thoracic cavity, the mediastinum is shifted toward the unaffected side, disrupting cardiovascular dynamics. Death may occur very rapidly due to the respiratory distress caused by the hypoplastic lung. Newborns who develop severe respiratory distress within the first 24 hr have a 50% mortality rate. Infants who survive on their own for more than 72 hr have survival rates approaching 100%.

DIASTOLIC PRESSURE: The arterial pressure when the ventricles are at rest and filling.

DIATHERMY: The use of high-frequency electromagnetic radiation to generate heat within a body part. See Cauterization.

DIATHESIS: A condition in which there is an enhanced susceptibility to disease. For example, hemophilia is a bleeding diathesis in which the propensity to hemorrhage is increased.

DIATOMACEOUS EARTH: See Gas chromatography.

DIAZEPAM: See Benzodiazepine.

DIAZOXIDE (HYPERSTAT IV): A derivative of the thiazides (but devoid of diuretic effect). It is used as an intravenous agent for the prompt treatment of hypertensive crisis. Diazoxide causes marked salt and water retention and, therefore, its clinical effect directly opposes many diuretic antihypertensive drugs.

DIBENZYLINE: See Phenoxybenzamine.

DIBUCAINE: See Local anesthetic.

DIBUCAINE NUMBER: A quantification of the inhibition of plasma cholinesterase activity (in breaking down succinylcholine) by dibucaine. At least two types of plasma cholinesterase (pseudocholinesterase) enzymes exist: normal and atypical. The difference between them is evident clinically only after the injection of succinylcholine. A person with the normal enzyme is able to hydrolyze the succinylcholine rapidly whereas the one with the atypical enzyme cannot. (A heterozygous individual, i.e., one with a normal and an atypical enzyme gene, hydrolyzes the drug much less efficiently than normal individuals.) In the dibucaine test, if a plasma sample has a high normal enzyme content, it will be inhibited by dibucaine and will have a high dibucaine number. Patients with a low dibucaine number will have low levels of normal plasma cholinesterase; however, patients with low levels of normal plasma cholinesterase will not necessarily have a low dibucaine number. The low enzyme level may be due to malnutrition and liver damage and not to an atypical gene. If the presence of an atypical gene is verified, however, other family members may be prone to the same response to succinylcholine and should be forewarned. Evidence exists for a second gene, a fluoride gene, which also determines plasma cholinesterase activity. The fluoride number and the dibucaine number may differ in individuals, i.e., one may be normal and the other abnormally low. An abnormal homozygous fluoride gene (low fluoride number) gives a moderately prolonged response to succinylcholine. A third gene, the "silent gene," which also determines plasma cholinesterase activity, has been identified. Patients with this gene show total plasma cholinesterase inhibition and therefore have a prolonged response to succinylcholine. See Pseudocholinesterase, Succinylcholine.

DICHLOROACETYLENE (C_2Cl_2): A toxic breakdown product of the obsolete anesthetic trichloroethylene (Trilene, $2C_2 HCl_3$). Trilene decomposes in the presence of elevated temperatures and soda lime and therefore should never be used in rebreathing circuits. Dichloroacetylene causes cranial nerve damage and decomposes into phosgene and CO. See Phosgene.

DICHLORODIFLUOROMETHANE: See Freon.

DICROTIC NOTCH: The cleft seen in the descending portion of the aortic pressure trace caused by the sharp deceleration of blood flow and the abrupt closure of the aortic valve. If observed in a radial artery tracing, the notch seen is an artifact of pressure wave reflexion from the arterioles. See Peripheral vascular resistance, Pulse pressure tracing.

DIELECTRIC: The medium that acts as an insulator between the two plates of a capacitor.

DIELECTRIC HEATING: A technique for heating an insulator by compressing it between two conducting plates or electrodes and applying a high-frequency current.

DIELECTRIC STRENGTH: A measurement of the maximal electric difference that an insulator can withstand without breakdown.

DIETHYL ETHER (ETHER): A highly flammable general anesthetic. It has a slow induction and emergence period, and its vapors are a respiratory irritant which induce copious secretions. It provides excellent cardiovascular stability. At low concentrations it is a good analgesic agent. A wide margin of safety exists between the anesthetic and toxic dose. Major contraindications of diethyl ether include postoperative nausea and vomiting and its potential flammability.

DIFFERENTIAL BLOCK: The phenomenon which occurs when a local anesthetic is injected close to a nerve trunk containing many different sized nerve fibers. Differential blockade occurs because of the variations in fiber diameter, myelin covering, and position in the mixed nerve. Some fibers are completely or partially blocked, while others are not blocked at all. The general order in which differential blockade occurs is B fibers, then A-delta fibers, and C fibers. The A-alpha fibers may be totally unaffected. Clinically, therefore, there is analgesia to a pinprick but motor activity may be preserved. (The large fibers also convey touch and light pressure sensations which may be misinterpreted by the patient as pain.) An alternate (and possibly equally valid) explanation of the differential blockade phenomenon is that local anesthetic agents first block those nerves which carry the heaviest number or the highest frequency of action potentials. Pain sensation is a high-frequency transmission and this may explain why it is blocked before the low-frequency motor nerves are blocked. It is thought that high-frequency transmission keeps more sodium channels open for longer time periods, allowing rapid entry of the local anesthetic molecule which acts on the inside opening of the sodium channel. Differential blockade may be deliberately induced by using a very low concentration of local anesthetic to block sympathetic fibers without blocking sensory or motor fibers. See Nerve fiber, anatomy and physiology of.

DIFFUSION: The process by which gases, fluids, and solids intermingle, due to the kinetics of their constituent atomic particles. Mixing is complete unless one set of particles is much heavier than the other; in this case gravitational effects will cause sedimentation of the heavier particles.

DIFFUSION BLOCK: See Alveolar end capillary difference.

DIFFUSION CAPACITY OF THE LUNG: A measurement of the ability of the lung to transfer alveolar gas to capillary blood without significant delay during passage of the gas through the alveolar capillary membrane. Diffusion capacity is affected by the area, thickness, and diffusion properties of the aveolar membranes and the solubility (in the alveolar membrane) of the gas concerned. Carbon monoxide (CO) is used to measure diffusion capacity because its transfer from the alveolus into the blood is diffusion-limited rather than perfusion-limited. (The combination of hemoglobin with CO occurs so readily that all CO in low concentrations will be absorbed into blood even if blood flow past the alveolus is slowed to nearly zero.) Measurements of diffusion capacity using CO (D_{CO}) can be made by the single-breath method, steady-state method, rebreathing technique, and fractional CO uptake technique. The D_{CO} is affected by many variables. It increases with increasing lung volume and exercise. Body position affects the D_{CO}: it is highest if the body is in a supine position and higher in a sitting rather than standing position. The D_{CO} varies in direct proportion to body size. Within the physiologic range of O_2, diffusion capacity decreases insignificantly with inspired O_2 tension and increases with increased CO_2 tension. The normal value (at rest) for D_{CO} is approximately 17-25 ml/min/mmHg of P_{CO}.

DIFFUSION CONSTANT: The specific quantity necessary to determine accurately the transfer of gas across a membrane. The constant is directly proportional to the solubility of the gas and is inversely proportional to the square root of the molecular weight of the gas. See Fig.

DIFFUSION HYPOXIA: A phenomenon which can be produced after prolonged anesthesia with high concentrations of N_2O/O_2. If the patient is allowed to breathe room air at the termination of the anesthetic, the outflow of N_2O/O_2 from blood will dilute the O_2 in the alveolus, lowering its partial pressure below the 21% normally seen in room air. This can cause some arterial O_2 desaturation. While this phenomenon is of little significance in the normal patient, it may become extremely important in the patient with marginal oxygenation. The anesthetist may avoid this occurrence by adding high concentrations of O_2 instead of room air at the termination of anesthesia. See Concentration effect.

DIFFUSION LIMITATION: The concept that a barrier to diffusion across the alveolar capillary membrane can limit uptake of alveolar gas by the blood (alveolar-capillary block). See Alveolar end capillary difference, Diffusion capacity of the lung.

DIFFUSION RESISTANCE: The relative impedance by a given membrane to gas transfer. See Diffusion capacity of the lung.

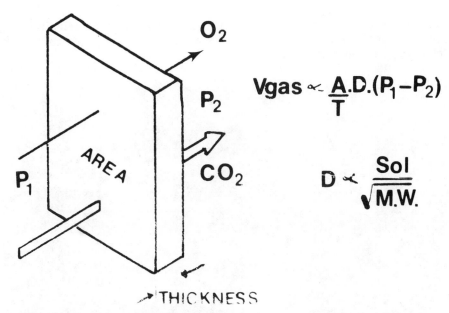

$$Vgas \propto \frac{A.D.(P_1 - P_2)}{T}$$

$$D \propto \frac{Sol}{\sqrt{M.W.}}$$

THICKNESS

Diffusion Constant: Gas diffusion through a tissue sheet. The amount of gas transferred is proportional to the area of the tissue, a diffusion constant, and the difference in partial pressure across the surfaces of the tissue, and inversely proportional to the tissue thickness.

DIFFUSION RESPIRATION: See Apneic oxygenation.

DIGITAL BLOCK (FINGER BLOCK): The direct injection of local anesthesia into an individual finger at the base of the proximal phalanx.

DIGITAL COMPUTER: See Analog computer.

DIGITAL DATA: See Binary code.

DIGITALIS: See Cardiac glycosides.

DIGITOXIN: See Cardiac glycosides.

DIGOXIN: See Cardiac glycosides.

DIHYDROHYDROXYMORPHINONE; OXYMORPHONE (NUMORPHAN): A semisynthetic morphine derivative. See Narcotic.

DILANTIN: See Diphenylhydantoin.

DILATATION: The stretching of an orifice or tube beyond its normal dimensions.

DILAUDID (DIHYDROMORPHINONE): See Narcotic.

DIMETHYL TUBOCURARINE CHLORIDE (TUBARINE): See Tubocurarine chloride.

DIMETHYL TUBOCURARINE IODIDE (METUBINE): A synthetic derivative of d-tubocurarine (curare) two to three times more potent. See Neuromuscular blocking agent, Tubocurarine chloride.

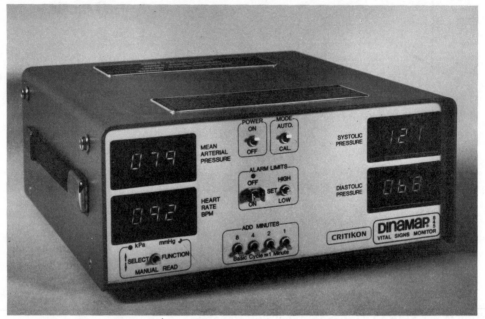

Dinamap^tm: Dinamap^tm automatic blood pressure device.

DINAMAP^tm: The brand name for an automatic device which uses the oscillometric method to determine blood pressure. See Fig.

DIPHENHYDRAMINE (BENADRYL): An antihistamine useful in oral and parenteral form. It antagonizes the action of histamine at its receptors and may cause some central nervous system depression. See Antihistamine.

DIPHENYLHYDANTOIN; PHENYTOIN (SODIUM DILANTIN): An anticonvulsant drug used in treating epileptic and psychomotor seizures. It appears to exert specific antiepileptic actions without causing general depression of the central nervous system. Its therapeutic effectiveness and toxicity may be correlated with the plasma concentration of the drug: low levels are ineffective and high levels produce neurotoxicity. Common side effects of the drug are ataxia, nystagmus, double vision, excitement, tremors, and gingival hypertrophy. Diphenylhydantoin is also useful in treating digitalis-induced tachyarrhythmias.

2,3-DIPHOSPHOGLYCERATE: See Oxygen-hemoglobin dissociation curve.

DIPOLE: An object with two equal and opposite charges located close to each other. For example, a small magnet constitutes a magnetic dipole.

DIRECT FETAL ELECTROCARDIOGRAPHY: The technique for recording fetal heart activity during labor by placing an electrode onto a presenting part. The electrode contains a stainless steel coil which penetrates the skin. Sterile technique is required.

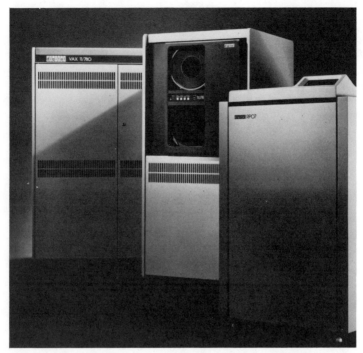

Disc Drive: Large-capacity disc drive capable of storing 516 megabytes of information.

DISC DRIVE (TAPE DRIVE): The mechanism which moves a magnetic disc or tape past the sensing unit (read/write head), usually in either direction at high speed. (It is sometimes referred to as a transport unit.) See Fig. See Disc, magnetic.

DISC FLOAT: The type of indicator used in older flowmeters. It consists of a thin horizontal disc with a long protruding stem. The disc and the stem are pushed upward in the tapered tube as in modern flowmeters; however, the disc is the only portion of the float which acts as an obstruction to flow. The tip of the stem moves upward behind a calibrated scale to indicate the amount of flow.

DISC, MAGNETIC: A distinct type of storage device for computers in which information is recorded on the magnetized surface of a rotating disc. The read/write arm, a mechanical device, either detects (while reading) the magnetic fields already on the disc or imposes (while writing) magnetic fields on it. Disc files and disc packs are variable combinations of discs and read/write heads. Discs are rated according to information capacity and size.

DISINTEGRATION SCHEME: A line drawing showing the products of decay of a radioactive atom including the forms of energy released, types of particles released, and final stable nucleus.

DISPERSIVE ELECTRODE (GROUND OR INDIFFERENT ELECTRODE): The electrode by which radiofrequency energy is returned to an electrosurgery machine. It must provide a wide area of contact with the patient's skin so that the density of radiofrequency energy over any particular square centimeter of tissue is below the level which will heat the tissue. Factors in the design or development of the dispersive electrode include the area of the electrode, medium for maintaining contact

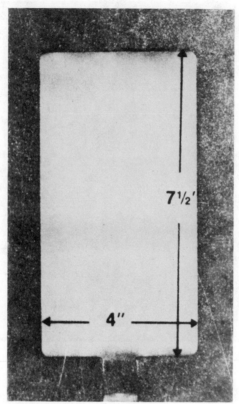

Dispersive Electrode: Disposable dispersive electrode.

(i.e., gelled or ungelled), and geometric shape of the electrode. Even with the best contact and optimal pattern, current flow under the surface of the electrode is not uniform due to skin variations. See Fig.

DISSEMINATED INTRAVASCULAR COAGULATION (DIC): A clotting disorder which is almost invariably catastrophic. It is seen in trauma patients or obstetric patients after amniotic fluid embolization. It is characterized by the continuous consumption of clotting factors and platelets, formation of fibrinogen thrombi, decrease in platelet count, and activation of the fibrinolytic system. This process is diffuse, occurring throughout the body. The patient with DIC may present with either massive bleeding (bleeding from every needle stick), which is the more usual presentation, or thrombotic symptoms, or a combination of the two. No single laboratory test will diagnose DIC. It has been suggested that the test criteria are lengthened prothrombin time, low platelet count, and low fibrinogen level. While heparin has been used for DIC, treatment of underlying cause(s) should be done first. See Fig. See Primary fibrinolysis.

DISSOCIATION CONSTANT (pK_a): The pH at which a given acid or base is 50% ionized and 50% nonionized. The pK_a of a drug is important because in most biologic systems it is only the nonionized drug which can cross cell membranes easily. (The lower the pK_a of a drug, the stronger the acid; the higher the pK_a of a drug, the stronger the base.) See Fig. See Henderson-Hasselbalch equation, Local anesthetic.

Disseminated Intravascular Coagulation: Diagnostic criteria for disseminated intravascular coagulation (DIC).

1. Decrease in platelet count
2. Abnormal serial thrombin test
3. Normal clot lysis time
4. Decrease in fibrinogen
5. Positive test for split products of fibrinogen, i.e., positive protamine test, positive Fi test (fibrinogen degradation products)

Dissociation Constant: Dissociation constants of local anesthetics.

Local Anesthetic	pK_a
Mepivacaine	7. 6
Etidocaine	7. 7
Lidocaine	7. 9
Prilocaine	7. 9
Bupivacaine	8. 1
Tetracaine	8. 5
Procaine	9. 1
Propoxycaine	Unknown

DISSOCIATIVE ANESTHESIA: A pharmacologic state in which the patient does not lose consciousness but is emotionally detached from and disinterested in the environment. The patient shows no desire to change position or move about. The term is often used interchangeably with neuroleptanesthesia. The only difference between the two appears to be that neuroleptanesthesia is caused by drugs such as droperidol and fentanyl in combination (Innovar), whereas dissociative anesthesia is induced by ketamine. Since increasing the dosage of these agents or adding the proper concentrations of N_2O produces a state indistinguishable from general anesthesia, these terms appear to be somewhat arbitrary.

DISSOLVED OXYGEN: The O_2 which is dissolved in blood. The O_2 obeys Henry law, which states that the solubility of a gas in a liquid solution is proportional to the partial pressure of the gas. Normal arterial blood with a PaO_2 of 100 mmHg contains 0.3 ml O_2/100 ml blood.

DISTORTION: A change, usually undesirable, in the shape of a waveform caused by either mechanical or electric interference. In an electrocardiograph displayed on a poorly adjusted oscilloscope, for example, the upstroke of the electric complexes may be overextended enough to indicate nonexistent ventricular hypertrophy. See Electrocardiogram.

DIURESIS: The increased excretion of urine. Diuretics cause diuresis.

DIURNAL RHYTHM: See Circadian rhythm.

DIVER PARALYSIS: See Caisson disease.

DOLOPHINE: See Methadone.

DOPAMINE HYDROCHLORIDE (INTROPIN): A naturally occurring precursor of epi-nephrine and norepinephrine which is used as a chemical messenger in certain parts of the central nervous system. When given as a continuous infusion for cardiovas-cular support (depending on dosage), cardiac contractility, cardiac output, and re-nal blood flow all increase. Dopamine is useful in the management of various types of shock. It may cause serious cardiac arrhythmias.

DOPAR: See Levodopa, L-dopa.

DOPING: A technique for creating semiconductors. See Semiconductors.
ing a medical student with misinformation. See Semiconductors.

DOPPLER BLOOD PRESSURE MEASUREMENT: See Doppler effect.

DOPPLER EFFECT: The apparent shift in the frequency of sound or light waves

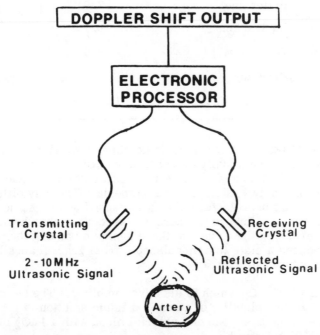

Doppler Effect: Mechanism for determining arterial wall movement and subsequent measurement of blood pressure by means of the Doppler ef-fect. Sudden vibrations in the arterial wall when the cuff pressure falls slightly below systolic pressure cause variations in the reflected ultra-sonic signal frequency. An electronic processor compares the trans-mitted and reflected frequencies and from their differences generates a Doppler signal.

when the wave source is moving in relation to the observer. The classic example of this phenomenon concerns a train with a constant pitch whistle. As it approaches the stationary observer, the pitch of the whistle is perceived as higher (up Doppler) than it is, and lower (down Doppler) as the train recedes. The amount of observed change is proportional to the speed of the train. A doppler device can be used to determine blood pressure. Arterial wall movement changes the frequency of the sound wave produced by the transmitting crystal. This change is detected by the receiving crystal and is used with a known cuff pressure to determine arterial pressure. See Fig.

DOSE RESPONSE CURVE: The graphic representation of the relationship between the amount of an administered drug and the biologic effect observed. (The X axis represents the drug amount; the Y axis represents the effect.) A flat response curve indicates that major changes in dosage produce little biologic effect, whereas a steep response curve demonstrates that minor changes have a significant effect.

DOSIMETRY: A measurement technique for quantitating a radiation dose. The x-ray film badge, worn by those occupationally exposed to radiation, is analyzed by dosimetry.

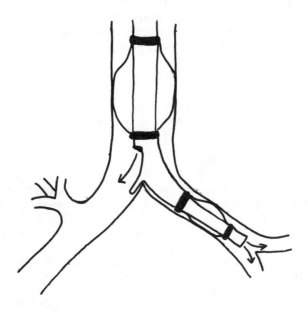

Double-Lumen Tube: Carlens double-lumen tube seated in the trachea. The arrows indicate the direction of gas flow.

DOUBLE-LUMEN TUBE: A type of tube available for selective control of either lung during anesthesia. Each lung can be ventilated separately or blocked off from the other. Because these tubes have two lumens, the cross-sectional area of each is small and resistance is high. There are three types of double-lumen tubes: the Carlens, Bryce-Smith, and Robert Shaw. Each has a tracheal cuff and a cuff to be inflated in the intubated bronchus. The latter two tubes come with either right or left configurations depending on the mainstem bronchus to be intubated. See Fig. See Endobronchial intubation, Intubation.
bation, Intubation.

DOWN TIME: The period of time during which a system, particularly a computer, is malfunctioning and cannot meet its operational requirements. This also refers to the time period when an operating room is not functioning.

DOXAPRAM (DOPRAM): A respiratory stimulant used to treat postoperative respiratory depression. It tends to activate carotid chemoreceptors and has a wide margin of safety.

dP/dt: The rate of change of pressure (P) in the ventricle (usually measured in the left) with respect to time (t). The maximum dP/dt is reached at the same time as the peak positive deflection in an apexcardiogram. It has been advocated as a measurement of cardiac contractility.

DRAMAMINE (DIMENHYDRINATE): See Antihistamine.

DRAW-OVER VAPORIZER: A device which vaporizes liquid anesthetic into a stream of gas being drawn or pulled over the surface of the anesthetic, usually by spontaneous respiration of the patient. Although a wick may be used to increase surface area, no attempt is made to regulate vaporization except that the process of rapid vaporization cools the liquid anesthetic, thus lowering its vapor pressure and thereby inhibiting further vaporization. It is often confused with a flow-over vaporizer, which vaporizes anesthetics into a gas stream moved by a machine rather than the patient. See EMO inhaler, Vaporizer, draw-over; flow-over; bubble-through.

DRIVE, DISC OR TAPE: See Disc drive.

DRIVER: An electric circuit in which the output is used to provide input for one or more other circuits. Commonly, the amplifier stage immediately preceding the output stage of a transmitter or receiver "drives" the speakers.

DROMRAN: See Levorphanol tartrate.

DROPERIDOL (INAPSINE): A butyrophenone related to haloperidol. It is used in combination with the potent narcotic fentanyl to produce neuroleptanesthesia. Used alone as a predmedicant for its antianxiety effect, it is also employed clinically for its antiemetic and antinausea actions. See Dissociative anesthesia, Innovar.

DROWNING: The suffocation by submersion, especially in water. For medical purposes (since drowning implies death), two further categories are defined: near-drowning with aspiration and near-drowning without aspiration. It is estimated that approximately 10% of drowning victims die without aspirating water. It appears that death in these patients is caused by laryngospasm and acute asphyxia. Animal studies have shown that in acute asphyxia arterial O_2 tension drops from a control value of approximately 100 torr to 40 torr in 1 min, 10 torr in 3 min, and 4 torr in 5 min. It is this hypoxia which causes death since an increase in CO_2 tension high enough to cause death could not take place in such a short time period. With aspiration, a distinction is made between those individuals who aspirate fresh or salt water. In fresh water (hypotonic compared to plasma) aspiration, the water is rapidly absorbed into the circulation causing dilution of the blood (hemodilution). In sea water (hypertonic compared to plasma) aspiration, plasma water leaves the circulation, further filling the alveoli and simultaneously causing hemoconcentration. While these two conditions both lead to derangement in serum ion concentration, they are rarely of sufficient magnitude to cause death.

DRUG C-5: See Pentolinium.

DRUG C-6: See Hexamethonium.

DRUG C-10: See Decamethonium.

DRUG DEPENDENCE: A state of tolerance or psychologic and/or physiologic need for a drug as a result of periodic or continued use of that drug. The specific characteristics of dependence vary for different drug classifications. Whereas psychologic dependence may be altered by subjective and behavioral factors, physiologic dependence and tolerance are pharmacologically based in that normal body functions are maintained only in the continued presence of the drug. Abrupt withdrawal of the agent results in the adverse physiologic changes of withdrawal syndrome. See Tolerance.

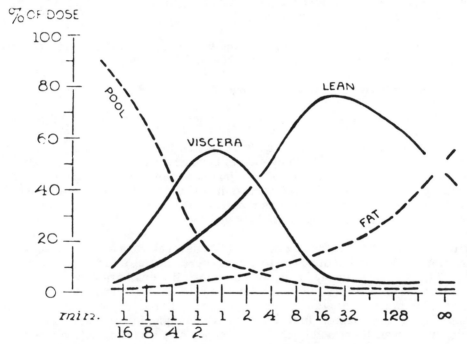

Drug Distribution: Distribution of thiopental in different body tissues and organs at various times after its intravenous injection.

DRUG DISTRIBUTION: The concept that drugs introduced into the body tend to accumulate in or avoid various locations depending on dose, tissue absorption, blood flow, and time. See Fig.

DRUG INTERACTION: A change in the performance of one drug when combined with the administration of another drug. Most drug interactions involve one drug changing the rate of excretion or metabolism of another drug or its tissue binding. Major drug interactions are quite rare and may involve physical incompatabilities between two or more compounds. For example, injectable diazepam cannot be added to common intravenous solutions because it will precipitate. See Synergism.

DRUG LEVEL MONITORING IN SERUM: The laboratory determination of the amount of drug present in a sample of the patient's blood. This measurement is particularly useful in evaluating drug levels which cannot be readily monitored by clinical observation. Since patients' responses vary to specific drugs due to concurrent illnesses or conditions and drug tolerances, dosages may have to be adjusted for each patient in order to achieve the desired response. Serial serum level measurements are more accurate than a single determination.

DRUNKEN SAILOR EFFECT: A metaphor for intermittently controlling ventilation such that the $PaCO_2$ drifts back and forth around the normal level. First the patient is hyperventilated by the anesthetist and becomes alkalotic. Then controlled respiration is stopped and the patient becomes acidotic as $PaCO_2$ builds up until spontaneous respiration begins again. Controlled ventilation is then resumed. The drunken sailor effect is also a metaphor describing an inexperienced anesthetist trying to establish the proper required depth of anesthesia. He or she acts much like a drunken sailor trying to navigate a straight line and lumbering first to one side and then to the other, overcorrecting at each extreme.

DRY CELL: A primary cell or battery in which the active ingredients are absorbed in a solid material so they will not spill out when the cell is tipped.

D-TUBOCURARINE: See Tubocurarine chloride.

DUAL BLOCK: See Phase II block.

DUALITY OF PAIN TRANSMISSION: The two systems for the transmission of pain sensation which appear to occur side by side in humans. One transmission pathway is comparatively fast and comprises the myelinated A-delta fibers. The other pathway is made up of the slow-conducting nonmyelinated C fibers. The A-delta fibers and the C fibers are roughly equally sensitive to local anesthetics. See Gate theory of pain, Nerve fiber, anatomy and physiology of.

DUMP (DUMPING): A term which can be used in several ways. It is the accidental or intentional interruption of power to a computer. Because of the monumental difficulties this can cause, many large computer installations have uninterruptable power supplies. It also refers to spilling the contents of all internal memories at a particular point in time onto tape or onto hard copy in order to detect some error in programming or functioning. In medical slang, dumping is transferring a patient from one service to another to rid one's own service of a social or behavioral problem.

DUPACO INCORPORATED: A company which currently manufactures many anesthesia-related items including anesthesia machines. It is a division of American Hospital Supply Corporation and is located in San Marcos, California.

DURAL PUNCTURE: The penetration of the dura, the covering over the spinal cord and brain, usually with a needle. It is a necessary prerequisite for the induction of spinal anesthesia.

DUST CELL: See Macrophage.

DUTY: A legally enforced obligation which requires one person to act in a particular way with respect to another person.

DYE DILUTION: See Cardiac output.

DYNAMIC COMPRESSION: The condition of airway resistance which occurs during forced expiration. High intrapleural pressure is applied to the alveoli and to the outside walls of the airways as a forced effort is made to empty them. This pressure can cause the airways to collapse. This paradoxical situation flattens expiratory flow rate independent of respiratory effort (with a greater effort more of the airways collapse, thereby impeding flow).

DYNAMOMETER (TORQUEMETER): A device for measuring the rotational force of an engine or motor.

DYNE: A unit of force in the centimeter-gram-second (CGS) system. It is equal to the force acting on a 1-g mass to give it an acceleration of 1 cm/sec. One dyne is the equivalent of 10^{-5} newtons.

DYRENIUM: See Triampterene.

DYSBARISM: See Caisson disease.

DYSESTHESIA: A sensation which is both unpleasant and abnormal, usually pertaining to the sense of touch.

DYSPNEA: A condition in which there is difficult or labored breathing. It may be a subjective sensation in the patient which is usually defined as an awareness of respiration which is distressful. It should not be confused with shortness of breath since the latter is usually explained by physical causes, e.g., exercise.

DYSTOCIA: A condition of difficult or abnormal labor and delivery. It can occur because of multiple antecedent conditions but is usually seen as a result of cephalopelvic disproportion (CPD) (a generalized term for a mismatch between the cross-section measurement of the fetal head and the cross-section diameter of the pelvic outlet).

E

E: The unit charge of an electron. It is equal to 1.60210×10^{-9} coulomb.

ECHOTHIOPHATE IODIDE (PHOSPHOLINE): A topically applied ophthalmic drug used in the treatment of glaucoma. It is a cholinesterase inhibitor of the organo-phosphorus class. It is possible for enough Phospholine to be absorbed, via the cornea, into the systemic circulation to seriously depress serum cholinesterase activity. This, in turn, can significantly prolong neuromuscular blockade caused by succinylcholine.

ED_{50} (EFFECTIVE DOSE 50%): The dose of a pharmacologic substance which produces an effect in 50% of the subjects given the substance. The greater the difference between the ED_{50} and the LD_{50} (lethal dose 50%), the safer the substance. See LD_{50}, Therapeutic index.

EDECRIN: See Ethacrynic acid.

EDEMA: The accumulation of excessive amounts of fluid in the interstitial spaces. Edema may be due to congestive heart failure, venous obstruction, inadequate lymphatic drainage, and renal or hepatic disease. Generalized massive edema is known as anasarca whereas the accumulation of fluid in lung tissue and air spaces is known as pulmonary edema. See Pulmonary edema.

EDIT: To modify, rearrange, delete, or expand data or information.

EDROPHONIUM (TENSILON): A cholinesterase inhibitor which, in appropriate dosages, is shorter acting than neostigmine or pyridostigmine. In the patient who is not receiving anticholinesterase therapy, a small dose of edrophonium can be used as a diagnostic test for myasthenia gravis. (The disease is strongly suspected if muscle strength improves after drug therapy.) Edrophonium is also a potent antagonist to curare-like agents. See Myasthenia gravis, Neostigmine, Pyridostigmine.

EDUCATED HAND: The concept that the hand of the trained anesthetist could, by feeling the breathing bag, detect beginning attempts at respiration, bronchospasm, breath holding, and, in general, any changes in lung compliance, and could thereby monitor indirectly the depth of anesthesia. The further idea that the "educated hand" could, breath after breath, deliver the same tidal volume over a prolonged period of time has been discredited.

EFFACEMENT: The process by which the cervix is progressively thinned and the os dilated (during the first stage of labor) until only the thinned, external os remains.

EFFERENT: Going or moving away from the center. For example, efferent motor nerves transmit signals away from the central nervous system to muscle causing contractions.

EFFICACY: The relative ability of a drug to cause a specific biologic effect. For example, barbiturates are more efficacious than narcotics in decreasing cerebral electric activity. Efficacy is dependent on uptake and distribution, receptor site availability, and the development of intolerable side effects.

EFFICIENCY: The ratio (in mechanical terms) of energy output to input, usually expressed as a percentage.

EINTHOVEN TRIANGLE: The conventional way of describing the skin surface projections of the electric activity of the heart, named after the first electrocardiographer. The triangle is drawn from right shoulder to left shoulder, to left leg, and back to right shoulder. Lead I connects left shoulder to right shoulder, lead II connects left leg to right shoulder, and lead III connects left leg to left shoulder. Each lead records the difference in potential between the two connected limbs. If these points are connected, the electric axis of the heart lies parallel to lead II. This

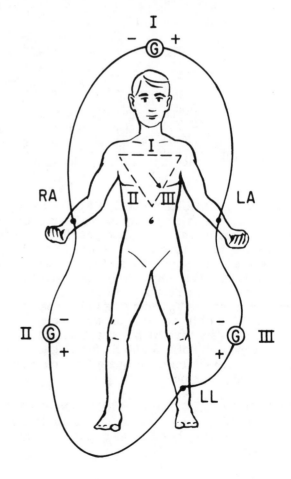

Einthoven Triangle: So-called Einthoven equilateral triangle as shown on the anterior chest wall indicating the relationship of the first three leads of the electrocardiograph.

means that in the normally positioned heart, lead II will have the highest QRS volt-age. Lead II is equal to the sum of the corresponding complexes in leads I and II (Einthoven law). See Fig. See Electrocardiogram, QRS complex.

EISENMENGER SYNDROME: A congenital heart condition characterized by pulmonary hypertension with reversed or bidirectional shunt through either a ventricular or atrial septal defect or a patent ductus arteriosus. There is an elevation of the pulmonary vascular resistance. Signs and symptoms of this syndrome include dyspnea, feeding difficulty, fatigue, cyanosis, and failure to gain weight. See Atrial septal defect, Patent ductus arteriosus, Ventricular septal defect.

ELASTOMER: A huge variety of materials distinguished from other "plastics" because of their extensibility. To be officially classified as an elastomer, a material must be able to be stretched to at least twice its initial length at room temperature and return quickly to its original length on release. Elastomers are also categorized as synthetic rubbers. A common brand name is Neoprene. Elastomers are capable of resisting chemical attack, extremes of use, and abrasion.

ELECTROANESTHESIA: See Electronarcosis.

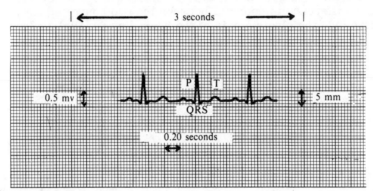

Electrocardiogram: Some of the standard parameters of the ECG shown in lead II.

ELECTROCARDIOGRAM (ECG, EKG): The recording, by means of electrodes or leads, of the electric activity of the heart. Conventionally, three electrode lead systems are used in which standard positions for electrode placement exist. These are known as (1) three limb leads, in which lead I connects right and left arm; lead II, right arm and left leg; and lead III, left arm and left leg; (2) three augmented unipolar limb leads, aVR (right arm), aVL (left arm), and aVF (left leg); and (3) six precordial leads, which connect different areas on the anterior chest to a limb and are known as leads V_1-V_6 according to the specific placement along the intercostal spaces. Each of these leads shows the electric activity of the heart on the side nearest the respective limb. The American Heart Association recommends a frequency band width of 0.5-100 Hz for diagnostic ECG recording. A much narrower band width of 1-50 Hz is adequate for monitoring purposes. See Fig. See Electrocardiography, His bundle.

ELECTROCARDIOGRAPHIC FREQUENCY SPECTRUM: The sum of the individual electric oscillations that make up the clinical electrocardiogram. These extend from 0.5 to 100 Hz when heart rates below 200 beats/min are considered. See Fourier analysis.

ELECTROCARDIOGRAPHY, HIS BUNDLE: A method of recording electric heart activity, specifically that of atrioventricular conduction. An electrocardiograph lead is placed through an intravenous catheter into the right side of the heart.

ELECTROCAUTERY: See Cauterization.

ELECTROCONVERSION: See Cardioversion.

ELECTROCONVULSIVE THERAPY (ECT); ELECTROSHOCK THERAPY: A treatment modality used in psychiatry for severe depressive disorders. The end point of the technique is the creation of an artificial grand mal seizure which causes (as yet poorly explained) a decrease in the degree of depression. Frequently, a patient may receive a series of ECT treatments and the only overt effect is some loss in recent memory function. Electroconvulsive therapy has replaced the older pharmacologic convulsive therapies such as intravenous (IV) atropine, scopolamine (in a dosage range of 50-100 mg IV push), or insulin. (Insulin causes deliberate hypoglycemic shock and convulsions, promptly terminated by glucose.) Modern ECT machines generate a voltage greater than 150 V, have a frequency range of 50-70 Hz, and have a current output ranging from 200 to >1500 mA. General anesthesia, a requirement for this therapy, is usually administered by IV barbiturate plus succinylcholine, the latter being given to prevent stress fractures, particularly of the vertebral column, due to the tremendously strong muscle contractions which accompany the generated seizures. See Defibrillation, Electronarcosis.

ELECTRODE: A device which emits, collects, or deflects electric charge carriers. An anode is an electrode carrying a positive charge and a cathode is an electrode carrying a negative charge.

ELECTROENCEPHALOGRAM (EEG): The recording, by means of electrodes (usually placed on the scalp), of the electric activity generated by the brain during its normal functioning. (Normal EEG signals recorded on the scalp are on the order of 10-100 μV.) The standard EEG is usually measured in at least eight separate channels which record the activity of the brain in its many subdivisions. See Fig. See Fourier analysis.

ELECTROMAGNET: A coil of wire which produces a magnetic field when an electric current is passed through it. The strength of the magnet depends on whether or not a metallic core is placed within the windings, the number and spacing of the turns, and the current flow.

ELECTROMAGNETIC FLOWMETER: See Blood flow, methods for measuring.

ELECTROMAGNETIC RADIATION: A form of energy which is generated by the acceleration of charged particles. It consists of electric and magnetic fields vibrating transversely, longitudinally, and at right angles to both the direction of motion and each other. The waves require no medium for propagation and can therefore traverse a vacuum at a uniform velocity of $2.997\,925 \times 10^8$ m/sec (i.e., the velocity of light). The characteristics of electromagnetic radiation are solely dependent on the frequency of the wave motion. Most phenomena connected with electromagnetic radiation, such as reflection or refraction, can be explained by wave motion. Certain other effects, however, require that electromagnetic radiation be explained as particles. This latter concept is the basis for the quantum theory, in which electromagnetic radiation consists of particles or quanta (photons) which travel at the speed of light and have zero rest mass.

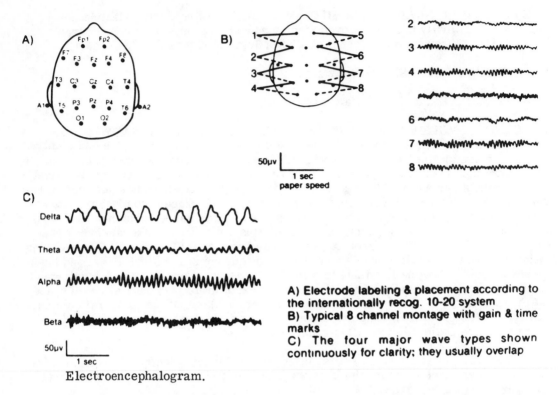

A) Electrode labeling & placement according to the internationally recog. 10-20 system
B) Typical 8 channel montage with gain & time marks
C) The four major wave types shown continuously for clarity; they usually overlap

Electroencephalogram.

ELECTROMAGNETIC SPECTRUM: The range of frequencies over which electromagnetic radiation can be propagated. The order of frequencies (from lowest to highest) are radio waves, infrared radiation, light, ultraviolet radiation, x-rays, and gamma rays. See Fig.

ELECTROMECHANIC SYSTOLE (EMS): See Systolic time intervals.

ELECTROMYOGRAM (EMG): The recording, by means of electrodes (surface or needles), of the electric activity of contracting skeletal muscle.

ELECTRON: An elementary particle usually found orbiting the nucleus of an atom. It has a negative charge of $1.602\ 192 \times 10^{-19}$ coulomb and a mass of $9.10\ 956 \times 10^{-31}$ kg. A moving electron (i.e., a free electron, one not circling a particular nucleus) constitutes an electric current. See Carrier, electric.

ELECTRONARCOSIS: A technique for producing anesthesia by passing an electric current through the brain via electrodes placed on the temples. The current is clearly below that which would produce convulsions. The efficacy of this technique is questioned in the United States; however, it is reported to be used widely in the Soviet Union.

ELECTRON GUN: A device used to produce a beam of electrons. This is usually accomplished by heating a wire (emitter) which causes the emission of electrons in all directions. These electrons are then focused and formed into a beam by magnetic or electric fields surrounding the emitter. The electron gun is also called a cathode because it is the source of negative charges. See Cathode ray tube.

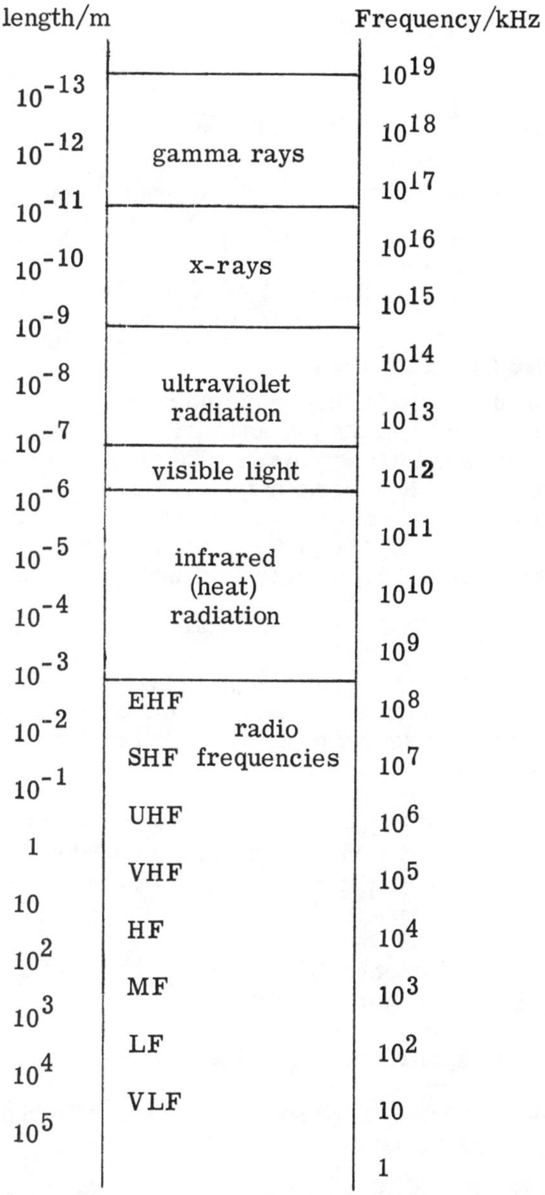

Wavelength/m   Frequency/kHz

Wavelength/m		Frequency/kHz
10^{-13}		10^{19}
10^{-12}	gamma rays	10^{18}
10^{-11}		10^{17}
10^{-10}	x-rays	10^{16}
10^{-9}		10^{15}
10^{-8}	ultraviolet radiation	10^{14}
10^{-7}		10^{13}
10^{-6}	visible light	10^{12}
10^{-5}	infrared (heat) radiation	10^{11}
10^{-4}		10^{10}
10^{-3}		10^{9}
10^{-2}	EHF	10^{8}
10^{-1}	SHF radio frequencies	10^{7}
1	UHF	10^{6}
10	VHF	10^{5}
10^{2}	HF	10^{4}
10^{3}	MF	10^{3}
10^{4}	LF	10^{2}
10^{5}	VLF	10
		1

Electromagnetic Spectrum: Spectrum of electromagnetic radiation.

ELECTRON MULTIPLIER: An electron tube which amplifies single-electron effects. The original electron hits an electrode which, in turn, releases more electrons (secondary emission) on impact. The resulting electrons are then accelerated to another electrode where the process is repeated. Electron multipliers are the basis for various instruments, such as scintillation counters and night vision scopes. See Fig.

ELECTRON VOLT: An energy unit employed in atomic physics. It signifies the energy acquired by an electron while falling freely through a potential difference of 1 V. It is equal to 1.602×10^{-19} joule.

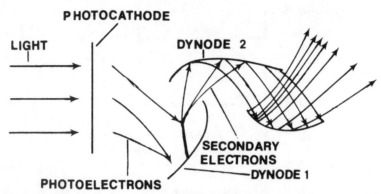

Electron Multiplier: Operating principle of the electron multiplier. Light rays approach from the left and strike the photocathode. The photocathode emits electrons which strike the first dynode. This dynode emits more than one electron for each electron hitting it. Magnetic fields direct these electrons to dynode 2 which has the same characteristics as dynode 1. The process continues with an ever larger cascade of electrons being reflected from dynode to dynode.

ELECTRO-OPTICAL COUNTER: See Automated cell counter.

ELECTROPHORESIS: The movement of small particles suspended in a liquid when an electric field is applied across the liquid. This technique is used extensively in laboratory work to separate serum proteins. Each protein migrates at a different rate due to minor differences in electric charge.

ELECTROPHRENIC RESPIRATION: The diaphragmatic respiration of a patient caused by electrically induced rhythmic stimulation of the phrenic nerves. This technique is most often used on patients who have suffered high cervical injuries and who would otherwise be apneic.

ELECTROPLATING: The process of coating, by means of electrodeposition, the surface of one metal with another for protection.

ELECTROSHOCK: See Electroconvulsive therapy.

ELECTROSPINOGRAM: The recording, by means of electrodes, of the electric activity of all or part of the spinal cord.

ELECTROSTATIC UNIT: The measurement of electrostatic charge in the centimeter-gram-second (CGS) system. It is defined as the charge which, if concentrated at one point in a vacuum, would repel with a force of 1 dyne a similar charge placed 1 cm away. See Dyne.

ELECTROSURGERY: See Coagulation current.

ELEMENTARY PARTICLE (FUNDAMENTAL PARTICLE): Any bit of matter which is a fundamental building block of the universe and cannot be subdivided into smaller particles. The only stable elementary particles are photons, electrons, neutrinos, and protons. (The neutron, another elementary particle, is only stable when it is bound in a nucleus.) All other subatomic particles ultimately decay into combinations of these particles.

ELIMINATION, DRUG: The processes that terminate the action of a drug in the body. Drugs may be eliminated or excreted unchanged or they may undergo biotransformation, i.e., a change in molecular structure.

EMBARRASSMENT: An action or device which impedes or obstructs normal functioning.

EMBOLISM: The sudden obstruction of a blood vessel by an abnormal clot, air, or foreign material circulating in the blood. The major target for embolization is the lungs as they are the only organs to receive the total cardiac output per minute. See Air embolus.

EMERGENCE: The period of time between the termination of an anesthetic (particularly a general anesthetic) and an appropriate patient response to direct commands. It is a particularly dangerous period since there may be a tendency on the part of the anesthetist to relax vigilance as the anesthestic administration is complete and the patient may appear to have adequate upper airway reflexes when, in fact, he or she does not.

EMESIS: See Antiemetic.

EMO INHALER (EPSTEIN, MACINTOSH, OXFORD): A sophisticated draw-over vaporizer used in the administration of diethyl ether. The inhaler contains a water bath which prevents sudden temperature changes in the anesthetic, has an integral bellows for intermittent positive pressure ventilation, and can be equipped to initially vaporize a small amount of halothane before switching to ether in order to speed induction. It is a particularly useful anesthesia administration device where limited facilities exist. See Fig.

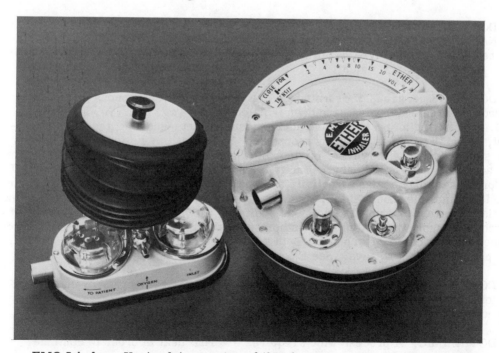

EMO Inhaler: Up-to-date version of this famous anesthetic device with attachment for assisted ventilation.

EMPHYSEMA: See Chronic obstructive pulmonary disease.

EMPYEMA: An infection of the pleural space, usually leading to abscess, which can be local or generalized.

ENCEPHALITIS: An inflammation of the brain. When possible, encephalitis is classified by naming the causative agent, such as measles encephalitis or herpes encephalitis.

ENCEPHALOCELE: A congenital malformation in which a portion of the brain substance is contained in an outpocketing of the meninges which protrude through a skull defect. This is a midline lesion.

ENCEPHALON: See Brain.

ENCEPHALOPATHY: Any disease of the brain.

ENDOBRONCHIAL ANESTHESIA: See Double-lumen tube.

ENDOBRONCHIAL INTUBATION: The deliberate or inadvertent insertion of a tube into the bronchus. When deliberate, bronchial intubation is performed to therapeutically deflate or lavage (as for pulmonary alveolar proteinosis) one lung. When inadvertent, it is the unfortunate placement of the tip of the endotracheal tube into a bronchus (usually the right). This may occur when altering the position of the head and may lead to obstruction of the other bronchus and ultimately to the collapse of the nonventilated lung, a shift of the mediastinum, and the progressive embarrassment of both respiratory and circulatory functions. See Pulmonary alveolar proteinosis.

ENDOCARDIAL CUSHION DEFECT (PERSISTENT COMMON ATRIOVENTRICULAR CANAL): A congenital cardiac abnormality characterized by an atrial septal defect of the ostium primum type resulting from imperfect fusion of the endocardial cushion. See Atrial septal defect.

ENDORPHINS: A group of drugs which are thought to be endogenous opiate-like compounds. Three endorphins have been isolated: alpha (α), beta (β), and gamma (γ), each having a specific amino acid sequence. Beta-endorphin is the most potent, being 10 times as active as morphine. The specific functions of endorphins are still speculative; however, in vivo, beta-endorphin, which is broken down slowly, acts as a modifier of neuronal activity and alters responsiveness for hours. The endorphins display analgesic activity and seem to play a role in temperature homeostasis and muscle tonus. It appears that endorphins possess the same addictive potential as narcotics and all effects are abolished (in vivo) by the administration of a narcotic antagonist. Enkephalins comprise another group of opiate-like compounds somewhat similar to endorphins. Both groups are indistinguishable from morphine in opiate-binding bioassays. See Enkephalins.

ENDOSCOPY: The visual inspection of the interior of a body organ or canal with the aid of a light-carrying instrument inserted within it. Examples are laryngoscopy, bronchoscopy, esophagoscopy, colonoscopy, and cystoscopy.

ENDOTHERMIC: A process which requires external heat in order to continue.

ENDOTRACHEAL TUBE: The semiflexible plastic catheter used to deliver anesthetic gases directly into the trachea of a patient. By proper sizing or by means of an inflatable cuff, the tube protects the airway against foreign matter when protective airway reflexes are obtunded. The tube also decreases anatomic dead space by traversing the oropharynx and nasopharynx which contribute to the dead space. The overwhelming majority of tubes currently in use are single-use disposable items made out of polyvinylchloride. The uncuffed type is simply a tube of semiflexible polyvinylchloride which is delivered in a sterile package and most frequently used in pediatric anesthesia. The cuffed endotracheal tube has a balloon or cuff approximately 1 cm from the distal end which can be inflated by a pilot line running down in the sidewall of the tube, topped by a one-way valve and a pilot or indicating balloon. The cuff permits a tight fit, preventing gas escape around the tube. Two subcategories of cuffed tubes are available. One is the high-volume, low-pressure cuff which, when inflated, is generally sausage-shaped and has a large contact area with the tracheal mucosa and a low pressure per unit area of tracheal contact. The other is a low-volume, high-pressure cuff which, when inflated, is elliptical in shape, has a small area of contact with the tracheal mucosa, and exerts relatively high pressures on the area of the trachea it contacts. As a generality, the high-volume, low-pressure cuffs may cause more postoperative sore throats in a short period of time, but can be left in place much longer than the high-pressure, low-volume cuffs. These cause fewer sore throats postoperatively, but when left in place for a long period of time cause moderate to severe mucosal erosion. Tubes can also be manufactured from Silastic, which has a high degree of tissue compatibility but is quite expensive. Most commonly, the size of an endotracheal tube is designated by its inside diameter. (The French system assigns each tube a number derived by taking the external diameter measured in millimeters and multiplying by 3. This system is no longer used.) The distal end of the endotracheal tube is beveled and rounded to cause the least amount of trauma. Specific tube modifications exist such as the Kamen-Wilkinson tube in which a foam rubber cuff is deflated for insertion by applying a negative pressure to the pilot line. Murphy endotracheal tubes have a hole through the tube wall opposite the beveled end. Those tubes which do not have this accessory hole are Magill tubes. Two special tubes which are found most frequently in pediatric practice are the Cole tube, which has a tapered end, and the Rae tube, which has a fixed curvature to facilitate access to the head and neck during surgery. Although most single-use endotracheal tubes look alike, the degree of curvature of the tube may be used to designate it as orotracheal or nasotracheal depending on the intended route of entry. The nasotracheal tube has more of a curve. See Figs.

ENDPLATE: See Neuromuscular blockade, assessment of.

END TIDAL CARBON DIOXIDE MEASUREMENT (F_{ET} CO_2): A technique of measuring the CO_2 content just as air movement ceases in expiration. A sample taken at this time is considered to come from the alveoli as the dead space gas has been swept past the detectors. It is used clinically as a technique for detecting air embolization which has occurred in the pulmonary circulation. The principle involved is that before embolization has become florid enough to cause blood pressure changes, a significant portion of the pulmonary vessel may become blocked, raising the dead space volume. This dilutes expired CO_2 with dead space air.

ENERGY: The capacity for performing work (actual or potential). Energy is quantified in joules.

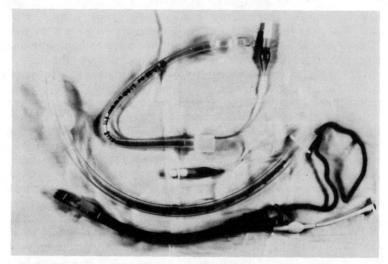

I

OUTSIDE DIAMETER mm	FRENCH SCALE	MAGILL NUMBER	DAVOL NUMBER
	10		
	11		
4	12		0
	13		
	14	00	
5	15	0A	1
	16		
	17	0	
6	18		
	19	1	2
	20		
7	21	2	
	22		3
	23		
8	24	3	
	25	4	4
	26		
9	27	5	5
	28	6	6
	29		
10	30		
	31	7	7
	32	8	
11	33		
	34		8
	35	9	
12	36		9
	37		
	38	10	
13	39		
	40		10
	41		
14	42		

II

Endotracheal Tube: (I) Assortment of endotracheal tubes. (II) Common numbering systems for endotracheal tubes.

$$H-\underset{\underset{\text{Cl}}{|}}{\overset{\overset{\text{F}}{|}}{C}}-\underset{\underset{\text{F}}{|}}{\overset{\overset{\text{F}}{|}}{C}}-O-\underset{\underset{\text{F}}{|}}{\overset{\overset{\text{F}}{|}}{C}}-H$$

Enflurane.

ENFLURANE (ETHRANE): A nonflammable liquid which is one of the most frequently used inhalation agents for general anesthesia. It is extremely stable chemically and does not require a preservative. Postoperative side effects such as nausea, shivering, and vomiting may occur, but to a lesser extent than with other agents such as halothane. High concentrations of enflurane, however, are associated with respiratory and circulatory depression and may produce seizure-like activity even in the neurologically normal patient. The vapor pressure of enflurane (2-chloro-1, 1,2-trifluoroethyldifluoromethyl ether) at 20 torr is 175. See Fig.

ENGINE: A machine for turning heat energy into mechanical work.

ENHANCEMENT: The increase in value or in quantity. Radiographs taken with low levels of x-rays can be enhanced by a computer, sparing patients an increased radiation dose.

ENIAC: An acronym for Electronic Numerical Integrator And Calculator. It was a computer that was designed and developed by scientists at the University of Pennsylvania during World War II. (It was considered by many to be the first computer.) A prior claim to developing the first computer, however, belongs to a British code-cracking group which built an electronic machine in the early 1940s to break the German Ultra Code. It is interesting to note that the capabilities of ENIAC were essentially duplicated in a hand-held calculator in 1976.

ENKEPHALINS: A group of endogenous opiate-like compounds composed of penta-peptides such as met-enkephalin and leu-enkephalin. They are synthesized in brain tissue and appear to function as neurotransmitters. They display a weak analgesic action and are broken down rapidly. The enkephalins are somewhat similar to endorphins and both are indistinguishable from morphine in opiate-binding bioassays. See Endorphins.

ENTEROHEPATIC RECIRCULATION: The pathway by which drugs excreted in bile return to the body by being reabsorbed further in the intestine. This is clinically significant when it involves drugs which have toxic effects remanifesting themselves after a period of apparent recovery as the initial drug or its active metabolites return to the circulation from the intestine.

ENTHALPY: The heat content of a system.

ENTROPY: A measure of the disorder of a system. The human body can, under normal circumstances, be considered to have low entropy. As the body ages and control mechanisms become less precise, entropy is increased; as random or uncontrolled activity increases, so does entropy.

ENZYME INDUCTION; ENZYME INHIBITION: The enhancement or retardation of an enzymatically mediated drug breakdown. For example, the drug phenobarbital (and, to some extent, other barbiturates) increases the effectiveness of liver enzymes in metabolizing a broad spectrum of other drugs. Cytochrome P-450, often involved in drug metabolism, is one of the enzyme systems most frequently affected by phenobarbital. Enzyme inhibitors which decrease drug metabolism include such drugs as chloramphenicol and some of the phenothiazines.

EPHEDRINE: A naturally occurring compound known to Chinese medicine for thousands of years and introduced to Western clinical practice in the 1920s. Ephedrine is classified as a sympathomimetic drug. It stimulates both alpha and beta receptors and is used in those conditions in which both central and peripheral cardiovascular stimulation is desired. It has a positive inotropic effect on the heart while at the same time constricting peripheral vasculature. In anesthetic practice it is often used as the drug of choice to counteract the pressure drop seen with epidural and spinal anesthetics.

EPIDERMOLYSIS BULLOSA: A genetically determined disorder of the skin. It is characterized by the appearance of blisters, which can occur both spontaneously and at the site of even insignificant trauma. This clinical history is important for the anesthetist because rapid obstruction of the airway may occur following any manipulation of the area during anesthesia.

EPIDURAL ANESTHESIA (PERIDURAL ANESTHESIA): A type of regional anesthesia induced by the injection of a local anesthetic agent into the epidural (extradural) space, thus blocking the spinal nerve trunks. The block occurs both by diffusion of the drug through the dura and by direct contact with the nerves as they exit the dural sleeves. The percentage contribution from each pathway is controversial. Compared to subdural (spinal) anesthesia, epidural anesthesia (1) requires greater volumes of anesthetic agent (5-10 times more depending on the effect desired), (2) is not as dependable, (3) has a slower onset, and (4) has a greater incidence of differential blockade.

EPIDURAL NEEDLE: A needle used to place either a catheter or a dose of local anesthetic into the epidural space. Many types of epidural needles exist. See Hustead epidural needle, Spinal needle.

EPIDURAL PATCH (BLOOD PATCH): A technique for the relief of severe spinal headache. A fluid, usually autologous blood, is injected into the same vertebral level as the previous puncture site in the dura. Relief of the headache is accomplished by sealing this hole, thereby preventing leakage of cerebrospinal fluid (CSF). Since the brain normally floats in and is supported by CSF, the loss of this fluid may produce the headache. This proposed mechanism does not explain a number of clinical cases in which the patient experiences immediate relief after placement of the patch, long before CSF pressure could have been built up. Although essentially without major morbidity, back pain and signs of meningeal irritation have been noted in the patient after employment of this technique. See Spinal headache.

EPIDURAL PRESSURE SWITCH: A pressure-sensing device used to detect changes in intracranial pressure (ICP). It is applied to the dura through a burr hole in the skull and generates a signal proportional to the pressure of the dura against the tip of the switch. This technique lacks long-term stability and has a poor response speed; it does not, however, require a dural puncture and therefore is theoretically safer than other ICP detection techniques.

EPILEPSY: A recurrent disorder of brain function affecting either the entire central nervous system or only a part of it. It is manifested by altered consciousness and abnormal motor and sensory activity. The classification of epilepsies now distinguishes primary generalized epilepsy from partial (focal) epilepsy. Malfunction of the central, brain-integrating mechanism is the direct cause of primary generalized seizures (centrencephalic epilepsy). The terms petit mal and grand mal are imprecise and are no longer used to describe a seizure. Approximately 10% of seizure patients have primary generalized epilepsy which is a specific hereditary disease. Seizures of this type consist of (1) typical absence attacks (true petit mal), (2) generalized convulsive seizures (true grand mal), and (3) myoclonic and akinetic seizures. Typical absence attacks are precipitated by repetitive flashes of bright light and by forced hyperventilation (the latter being a diagnostic test because primary generalized epilepsy is the only seizure disorder precipitated this way). The patient, usually a young child, during an attack does not respond to stimuli or verbal commands. Rapid eye blinking, blank stares, and upper extremity muscle twitching may be present as well. These attacks may last only a few seconds and may go unnoticed. They are followed by a complete return to consciousness and the patient may deny the entire episode. Generalized convulsive seizures usually develop in adolescence or young adulthood. The attacks occur without warning as the patient suddenly becomes unconscious and falls. During the tonic phase of this seizure, the patient is rigid for approximately 30 sec, the face is contorted, and the skin appears purplish. The tongue may be severely bitten during this phase. As the seizure progresses, the tonic phase is followed by repetitive symmetric clonic jerks of the arms and legs. As the patient recovers and takes some breaths, the cyanotic appearance disappears. This is followed by a confused, restless state, and then sleep. The patient will have no memory of the events. Myoclonic and akinetic seizures consist of small symmetric rhythmic jerking movements of the upper extremities. The patient does not lose consciousness. The other type of seizure disorder, partial (focal) epilepsy, occurs in nearly 90% of patients with seizures. The etiology is usually related to trauma, anoxia, infection, vascular disease, tumor, or some specific metabolic disease; the seizures are merely symptoms of the underlying brain abnormality. The manifestation of the focal seizure depends on the site of brain damage and not the pathologic process that caused it. The ultrashort-acting barbiturate Brevital is a specific provoking agent for psychomotor seizures, a subcategory of partial seizures. Airway maintenance may be critical during seizure activity. See Status epilepticus.

EPINEPHRINE: A naturally occurring catecholamine which is one of the most potent vasopressors and cardiac stimulants known. It is normally produced by the adrenal medulla and reaches its sites of action through the circulation. It stimulates metabolism and promotes blood flow to skeletal muscles to prepare the body for the "flight-or-fight" response. Because of its extremely powerful effects, it is the drug of choice during resuscitation because it increases cardiac contractility and peripheral resistance. It can also be used under less extreme circumstances as an intravenous drip to support circulation. At times it is used in local anesthetic preparations to promote vasoconstriction, thereby prolonging anesthetic action.

EPISTAXIS: A nosebleed.

EPOXY RESIN: A class of synthetic resin compounds which have a highly reactive ring consisting of an oxygen atom bonded to two adjoining carbon atoms. Epoxy resins are used as adhesives and coatings.

EPSOM SALTS (HYDRATED MAGNESIUM SULFATE): See Magnesium sulfate.

EQUALIZATION: An electronics term which refers to the use of various circuits to compensate for a known distortion.

EQUIPOTENTIAL: A term referring to a surface or body on which all points are at the same electric potential.

Equivalent System of Measurement: Conversion of milligrams percent to milliequivalents.

		To Convert mg% to Milliequivalents per Liter		To Convert Milliequivalents per Liter to mg%	
		Multiply by:	Divide by:	Multiply by:	Divide by:
Sodium	Na^+	0.435	2.30	2.30	0.435
Potassium	K^+	0.256	3.91	3.91	0.256
Magnesium	Mg^{++}	0.820	1.22	1.22	0.820
Calcium	Ca^{++}	0.500	2.00	2.00	0.500
Chloride	Cl^-	0.282	3.55	3.55	0.282
Bicarbonate	HCO_3^-	0.164	6.10	6.10	0.164

EQUIVALENT SYSTEM OF MEASUREMENT (MILLIEQUIVALENT): A system for quantitating an ionic solution by the number of electric charges that are contained per unit volume. The unit of measurement is the milliequivalent per liter (mEq/L), which is derived from the weight measurement of milligrams per liter (per ion) by the following equation: milliequivalents per liter = milligrams per liter X valence of the ion ÷ by the atomic weight of the ion. See Fig.

ERYTHROPOIESIS: See Anemia.

ESCAPE VELOCITY: The velocity that an object must achieve in order to escape a gravitational field.

ESERINE: See Physostigmine.

ESOPHAGEAL LEAD: An electrocardiograph lead inserted into the esophagus. It records electric activity posterior to the heart. This lead is particularly important to establish the relative timing of atrial contractions. It is also useful in obtaining additional information concerning individual atrial conduction.

ESOPHAGEAL REFLUX (STOMACH REFLUX): The reverse flow of gastric contents into the esophagus. This flow is usually a passive process whereas vomiting is an active process involving contraction of gastric and esophageal smooth muscle. In both processes, however, the esophageal sphincter must open for the liquid and solid matter to pass out of the stomach. In the normal individual, the lowest limit of pressure necessary to open the esophageal sphincter is approximately 15 cm of water.

ESSENTIAL HYPERTENSION: The elevation of arterial blood pressure with little or no symptomatology and with no discernible etiology. Hypertension can be called essential after all known causes of raised arterial pressure, such as restricted kidney blood flow, hormone-secreting tumors, inappropriate drug administration, etc., are ruled out. A resting diastolic pressure of 90 mmHg is considered the threshold of disease in an adult when determined on multiple occasions.

ETHACRYNIC ACID (EDECRIN): A potent diuretic believed to exert its major action in the loop of Henle. Overdosage can lead to circulatory collapse and severe hypokalemia.

ETHANOL (ETHYL ALCOHOL): The chemical name for alcohol. Although it may be the most popular molecule in history, its medicinal uses are severely limited. Intravenously, it has been used to control premature labor. Its use as a general anesthetic is restricted because of the proximity of its therapeutic and lethal dose.

ETHER: See Diethyl ether.

ETHER DOME: See Morton, William T. G.

ETHINAMATE (VALMID): A minor hypnotic-sedative drug which is short acting.

ETHRANE: See Enflurane.

ETHYL ALCOHOL: See Ethanol.

ETHYL CARBAMATE (URETHAN): An ester of ethanol used occasionally as an anesthetic in animals. It has no human anesthetic clinical use.

ETHYL CHLORIDE: A simple organic molecule used for many years as a rapid-induction, short-duration general anesthetic. Because of its tremendous rate of evaporation at room temperature, it is also used as a topical anesthetic to cool and numb the skin rapidly. Ethyl chloride as a general anesthetic is now obsolete because of its hepatotoxicity and the small difference between its therapeutic and toxic doses.

ETHYLENE: An organic molecule, gaseous at room temperature, formerly used as a substitute for N_2O in balanced anesthesia. Considered to be slightly more potent than N_2O, its chief disadvantages are that (1) it is explosive in clinical concentrations, (2) it is lighter than air (floating in the atmosphere of an operating room it may be detonated by the electric circuitry in the ceiling), and (3) it has a slightly sick-sweet odor. Its major uses outside the medical field are as a raw material for the manufacture of plastics and as an agent to ripen tomatoes on the way to market. This has led to an unusual number of conflagrations at vegetable depots around the country.

ETHYLENE OXIDE STERILIZATION: A method used to sterilize heat- or moisture-sensitive hospital equipment. Ethylene oxide (ETO), a highly toxic gas, penetrates some materials well, allowing items to be prepackaged in polyethylene or paper prior to sterilization. Long-term storage is then possible after the aeration process, which removes the residual ETO. The disadvantages of the ETO technique include (1) the extended time period needed for sterilization (up to 12 hr in some circumstances), (2) the possible complications of skin reactions and laryngotracheal inflammation (which are due to inadequate aeration of the sterilized items), and (3) the rigid controls necessary to keep ETO concentrations low in the work place.

ETHYL ETHER: See Diethyl ether.

ETHYLPARABEN: See Preservative.

ETHYL VINYL ETHER (VINAMAR): An obsolete variant of diethyl ether and vinyl ether no longer used in clinical anesthesia.

ETIDOCAINE (DURANEST): An amide-type local anesthetic. See Local anesthetic.

ETOMIDATE: A recently introduced intravenous anesthetic used primarily as an induction agent. However, this agent has no advantages over current induction agents and has a high incidence of pain on injection.

ETORPHINE: The most potent narcotic ever synthesized. It is 5000-10,000 times as potent as morphine and its effects on the central nervous system are more potent than those of lysergic acid. It is used primarily (in combination with a phenothiazine) as a large-animal immobilizing agent.

EUTONYL: See Pargyline.

EVAPORATION: The conversion of a liquid to its vapor at a temperature below its boiling point. This process causes cooling of the liquid because the fastest molecules escape the surface, thereby lowering the average kinetic energy of those remaining. See Vapor pressure.

EVIPAL: See Barbiturate, Hexobarbital.

EVOKED POTENTIAL (EVOKED-RELATED RESPONSE): An adaptation of electroencephalographic monitoring used to test the functional integrity of the brain. A stimulus is presented to the brain by visual, auditory, or somatosensory means, repeatable in intensity and time interval as often as necessary. The changes in neuroelectric activity occur in two parts. The first part, the primary or specific complex, occurs after each stimulus with a latency of less than 15 msec and is made up of a 10- to 15-msec surface-positive deflection followed immediately by a negative deflection. The combined positive and negative deflection lasts for less than 30 msec. The specific complex is followed by smaller, diffusely distributed positive

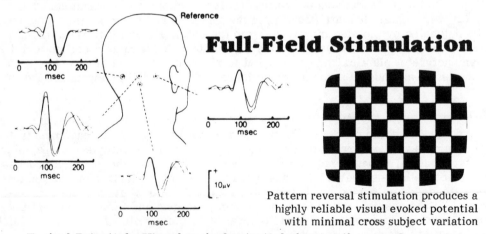

Pattern reversal stimulation produces a highly reliable visual evoked potential with minimal cross subject variation

Evoked Potential: Visual evoked potential showing the signal recorded from various locations on the back of the head.

and negative oscillations. Anesthetic agents have a minimal effect on the specific complex but greatly affect the late-occurring, diffusely distributed deflections. Primary or specific complex disappearance is more closely correlated with irreversible hypoxic cellular damage, although under certain circumstances it can be elicited when the spontaneous electroencephalogram is absent. To be of value, evoked potential monitoring must have the capability of recording and displaying a number of evoked potentials in series for comparison. See Fig.

EXCITABILITY: The state in which a tissue is capable of a rapid response to a stimulus. Nerve tissue and muscles, by their very nature, are excitable. The threshold of excitability can be raised or lowered by various methods.

EXCITATORY POSTSYNAPTIC POTENTIAL (EPSP); INHIBITORY POSTSYNAPTIC POTENTIAL (IPSP): The effects (excitatory and inhibitory) at synaptic junctions of the release of single quanta of neurotransmitters. The postsynaptic membrane is changed slightly to either facilitate or prevent the initiation of an impulse. Usually this change in potential is too small to cause postsynaptic membrane depolarization or the initiation of an action potential. See Neuromuscular transmission.

EXCRETION: The elimination of a substance from the body, e.g., in saliva, bile, urine, feces, or sweat.

EXHAUST SYSTEM: See Scavenger system.

EXPIRATION: The expelling of air from the lungs, usually due to the elastic recoil of the lungs and the thoracic wall. Although it can be aided by forceful contraction of the abdominal muscles, expiration is usually a passive process. Some older ventilators placed a negative pressure in the airway during the expiratory phase to aid and speed up expiration. (The reverse is the physiologic state in which airway pressure is slightly positive in relation to atmospheric pressure during respiration.) This procedure is no longer widespread, however, since negative pressure in the airway tends to promote the closure of small air passageways, thereby trapping air.

EXPIRATORY RETARD: A setting on a ventilator which can variably delay the amount of time expiration takes. The purpose of expiratory retard or its modification, expiratory plateau, is to maintain positive pressure in the airways as long as possible to prevent small-airway collapse and to improve ventilation perfusion. Expiratory retard is a step away from positive end expiratory pressure (PEEP), which has replaced it in ventilation therapy. See Continuous positive airway pressure, Positive end expiratory pressure.

EXPLOSIMETER: A device for measuring the combustion capabilities of a gas/air or gas/O_2 sample. It must be calibrated for individual gas mixtures.

EXPLOSION: A detonation which occurs in gaseous mixtures when the flame (propagating outward from the point of ignition) moves so rapidly that there is no time for the heat generated by the passage of the flame to be dissipated into the surroundings. The pressure in the flame front rises to very high values. This pressure wave interacts with the adjoining layer of fresh gaseous mixture and heats it by compression, which in turn raises the adjoining layer to well above its ignition temperature. If enough fuel/gas mixture is available, a narrow zone of high pressure traveling at supersonic speed is created which is called a shock wave. In a true explosion, the shock wave and the accompanying flame front behind it can reach speeds of 2000-3000 m/sec. The maximum temperature is in excess of 2500 degrees Celsius and maximum pressure is in excess of 20 atmospheres.

EXPLOSION LIMITS: See Detonability, limits of.

EXPLOSION PROOF: See Intrinsically safe device.

EXPRESSED CONSENT: A legal term denoting the expressed (either oral or written) permission by a patient for the performance of a procedure. See Implied consent.

EXTERNAL JUGULAR VEIN: See Jugular veins.

EXTRA-ALVEOLAR VESSEL: A blood vessel which is not exposed to alveolar gas although it is part of the pulmonary circulation. The caliber of the extra-alveolar vessels is greatly affected by lung volume since they are supported by and entirely surrounded by lung parenchyma.

EXTRACORPOREAL CIRCULATION: See Cardiopulmonary bypass.

EXTRACORPOREAL MEMBRANE OXYGENATION: See Membrane oxygenator.

EXTRAPOLATION: The estimation of a value for a variable from outside the range of those values already known.

EXTRINSIC PATHWAY: A mechanism for activating blood coagulation. It is initiated by the blood contacting extravascular structures. The "prothrombin time" (PT test) laboratory test evaluates this pathway. See Blood coagulation, Intrinsic pathway.

EXTUBATION: The process of removing an endotracheal tube. Never a casual process, extubation must be preceded by patient evaluation since removal of the endotracheal tube immediately increases the dead space and, in many instances, may leave the patient with some vocal cord incompetence. The degree of incompetence is related to the length of time the tube was in place. See Endotracheal tube.

EYE SIGNS DURING ANESTHESIA: An attempt to monitor depth of anesthesia by evaluating eyelid reflex, pupillary size, response to light, and eyeball activity. Of great value during ether anesthesia (with no premedication), it is considered to be unreliable with more rapidly acting agents, particularly when multiple premedications have been given. See Stages and planes of anesthesia.

$\mathcal{F}$

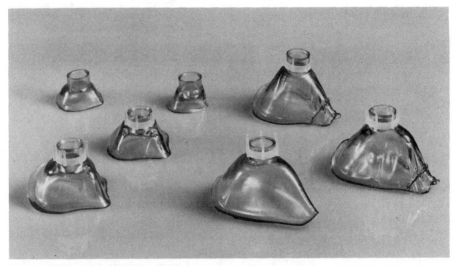

Face Mask: Series of clear plastic full face masks covering the pediatric to adult size range.

FACE MASK: A device used in the breathing of anesthetic gases and/or vapors. It is designed to maintain and form a gas-tight seal over the nose and mouth. Qualitative variations include shape, type of seal around the border, and opacity or clarity of the mask material itself. See Fig.

FACIAL NERVE: The seventh cranial nerve. See Cranial nerves.

FACULTY OF ANAESTHETISTS ROYAL COLLEGE OF SURGEONS OF ENGLAND (FARCS): The British counterpart of the American Board of Anesthesia. The Faculty of Anaesthetists was founded as the second faculty of the College of Surgeons in 1948. Fellowship in the Faculty is granted after an examination, and there are now approximately 4300 individuals who have the full title of Fellow, Faculty of Anaesthetists Royal College of Surgeons of England (FFARCS). The FARCS is located in Lincoln's Field, London.

FADE: See Neuromuscular blockade, assessment of.

FAHRENHEIT SCALE: A temperature scale in which the ice or freezing point of water is 32 degrees and the steam or boiling point is 212 degrees. In scientific usage it has been replaced by the Celsius scale.

FAIL-SAFE DEVICE: A device so designed and constructed that it cannot malfunction in a damaging or detrimental manner when it or the apparatus it controls ex-

F500 GAS CIRCUIT DIAGRAM

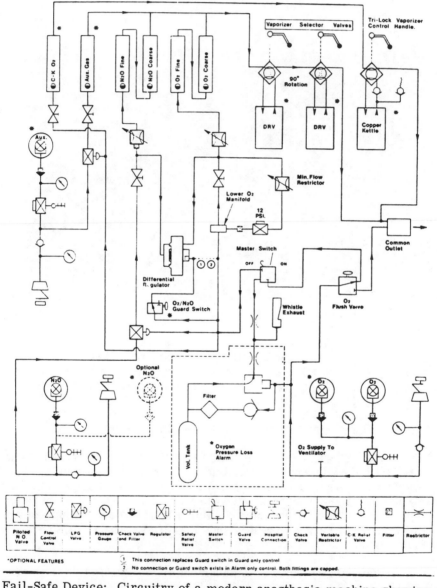

Fail-Safe Device: Circuitry of a modern anesthesia machine showing a fail-safe device, here called an LPG (low-pressure guardian valve). It shuts off all non-O_2 gas flows when O_2 pressure falls below a preset limit.

ceeds design limits. The most frequently encountered fail-safe system in anesthesia is the anesthesia machine valve which prevents the delivery of any gas other than O_2 when the pressure of the O_2 supply falls below a preset point. Fail-safe devices can be defeated by improper maintenance and inadequate understanding of their limits. See Fig.

FALLING INTO THE CRACKS (FALLING BETWEEN THE BOARDS): A slang phrase describing the situation in which a patient is attended by teams of specialists who concern themselves with their own discrete area of expertise and not with the patient as a whole. An example would be a brain-injured patient with kidney failure who is successfully dialyzed without any attention given to the effect of dialysis on the injured brain.

FAMILIAL PERIODIC PARALYSIS: A rare type of muscle disease which has a definite, although obscure, genetic basis. At least three distinct types have been described; hypokalemic, hyperkalemic, and normokalemic. The hypokalemic attack can be precipitated by large carbohydrate-containing meals and stress of any kind, including infection, surgery, or trauma. Paralysis is variable and can be asymmetric. The cardiac effects of hypokalemia can be demonstrated by electrocardiography. Muscles are unresponsive to even direct electric stimulation and the attack can be of such severity that the patient dies from respiratory insufficiency. For anesthetic purposes, patients who are so diagnosed must be exquisitely managed for fluid and electrolyte levels, and muscle relaxants are relatively contraindicated. The hyperkalemic form of the disease appears unrelated to high-carbohydrate meals with attacks occurring spontaneously after exercise or stress. This form is marked by a rise in serum potassium and the administration of potassium can provoke an attack. The cardiac effects of hyperkalemia can be demonstrated by electrocardiography. This form of the disease appears to exaggerate the action of depolarizing muscle relaxants. In normokalemic period paralysis the serum potassium remains unchanged during an attack although cardiac arrhythmias do occur. Attacks may be precipitated by stress or may occur spontaneously. Anesthetic management is aimed at preventing respiratory embarrassment, maintaining serum fluid and electrolyte balance, and avoiding neuromuscular blocking agents.

FARAD (F): A standard international unit which measures capacitance. One farad is the capacitance of a capacitor that acquires a charge of 1 coulomb when a potential difference of 1V is applied. This is far too large a unit to be used handily, as most common capacitors are in the pF, nF, μF, and mF ranges. See Capacitance, electronic.

FASCICULATION: The random contraction of part of a muscle mass due to uncoordinated stimulation of the motor end-plates. Most commonly seen in the normal individual in extreme muscle fatigue, fasciculations are also seen after the administration of a depolarizing muscle relaxant. These agents first stimulate and then block the motor endplate. This action does not occur over the whole muscle simultaneously because of local circulation differences. Because the external muscles of the eyes are the most highly innervated muscles in the body (thus having the most motor endplates), they fasciculate strongly when a depolarizer is administered. This raises intraocular pressure transiently and is of no consequence in the normal eye but can be catastrophic if the eye is disrupted by injury. The abdominal muscles can also fasciculate strongly and this may cause a transient rise in intragastric pressure. This pressure rise can theoretically cause esophageal reflux and can increase the danger of aspiration of gastric contents. Fasciculations caused by a depolarizing neuromuscular blocker can be almost totally prevented by giving a small dose of nondepolarizing drug first, but this effect is not 100% reliable.

FASTING: The abstinence from all food intake for a specified period of time.

FAULT CURRENT: The flow of electrons in an unintentional path resulting from a complete breakdown of the normal separation of circuit parts or current-carrying wires. A fault differs from a leak in that a fault will activate an overcurrent protector, whereas a leak usually will not. For example, a nail bridging two conductors is a fault, whereas a gradual degradation of insulation allowing a small current flow is a leak.

FEEDBACK: The process of returning a part of the output of a machine or system to the input. Negative feedback indicates that input energy is decreased whereas positive feedback indicates that input energy is increased. See Hormone.

FENTANYL (SUBLIMAZE): A popular synthetic narcotic which is approximately 80 times more potent than morphine. Onset of action is extremely rapid when administered intravenously. Combined with droperidol (a butyrophenone) and marketed as Innovar, it is useful as an adjunct to N_2O/O_2 administration to produce neuroleptanesthesia. Sufentanyl and alfentanyl, recently synthesized derivatives of fentanyl, have different potencies and half-lives and may soon be used clinically. See Narcotic, Neuroleptanesthesia.

FETAL CIRCULATION: The specialized system of blood flow in utero comprising the fetal heart, umbilical arteries and vein, foramen ovale, ductus arteriosus, and

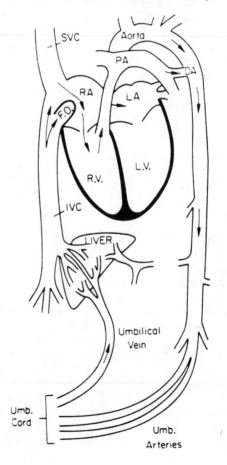

Fetal Circulation: Diagram of fetal circulation and circulatory changes at birth. The pulmonary vessels open up as the lungs expand; umbilical vessels close; foramen ovale closes when left atrial pressure exceeds right atrial pressure; ductus arteriosus closes as pulmonary artery resistance falls.

placental villi. The fetus must receive O_2 and excrete CO_2 through the placenta since the lungs are collapsed and nonfunctioning. With the first breath after birth, the lungs begin to expand and the pulmonary vascular resistance decreases. More blood goes to the lungs and is returned to the left atrium. This causes left atrial pressure to increase and the foramen ovale to close. Semi-independently, the umbilical vessels begin to close. The functioning lungs effectively raise the PO_2 in the aorta, and the ductus arteriosus also begins to close. See Fig.

FETAL HEART RATE (FHR) TERMINOLOGY: See Fig.

Fetal Heart Rate Terminology: Nomenclature for fetal heart rate variations.

Terms	Descriptions
Baseline FHR	Rate observed between contractions.
FHR Level	
Normal	120-160 beats per minute (BPM)
Mild bradycardia	100-119 BPM
Marked bradycardia	99 or less BPM
Mild tachycardia	161-180 BPM
Marked tachycardia	180 or more BPM
FHR Variability	
Short term	Beat to beat changes or interval differences between successive cardiac cycles.
Normal	5-15 beats interval difference.
Long term	Fluctuations described in terms of frequency in cycles per minute and amplitude of change in BPM.
Normal	2-6 cycles per minute with amplitude 6-10 BPM.
Periodic FHR	Rate observed during contractions.
No change	Rate maintains characteristics of preceding baseline FHR.
Acceleration	FHR increases in response to contractions.
Deceleration	FHR decreases in response to contractions.
Uniform patterns	Reflect shape of uterine contraction and are usually repetitive.
Early deceleration	Pattern usually has onset, maximal fall, and recovery which is coincident with onset, peak, and end of contraction. Synonyms are head compression (HC) and Type I dip.
Late deceleration	Pattern has onset, maximal fall, and recovery which is late in relationship to onset, peak, and end of contraction. Synonyms are uteroplacental insufficiency (UPI) and Type II dip.
Variable patterns	Patterns have variable time of onset, variable waveform, and may not be repetitive. Synonyms are cord compression (CC) and Type III dip.
Combined or mixed patterns	Patterns may be difficult to define and have characteristics of any of the other patterns.

FETAL MONITOR: A device used to continuously evaluate and record the effect of labor on the fetus. A gauge attached to the abdomen of the mother follows the force of uterine contractions and the pulse rate of the fetus by tracing fetal heart movement via Doppler ultrasound. Some sophisticated monitors record both fetal (by a scalp electrode) and maternal electrocardiograms.

FEV_1: See Forced expiratory volume.

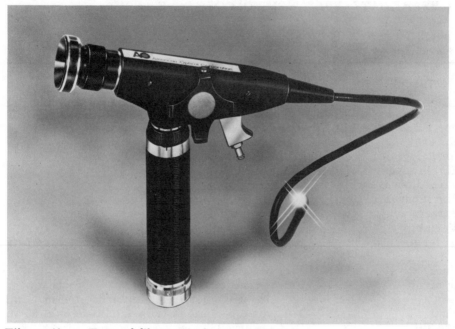

Fiberoptics: Type of fiberoptic laryngoscope.

FIBEROPTICS: The transmission of an image by means of coated glass fibers having special optical properties. Light, transferred by internal reflection along the length of the fibers, can traverse long distances with minimal attenuation. This process facilitates endoscopic examinations. See Fig. See Endosocopy.

FIBRILLATION, VENTRICULAR: See Ventricular fibrillation.

FIBRINOGEN DEGRADATION PRODUCTS (FDP): The substances which are produced by the action of fibrinogen (plasmin) on fibrin and fibrinogen.

FIBRINOLYSIS: The enzymatic breakdown of fibrin. During this process, the circulating protein (plasminogen) is activated to plasmin by tissue factors. Plasmin will destroy fibrin, fibrinogen, and clotting factors V and VIII. The plasmin activation system appears to be the method by which the body disposes of intravascular clots. See Disseminated intravascular coagulation, Primary fibrinolysis.

FICK LAW OF DIFFUSION: A principle which states that the amount of gas moving across a tissue is directly proportional to the tissue area and the difference in the partial pressure of gas between the two sides of the tissue. It is inversely proportional to the tissue thickness.

FICK PRINCIPLE: A means of calculating cardiac output and blood flow to an organ. The amount of a given substance taken up by a tissue or organ per unit time is equal to the arterial level of that substance minus the venous level, multiplied by the blood flow to the tissue or organ in question. Using O_2 uptake as the variable, cardiac output is calculated as follows: left ventricular output = body O_2 consumption (ml/min)   arterial O_2 (ml/L) - venous O_2 content of the normal human being (ml/L). In the pulmonary artery this is 250 ml/min   190 ml/L arterial blood - 140 ml/L venous blood in the pulmonary artery. This equals 5 L/min. (A mixed venous O_2 sample truly representative of venous oxygenation is difficult to obtain.) See Cardiac output.

FIELD BLOCK: A type of anesthesia technique in which a series of injections are used to encircle the operative site. It can be used in combination with any regional technique. See Block.

FIFTEEN/TWENTY-TWO STANDARD: The connectors with a 15-mm inner diameter and a 22-mm outer diameter which join anesthesia equipment, particularly hoses, bags, masks, and endotracheal tubes.

FILLING PRESSURE: The pressure recorded in the various chambers of the heart while they are being filled with blood.

FILTER: A device or program which separates particulate matter, data, or signals in accordance with selected criteria. It may be a porous membrane which acts as a sieve to separate minute particles from suspension. The efficiency of a filter is measured by the percentage of particles (of a preselected size and characteristic) trapped. Types of filters include electric (which stop random noise but allow coherent signals to get through), frequency (which block certain frequency bands while offering comparatively little resistance to others), bacterial (which block all particles of bacteria size or larger while allowing the passage of smaller particles), and optical (which permit the passage of certain spectral frequencies while suppressing the transmission of others). See Transfusion filter.

FINK VALVE: See Nonrebreathing valve.

FIRST ORDER PROCESS (FIRST ORDER KINETICS): The manipulation of a constant fraction or percentage of a particular molecular group per unit of time. For example, glomerular filtration (passive process) may filter 10% of a given drug/hr. If 100 mg of this drug circulate to the glomeruli in 1 hr, 10 mg will be filtered; in the next hour, of the 90 mg available, 9 mg will be filtered.

FISTULA: An abnormal passage between two internal organs or leading from an internal organ to the surface of the body. It is named according to the organs or parts with which it communicates, such as tracheoesophageal, bronchocutaneous, or bronchopleural.

FIXED ACID (NONVOLATILE ACID): An acid molecule which does not have a significant vapor pressure at body temperature. It must be metabolized or excreted in order to be eliminated from the body. Lactic acid is an example of a fixed acid.

FLAG: A term which refers to an identifiable marker denoting the beginning or end of a set of data. Flags may be inserted in a program to command a computer to stop in order that intermediate information may be communicated to the operator.

FLAGG CAN: A crude draw-over vaporizer which was often used to administer diethyl ether. This vaporizer is a can with several openings on the top. A mask or endotracheal tube is attached to the can by a hose and the ether vapor is picked up as air is blown back and forth by the patient's respiratory movements. This vaporizing method is obsolete.

FLAIL CHEST: A traumatic condition characterized by multiple rib fractures. A paradoxical motion of the chest wall with respiration is evident. There is inadequate pulmonary ventilation and frequently the patient will require mechanical ventilatory support with positive pressure respiration.

FLAME PHOTOMETER: An instrument for measuring the light emitted by a substance when made incandescent by a flame. It is useful in determining the concentration of sodium, potassium, and calcium ions in biologic solutions. Flame photometry is based on the principle that when an atom is exposed to a hot flame, its orbiting electrons are excited causing light emission at a specific frequency. Light intensity is proportional to ion concentration.

FLAME SPEED: The speed at which a self-propagating flame travels in a fuel/air or fuel/O_2 mixture. If the flame speed is too slow, there will be no deflagration in the mixture.

FLAMMABILITY: The capability of a substance or material to support combustion. A self-propagating flame may lead to deflagration. See Deflagration.

FLAMMABILITY LIMITS: The upper and lower limits of the ability of a gas or liquid to support combustion, i.e., a lean or rich fuel/air or fuel/O_2 mixture. Generally, the upper and lower limits of flammability for a given fuel are much higher with O_2 than with air.

FLASHOVER (SPARKOVER): The destructive formation of an arc or spark between two electric conductors.

FLASH POINT: The lowest temperature at which the vapors of a volatile combustible substance will ignite when exposed to flame.

FLAXEDIL: See Gallamine triethiodide.

FLEISCH PNEUMOTACHYGRAPH: See Pneumotachygraph.

FLIGHT-OR-FIGHT RESPONSE: See Epinephrine.

FLOW COMPARTMENTS: The subsections of organs which are characterized by the rate of blood flowing through them.

FLOW CONTROL VALVE (NEEDLE VALVE; PIN VALVE): The basic device used to adjust the amount of gas entering a flowmeter. It is usually located in the base of the flowmeter. As its stem is turned counterclockwise, it moves a pin which allows gas to escape into the flow column. A flow control valve is a precision device easily damaged by misuse, especially if it is overclosed thereby wearing out the pin. See Fig.

FLOW-LIMITED VENTILATOR: See Ventilator.

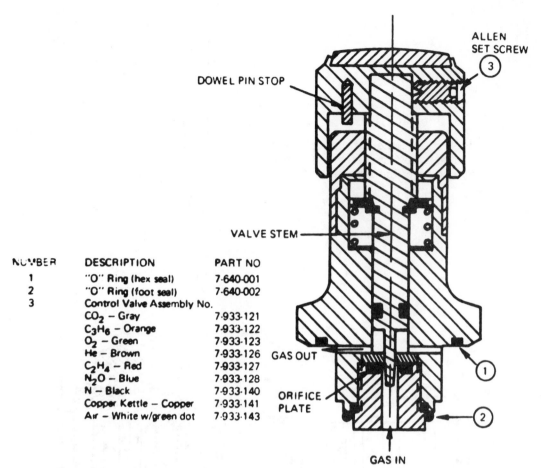

NUMBER	DESCRIPTION	PART NO
1	"O" Ring (hex seal)	7-640-001
2	"O" Ring (foot seal)	7-640-002
3	Control Valve Assembly No.	
	CO_2 – Gray	7-933-121
	C_3H_6 – Orange	7-933-122
	O_2 – Green	7-933-123
	He – Brown	7-933-126
	C_2H_4 – Red	7-933-127
	N_2O – Blue	7-933-128
	N – Black	7-933-140
	Copper Kettle – Copper	7-933-141
	Air – White w/green dot	7-933-143

Flow Control Valve: Cross-sectional view.

FLOWMETER: A device for measuring the flow rate (usually in milliliters or in liters per minute) of a gas passing through it. Modern anesthesia machines use flowmeters or flow columns of the variable orifice type (the Thorpe tube). A Thorpe tube is a transparent tapered tube which has a smaller internal diameter at the bottom than at the top. The tube contains an indicator (also called a ball, float, or bobbin) which floats freely inside the tube. When the flow control valve at the base of the tube is opened, gas entering at the bottom flows upward and lifts the float. Since the tube is tapered, the cross-sectional area of the opening between the float and the inner walls of the tube increases in size as the float goes higher in the tube. The float is buoyed in the gas flow when the pressure drop caused by the gas flowing past the float (which acts as a restriction to flow) equals the weight of the float. This pressure drop across the float tends to remain constant, irrespective of the location of the suspended float in the tube. When the needle valve is turned outward, more gas passes up the flowmeter tube and, for a very short period of time, a larger pressure drop occurs across the float. This pressure drop is greater than the weight of the float so the float moves higher until the pressure drop just equals the weight of the float again. Flowmeter tubes can be of the single-taper type (in which the internal diameter increases by uniform amounts from bottom to top) or the dual-taper type (in which the taper of the lower end increases more slowly than that of the upper part of the tube). See Figs. See Bernoulli law, Poiseuille law.

Flowmeter: (I) Schematic diagram of
a rib guide-type flowmeter. (II) Group
of flowmeters of the rotameter type.

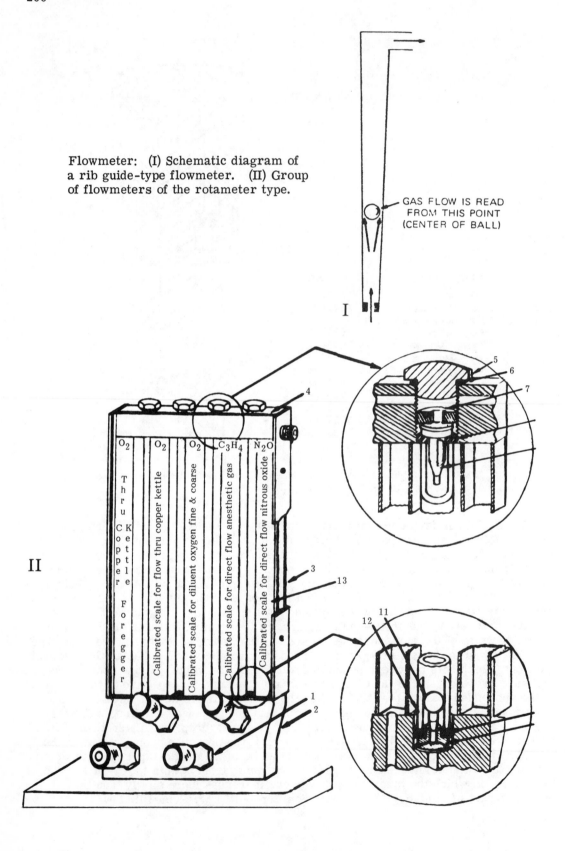

GAS FLOW IS READ
FROM THIS POINT
(CENTER OF BALL)

I

II

FLOW-OVER VAPORIZER: See Draw-over vaporizer; Vaporizer, draw-over; flow-over; bubble-through.

FLOW SHEET (FLOWCHART): A method of data recording and display which illustrates one or more parameters in relation to each other and to time. An example of a flow sheet would be recordings of arterial blood gases at 30-min intervals on a patient with concurrent recordings of respiratory function. A flow sheet can also indicate alternate or progressive pathways for routing messages or materials.

FLUID: An all-encompassing term for liquids and gases.

FLUIDICS: The technique of using pressurized jets of fluid in specially designed circuits performing tasks such as switching or amplifying, which are usually carried out by electronics. For example, a fluidic anesthesia ventilator used in the operating room is powered by high-pressure O_2 switching between inspiration and expiration cycles.

FLUOMAR: See Fluroxene.

FLUORESCENCE: The emission of light or electromagnetic radiation by a substance as the result of the absorption of energy of shorter wavelengths. When the material on the inside surface of a fluorescent tube is excited by ultraviolet (UV) radiation which has been generated when current passes through mercury vapor contained within the tube, it dissipates the UV energy by emitting visible light.

FLUORESCENT LAMP: A device which efficiently converts electric energy to light energy. It may consist of a glass cylinder which contains mercury vapor at low pressure. The inner surface of the lamp is coated with a phosphor. When an electric current is passed through the vapor, ultraviolet radiation is produced which in turn emits visible radiation as it strikes the phosphor. The circuitry which provides high voltage across the ends of the lamp in order to initially ionize the gas is referred to as a ballast.

FLUORESCENT SCREEN: A screen coated with a phosphor which fluoresces as a result of electron excitation. This type of screen is used on cathode-ray and television picture tubes. See Fluorescence.

FLUORIDE: The ionic form of fluorine. Fluoride ion is one of the degradation products of fluorinated hydrocarbon anesthetics and its production in the body has been implicated in renal toxicity, particularly with the drug methoxyflurane. See Methoxyflurane.

FLUORIDE NUMBER: See Dibucaine number.

FLUORINATED (HALOGENATED) HYDROCARBONS: The class name for the stable, nonflammable inhalation anesthetic agents (introduced in the 1950s) which are characterized by different halogen atoms added to a short carbon chain. Fluorine is frequently used for this purpose, being present in halothane, methoxyflurane, enflurane, and isoflurane. See Enflurane, Halothane, Isoflurane, Methoxyflurane.

FLUOROCARBON: A diverse group of chemically inert compounds containing both carbon and fluorine atoms as basic parts of the molecule. See Freon.

FLUOTEC MARK II: See Vaporizer, Fluomatic.

FLUOTHANE: See Halothane.

FLURAZEPAM (DALMANE): A benzodiazepine used as a nighttime sedative. See Benzodiazepine.

FLUOROTHYL: A volatile liquid with a mild, pleasant odor administered by inhalation to cause convulsions. It is an alternative to electroshock therapy but has little clinical use at the present time.

FLUOROXENE; TRIFLUOROETHYL VINYL ETHER (FLUOROMAR): A halogenated hydrocarbon, liquid at room temperature, which was introduced into clinical practice in the early 1950s as a general anesthetic. It is unique in that it is a flammable substance even though it is fluorinated. Because of this flammability the use of fluoroxene was discontinued in the 1970s.

FLUTTER: A defect in the reproduction of high-fidelity sound characterized by changes of more than 10 Hz in frequency.

FORANE: See Isoflurane.

FORCED EXPIRATORY VOLUME (FEV): The volume a patient exhales maximally following a complete inspiration. The amount exhaled in the first second is the FEV_1 whereas the total volume exhaled is the vital capacity (VC). In healthy individuals, the FEV_1 is approximately 80% of the VC. The FEV is a fairly sensitive pulmonary function test to detect obstructive diseases of the air passageways, in which a marked reduction of the FEV_1 is noted.

FORCE-VELOCITY RELATIONS (FORCE-VELOCITY CURVE): A basic method for investigating myocardial contractility. An inverse relationship exists between the force and the velocity of the contractions of cardiac muscle. The velocity decreases as the total load increases. The maximum velocity at which the muscle shortens is called the V_{max} and is considered a good measurement of contractility. Theoretically, at zero load V_{max} is optimal. Since these measurements are only easily made in a suspended intact papillary muscle, it is not a clinically applicable technique; however, it is useful in developing and testing inotropic agents. See Fig.

FOREGGER COMPANY: A manufacturer of anesthesia machines and equipment. Founded by Richard Foregger in 1914, its headquarters are in Langhorn, Pennsylvania. It has been a division of Puritan-Bennett Corporation since 1978.

FORMALDEHYDE (CH_2O): A colorless, pungent, irritant gas. It has some bactericidal activity in a 37-40% solution. It is routinely used as a tissue specimen preservative at a 10% concentration. These aqueous solutions of formaldehyde contain some methanol and are known as formalin. Formaldehyde has many industrial uses.

FOURIER ANALYSIS: The expression of a complex waveform as the summation of sine wave components. For example, both the electrocardiogram (ECG) and the electroencephalogram (EEG) can be broken down into sine wave components of various frequencies. The human EEG can be shown to represent the summation of multiple sine waves with frequencies ranging between 0 and 32 Hz. In fast Fourier analysis, a complex waveform is devolved into its components on line by a computer. This allows display of an EEG as an analyzed waveform a few milliseconds after its detection by scalp electrodes. See Figs.

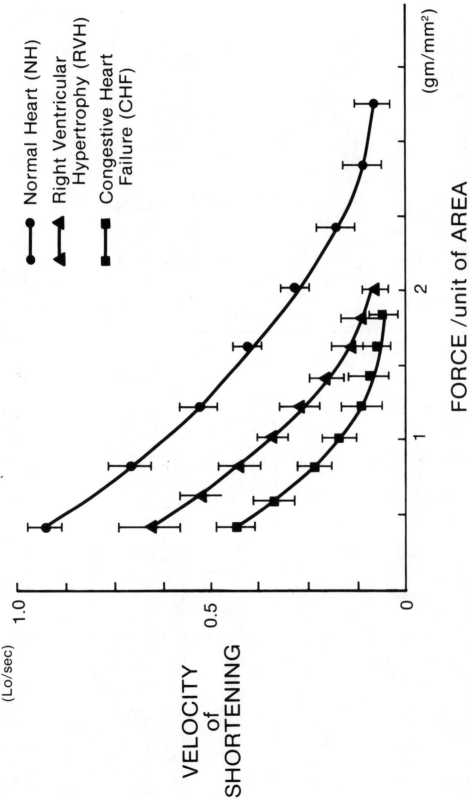

Force-Velocity Relations: Mean force-velocity curves obtained from isolated papillary muscles in the cat. Y axis: velocity of shortening expressed as a fraction of initial muscle length per second; X axis: force per unit of cross-sectional area in grams per square millimeter.

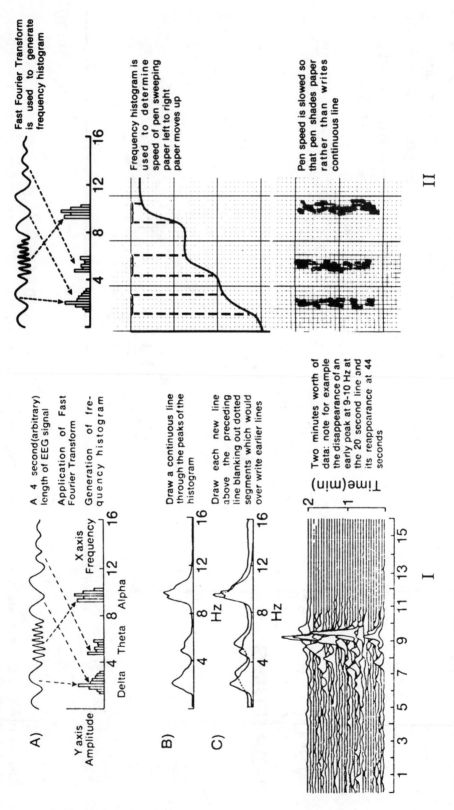

Fourier Analysis: Use of the fast Fourier transform to generate a frequency histogram from an EEG signal. (I) The frequency histogram is used in turn to generate a compressed spectral array. (II) The Fourier transform is used to generate a density modulated spectral array.

FRANGIBLE DISC: See Safety release device.

FRANK-STARLING LAW (STARLING LAW OF THE HEART): A principle which states that the force of cardiac contraction is related to presystolic length of the muscle fibers (and end-diastolic volume). The clinical significance of this observation is that the larger the volume at the beginning of systole, the larger the volume ejected. Practical limits exist in the ability of this mechanism to cope with increased filling volume and therefore this relationship progressively attenuates in the failing heart.

FRASER-HARLAKE COMPANY: A major manufacturer and distributor of anesthesia machines and related equipment based in Orchard Park, New York. The company developed from the merger of several interrelated companies which include Fraser-Sweatman Inc., Cyprane Ltd., and Harlake-Cyprane, Inc.

FREE (UNBOUND) DRUG: The portion of a drug which is not bound to plasma or tissue protein following administration. Typically it is this unbound (free) drug which is pharmacologically active and is available for metabolism and excretion.

FREE ELECTRON: An electron which is not permanently attached to an atom or molecule and can move under the influence of applied electric or magnetic fields.

FREEZE TRACE: See Shift register.

FREEZING POINT: The temperature at which the liquid and solid phases of a substance exist in equilibrium at a defined pressure.

FRENCH NUMBERING SYSTEM: See Endotracheal tube.

FREON: A trademark for a group of halogenated hydrocarbons which contain fluorine. They are widely used as refrigerants and propellants for aerosols. The most common is Freon 12 (dichlorodifluoromethane) which is inflammable in normal usage.

FREQUENCY: The number of complete oscillations or cycles in a unit of time (usually a second). The frequency is measured in hertz.

FREQUENCY CURVE: A method of presenting data in which each data point is plotted on a graph and is then joined by a continuous line. The curve most often encountered in biologic data is the bell-shaped curve (also called the symmetric, normal, or Gaussian distribution curve), in which data points on opposite sides of the central maximum point and equidistant from it have the same magnitude. Curves displaced to the left or the right are called skewed curves and are not symmetric. See Fig.

FREQUENCY DISTRIBUTION: A technique for organizing a complex signal into a series of components based on the frequency of the component. See Fourier analysis.

FRESNEL LENS: A type of lens which uses a series of cuts (or steps) to gain the magnifying qualities of a much thicker and heavier conventional lens.

FRUMIN VALVE: See Nonrebreathing valve.

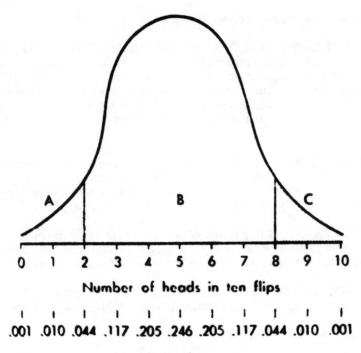

Number of heads in ten flips

.001	.010	.044	.117	.205	.246	.205	.117	.044	.010	.001

Probability of occurrence

Frequency Curve: Frequency curve showing the distribution of heads and tails when a coin is flipped 10 times and the probability of any particular outcome.

FUEL CELL: A device or machine which converts a chemical process, usually oxidation or reduction, into a flow of electricity. The requisite substrates or reagents are introduced continually from outside the cell and react together with the aid of a catalyst.

FUEL, RICH/LEAN MIXTURE OF: An evaluation of quantity of fuel mixed with O_2 or air. In a rich mixture fuel concentration is greater than in the stoichiometric mixture. Combustion will not be complete, i.e., there will be some fuel remaining. In a lean mixture all the fuel will be consumed but O_2 will remain and appear with the final products. See Stoichiometric mixture.

FUNCTIONAL RESIDUAL CAPACITY: The volume of gas remaining in the lungs after a normal expiration. It comprises the residual volume and the expiratory reserve volume. See Lung volumes and capacities.

FUROSEMIDE (LASIX): A sulfonamide which is related to the thiazides. It is, however, a more potent diuretic. Excessive diuresis with this agent can lead to severe hypokalemia and cardiovascular collapse.

FUSIBLE PLUG: See Safety release device.

G

G SUIT: An inflatable garment which can be wrapped around or zipped onto a patient. To achieve the greatest benefit, the suit must be adapted to the patient from the upper chest to the toes. When inflated, the suit places external pressure against the skin of the chest wall, abdominal cavity, and large muscle masses in the legs. The suit counteracts peripheral dilatation and has been found useful in transporting or maintaining patients with low circulating blood volumes or poorly responding sympathetic nervous systems.

GALANTHAMINE: A compound which acts as an antagonist to the nondepolarizing relaxants. It does not appear to be as potent as neostigmine in anticholinesterase activity.

GALLAMINE TRIETHIODIDE (FLAXEDIL): A nondepolarizing competitive muscle relaxant and vagal blocker. The actions of gallamine are very similar to those of tubocurarine, although they may be of slightly shorter duration. The effects of gallamine are dose-dependent. Gallamine is inappropriate for patients with poor renal function. It is metabolized very poorly by the body and excreted unchanged by the kidney. Gallamine also tends to produce tachycardia. See Tubocurarine chloride.

GALVANIC SENSOR: See Oxygen analyzer.

GALVANOMETER: An instrument which measures or detects small currents.

GAME THEORY: The mathematic analysis of conflicting interests to determine the best possible strategy to reach a particular outcome.

GAMMA-AMINOBUTYRIC ACID (GABA): A chemical constituent of the brain. It is a neurotransmitter which appears to be inhibitory as it causes hyperpolarization when released at a synapse. See Receptor/receptor site.

GAMMA CAMERA: A large and expensive gamma ray detection device for visualizing the distribution of radioactive compounds in the body. A radioisotope which is known to emit gamma radiation is administered to a patient. Abnormal concentrations are then detected by the gamma camera which scans the body. The particular radioisotope used depends on its affinity for different body tissues. For instance, phosphorus is used to outline the skeletal system and iodine is used to examine the thyroid gland.

GAMMA-ENDORPHIN: See Endorphins.

GAMMA-HYDROXYBUTYRIC ACID: An intravenous anesthetic agent introduced for clinical use in 1960. It has a slow onset but in appropriate doses deepens into an unarousable anesthetic-like state after which rapid awakening occurs. It does not appear, however, to be a true analgesic as, even during its deepest effects, surgical stimulation causes tachycardia, hypertension, and sweating. It is not currently in clinical use.

GAMMA RAY: An electromagnetic radiation spontaneously emitted from the nucleus of a decaying radioactive substance. Gamma rays constitute the extreme shortwave end of the electromagnetic spectrum. They are not deflected in magnetic or electric fields and have great penetrating power.

GANGLION: A collection of nerve cell bodies located outside the central nervous system. Ganglia are unmyelinated nerve cell bodies and are therefore masses of gray matter. A network of nerves is known as a plexus. Nerve fibers coming into a ganglion and synapsing with neurons contained within are preganglionic fibers. The fibers which leave a ganglion and are anatomically part of the ganglionic neurons are postganglionic fibers. Ganglia can multiply or amplify signals received from the preganglionic fibers, when those fibers synapse with many different neurons.

GARGLE: A technique for agitating a solution in the throat with air from the lungs (keeping the glottis closed). It is used for topical anesthesia of the upper airway in the cooperative patient.

GAS CHROMATOGRAPHY: A method of chemical analysis in which the components of a mixed substance are separated out using an inert gas to move it through a column packed with inert material (diatomaceous earth). As the substance moves along the column, the different constituents are individually slowed by the packing material in the column and therefore arrive at the column end at various intervals. The degree of separation depends on the length of the column, column temperature, type of packing, type of gas, and molecular size and charge of the constituents. Gas chromatography is extremely precise and accurate although it is slow when compared with mass spectrometry. Gas chromatography has been used to detect anesthetic concentrations clinically.

GAS CYLINDER: See Cylinder, gas.

GASEOUS ANESTHETIC AGENT (ANESTHETIC GAS): A pharmacologic agent which is a gas at room temperature and pressure. Included among these are N_2O, cyclopropane, and ethylene. These agents are in contrast to the volatile anesthetics which are liquids at room temperature and pressure, such as diethyl ether, halothane, and trichloroethylene.

GAS TRAP: See Scavenger system.

GASTROSCHISIS: A congenital defect of the abdominal wall which allows the intestines to protrude. The intestines are not covered by the peritoneal sac as they are in an omphalocele. The defect in the abdominal musculature is usually much smaller than with omphaloceles and therefore the musculature can usually be stretched to admit the extruding loop of intestine. The intestine usually takes several weeks to heal because of exposure to the irritating amniotic fluid in utero. Intravenous hyperalimentation is necessary for nutritional maintenance during this recovery period. See Omphalocele.

GATE: An electronic circuit with one output and two or more inputs. Whether an output signal is emitted is dependent on the combination of inputs. There are four basic gates: the "and," "or," "nand," and "nor." These refer to the possibilities in which either 1 and 2 equal x, 1 or 2 equals x, 1 but not 2 also equals x, or neither 1 nor 2 equals x. For example, an operating room has two thermostats, one in the room and one in the corridor. The two thermostats feed into an "and" gate. Both thermostat 1 and thermostat 2 must reach a critical temperature before the "and" gate will energize a heater. If the two thermostats operate an "or" gate, a signal from either thermostat will operate a heater. See Fig.

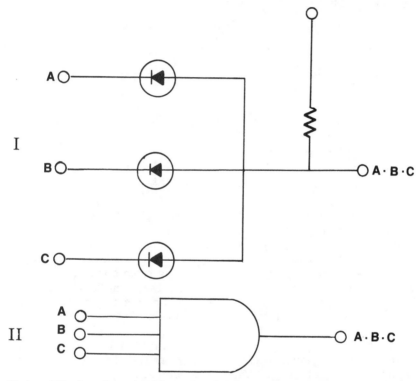

Gate: Electronic gate (I) made of three diodes called an AND gate along with the circuit symbol (II) for this gate. An output signal only occurs when inputs A, B, and C occur simultaneously.

GATE THEORY OF PAIN: The theory that an area of the central nervous system exists which acts like a "gate," i.e., it can block pain sensation from reaching the conscious levels of the brain when activated or "closed." Two observations have led to the formulation of the gate theory of pain control. (1) Stimulation of large sensory fibers from peripheral mechanoreceptors greatly depresses pain transmission in the spinal cord from either the same area of the body or from areas located many segments away. (2) Corticifugal signals (which begin in the cortex where the pain pathway terminates) decrease pain sensitivity by a feedback loop. The common action point of these two mechanisms appears to be in the substantia gelatinosa, a group of small neurons which are located near the tip of the dorsal horn of the spinal cord. This is where pain fibers terminate after they enter the spinal cord and

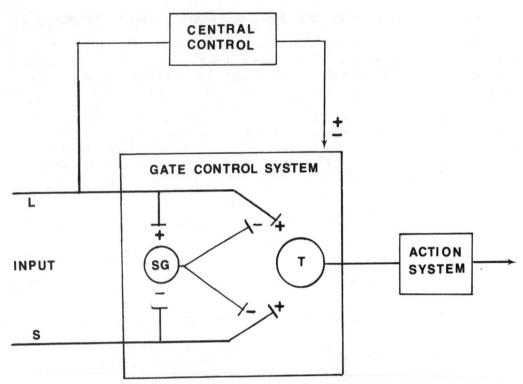

Gate Theory of Pain: Schematic of gate control of pain mechanisms: the large-diameter fibers (L). The fibers project to the substantia gelatinosa (SG) and the first central transmission (T) cells. The inhibitory effect exerted by SG on the afferent fiber terminals is increased by activity in L fibers and decreased by activity in S fibers. The central control trigger is represented by a line running from the large-fiber system to the central mechanisms; the mechanisms, in turn, project back to the gate control system. The T cells project to the entry cells of the action system. +, excitation; -, inhibition.

pass into the tract of Lissauer. It is believed to be in the substantia gelatinosa that the peripheral mechanoreceptor and corticifugal pathways can greatly suppress or prevent the upward travel of pain sensation in the spinal cord. See Fig.

GAUSSIAN CURVE: See Frequency curve.

GEIGER COUNTER: A device for detecting and measuring charged particle emission or electromagnetic radiation.

GENERAL ANESTHESIA: A physiologic altered state classically containing four progressive components: (1) analgesia, (2) amnesia, (3) muscle relaxation, and (4) unconsciousness. Areflexia (particularly of the autonomic nervous system) is now considered a goal of general anesthesia as well. The agents capable of producing these conditions may be administered by inhalation, intramuscularly, intravenously, or via the gastrointestinal tract. Light general anesthesia implies anesthesia with an absolute minimum depression of bodily functions from which the patient returns to normal as rapidly as possible. Deep general anesthesia implies total body depression to just before the point of deleterious reduction of vital signs requiring intervention and support. Light versus deep anesthesia is a continuum that depends on levels of surgical stress as well as dose of anesthetic. See Anesthesia, awareness during; Balanced anesthesia; Depth of anesthesia.

GENERATOR: A device for converting mechanical energy into electric energy.

GENERIC DRUG: A drug which is not protected by patent or trademark. The name usually describes the chemical structure of the agent. Most medications may be sold less expensively in the generic form.

GENTAMICIN (GARAMYCIN): An aminoglycoside antibiotic which inhibits protein synthesis in microorganisms. It has been implicated in augmenting neuromuscular blockade in anesthesia and is useful in treating serious gram-negative infections. It can be both nephrotoxic and ototoxic. See Antibiotic.

GEORGIA VALVE: A low-pressure relief valve found on breathing systems. When open, it allows for the passive escape of excess gas, but it closes rapidly when the pressure jumps to a high level as the bag is squeezed to assist ventilation. This is in contrast to the more common high-pressure relief valve (pop-off valve), which opens only when the preset limit of pressure on the system is exceeded. Both types of valves rid the system of excess gas and both have been used in a circuit at the same time. In general, the low-pressure relief valve is considered more difficult to use than the high-pressure one. See Pop-off valve.

GERIATRICS: The branch of medicine which concerns itself with the problems and diseases of the aged.

GIGA-: The prefix meaning 1 billion (10^9). It may be abbreviated G or B. See SI unit.

GLASS: An amorphous inorganic substance consisting of silicates combined with borates or oxides of boron and phosphorus. Ordinary glass transmits between 85 and 90% of the light striking it, whereas the best optical glass (highly refined with closely controlled impurities) can transmit up to 99%. Borosilicate glass (Pyrex) is known for its resistance to heat and thermal shock and for its low coefficient of thermal expansion.

GLAUCOMA: A disease of the eye characterized by increased intraocular pressure as high as 70 mmHg (normal range is 10-30 mmHg). The rise in pressure is due to the blockage of aqueous humor flow from the anterior chamber. Glaucoma leads to blindness due to atrophy of the optic nerve. Two types of primary glaucoma exist: chronic open-angle (wide-angle) (95% of cases) and acute or chronic angle-closure (narrow-angle) (5% of cases). These terms describe variations in the anatomy of the anterior chamber of the eye which appears normal in chronic open-angle glaucoma and, by contrast, shallow in acute or chronic angle-closure glaucoma. In the latter type, excess dilatation of the pupils may precipitate a worsening of the glaucoma condition. Large systemic doses of scopolamine or atropine may produce this effect.

GLENN SHUNT: An anastamosis of the superior vena cava to the right pulmonary artery. It is usually performed on older pediatric patients with tricuspid atresia in order to increase pulmonary blood flow.

GLOMERULAR FILTRATION RATE (GFR): The quantity of glomerular filtrate (similar to plasma but containing no significant amount of protein) formed per minute in the nephrons of both kidneys. In the glomeruli of the kidney, the filtrate passes through the walls of the glomerular capillaries into the renal tubules. In the tubules, some reabsorption of water and some secretion of solutes change this glomerular filtration fluid into urine. In order to measure the GFR, a substance, such as inulin, is required which will be freely filtered in the glomeruli and neither reabsorbed nor secreted in the tubule. The GFR in an average-sized adult male is approximately 125 ml/min. This is the equivalent of 180 L/day but the normal urine volume is approximately 1 L/day, indicating that more than 99% of the glomerular filtrate is reabsorbed in the tubules. It also means that in 1 day the kidney filters an amount of fluid equal to 4 times the total body water, 15 times the extracellular fluid volume, and 60 times the plasma volume.

GLOTTIS: The part of the larynx consisting of the true vocal cords and the opening between them. See Larynx.

GLUCONEOGENESIS: See Corticosteroid.

GLYCOLYSIS: The splitting of sugars into simpler compounds, such as pyruvate and lactate, usually for the purpose of energy production.

GLYCOPYRROLATE (ROBINUL): A long-acting, atropine-like agent used in anesthesia to dry the mouth and respiratory passageways. It also decreases the acidity and absolute quantity of gastric secretions and acts as an antispasmodic. Because its actions last longer than those of atropine or scopolamine, it can be matched with the longer acting anticholinesterases to reverse neuromuscular blockade.

GOLDMAN VAPORIZER: A universal flow-over vaporizer which does not contain a wick and can be used in or out of a breathing system. It has no temperature compensation and will volatilize many agents. The Goldman vaporizer is controlled by changing a variable bypass. It was originally designed for use in dentistry in conjunction with intermittent flow machines. See Boyle bottle.

GRAHAM LAW OF DIFFUSION: A principle stating that the rate of transfer of different gases through a fine membrane (when the gases are at the same temperature and pressure) is inversely proportional to the square roots of their densities.

GRAM-ATOMIC WEIGHT (GRAM-ATOM): The atomic weight of an element measured in grams.

GRAM-MOLECULAR WEIGHT (GRAM-MOLECULE; MOLE): The amount in grams of an element or compound which is numerically equivalent to its molecular weight.

GRATICULE: A network of fine lines set on a cathode ray tube or the eyepieces of a microscope or telescope which are in simultaneous focus with the object being viewed. They act as a convenient scale with which to measure the object.

GRENZ RAY: An x-ray of long wavelength which was used as a treatment for a wide variety of medical conditions in the past. Of low energy, its penetration through the body was very shallow; therefore, the radiation dose to the skin was quite high.

GROUND (EARTH): A conducting body (usually the earth) used to transmit electric current. The electric potential of the ground is arbitrarily set at zero. Conveniently, ground is usually a stake or cold water pipe directly thrust into the earth.

GROUND ELECTRODE: See Dispersive electrode.

GROUND FAULT CIRCUIT INTERRUPTER (GFCI; GFI): A device that interrupts the current flowing in a circuit when there is a discrepancy in the flow through the grounded and nongrounded conductors of that circuit. If the currents differ, the GFI opens the circuit so that current flow stops. The GFI acts as a safety device to prevent current from returning to ground through an unplanned path.

GROUNDING: A concept referring to the connection of electric equipment to an external common conductor. This provides a harmless pathway for electric current to flow. For instance, the grounding of an electrocardiograph machine is accomplished by connecting its case through the ground wire in its power cord to a conductor beyond the wall socket. This grounding provides for a current path in case the hot side of the power line makes contact with the case due to insulation breakdown or instrument malfunction. If the case is not grounded, the next individual touching the case and ground simultaneously would become the path to ground for the hot side and be shocked. See Ground, Hot versus cold electric circuits.

GROUND LOOP: An unwanted feedback of signal or current through the common ground of two or more instruments. Ground loops can be broken by ungrounding the instrument sensitive to the ground loop, although this is an unsafe alternative. Ground loops may also be broken by connecting the sensitive equipment at a different point to the common ground. The nature of the unwanted feedback signal can be determined and a specific remedy applied, such as inserting an inappropriately sized blocking capacitor into the path to ground.

GUANETHIDINE (ISMELIN): An antihypertensive agent which appears to block postganglionic adrenergic receptor sites and deplete the store of catecholamines. It is useful in the management of severe hypertension. Its actions are similar to reserpine's but guanethidine's advantage is that it does not cross the blood-brain barrier. See Reserpine.

GYVE: A shackle or restraint, particularly for the leg.

$\mathcal{H}$

HALDANE APPARATUS: A device used for measuring CO_2 in a sample. It works by measuring the volume change in a solution which is known to expand upon absorption of CO_2.

HALDANE EFFECT: The phenomenon in which the deoxygenation of the blood increases its ability to transport CO_2. The binding of O_2 with hemoglobin (Hb) tends to displace CO_2 from Hb. When Hb combines with O_2 it becomes a stronger acid than in its uncombined form. The increase in hydrogen ions from the stronger acid drives the reaction of hydrogen and bicarbonate ions toward the formation of carbonic acid which, in turn, dissociates to CO_2 and H_2O. Thus, the Haldane effect causes an increased removal of CO_2 from the periphery due to O_2 being removed from Hb. In the lungs, CO_2 release is enhanced by Hb binding with O_2. The Haldane effect is more important in CO_2 transport than the Bohr effect in O_2 transport. See Bohr effect, Carbon dioxide dissociation curve.

HALDOL: See Haloperidol.

HALF-CELL: An electrode of an electrolytic cell and the electrolyte with which it is in contact.

HALF-LIFE: The time in which the original quantity of a radioactive isotope decays to half its original amount. Decay rates are constant for a given radioactive nuclide. Half-life also refers to the time required for the serum concentration of a particular drug to be reduced by 50%.

HALF-VALUE THICKNESS (HALF-THICKNESS): The thickness of a uniform sheet of material which will reduce the intensity of radiation passing through it by one-half. The term is commonly used when comparing the ability of various materials to shield against radiation.

HALLUCINATION: A perception of stimuli, whether visual, auditory, or tactile, which do not actually exist. See Anesthesia, awareness during.

HALOGEN: An atomic group made up of the elements fluorine, chlorine, bromine, iodine, and astatine. In elemental form, halogens can be very toxic to tissues. When organic molecules are combined with halogens, they become stabilized and their susceptibility to flame, degradation, and metabolism is decreased.

HALOPERIDOL (HALDOL): An antipsychotic agent of the butyrophenone series. Its pharmacologic actions are similar to those of the phenothiazines. See Butyrophenone, Phenothiazine.

HALOPROPANE: An experimental halogenated hydrocarbon anesthetic. Clinical studies on halopropane revealed a tendency to cause myocardial irritability and its use was therefore abandoned.

Halothane.

HALOTHANE (FLUOTHANE; $C_2HBrClF_3$): The first halogenated hydrocarbon to find wide clinical acceptance as an anesthetic. It is currently the most popular inhalation anesthetic agent worldwide. Both a cardiovascular and central nervous system depressant, overdose usually leads to cardiovascular collapse. Induction and recovery is relatively rapid with this agent. Halothane is readily vaporized. It has been implicated in the condition known as halothane hepatitis, a progressive liver failure seen in a very small percentage of patients who receive halothane. The incidence of this disease is given variously as 1:50,000 or 1:14,000 halothane administrations. Usually seen following the second or third exposure, it has occurred in some individuals after their first exposure. Halothane hepatitis has a high mortality rate when florid, and no specific treatment has been found. An aphorism in the anesthesia world states that before the invention of halothane, there were many causes of postoperative jaundice. After the drug was introduced into clinical practice, only one cause remained. See Fig.

HALOTHANE ANALYZER: A device for the quantitative measurement of halothane vapor concentration. There are two principal types. One relies on ultraviolet light and the other on infrared light. Both depend on the fact that halothane absorbs ultraviolet and infrared rays, thereby decreasing the intensity of a light beam in proportion to its concentration. The ultraviolet device is cheaper, has a slower response time, and is accurate to approximately 0.1%. The device measures only halothane. In contrast, the infrared analyzer is very quick and extremely accurate; however, it is sensitive to the presence of N_2O and other halogenated agents and is considerably more expensive. Other methods to detect halothane exist. See Gas chromatography, Mass spectrometer, Narkotest.

HALOTHANE HEPATITIS: See Halothane.

HAND GRIP STRENGTH: A crude test for determining residual neuromuscular blockade. The patient grips the examiner's hand and the strength of grip is estimated. The efficacy of the exam depends on the experience of the examiner.

HARD COPY: Any information recorded in some permanent manner which can be directly read by individuals.

HARD RADIATION: The type of ionizing radiation that has a high degree of penetration. This designation is most commonly applied to x-rays (of short wavelength) and gamma rays.

HARDWARE, COMPUTER: The physical components of a computer system.

HEAD RAISE TEST: A sensitive test to determine recovery from neuromuscular blockade. The supine patient is asked to lift and hold up his or her head. Inability to sustain the head raise indicates incomplete recovery.

HEART, CONDUCTION SYSTEM OF: The intrinsic regulating system of the heart composed of specialized muscle tissue which is responsible for initiating and conducting the electric stimuli that trigger myocardial contraction. These structures are sinoatrial (SA) node, atrioventricular (AV) node, AV bundle (His bundle), internodal atrial pathways, and Purkinje fibers. The SA node, known as the cardiac pacemaker, has the most rapid rate of depolarization. (Its rate of discharge determines the heart rate.) It is located in the right atrium inferior to the opening of the superior vena cava. Once an electric impulse is initiated by the SA node, the impulse spreads outward over both atria causing them to contract. This depolarizes the AV node. The AV node is located near the inferior portion of the interatrial septum and is one of the last portions of the atria to be depolarized. The internodal atrial pathways (anterior, middle, and posterior) conduct impulses from the SA node to the AV node. Projecting from the AV node is the His bundle which descends along the posterior margin of the membranous interventricular septum. The His bundle continues as the right and left bundle branches. It distributes electric impulses over the medial surface of the ventricles. The actual contractions of the ventricles are stimulated by the Purkinje fibers that emerge from the bundle branches and enter the myocardium.

HEAT: The amount of energy (measured in joules) associated with the random movement of the atoms and molecules which make up a substance. When a material contains no heat energy, the molecules would theoretically be at rest and this point is used as a zero point in the Kelvin temperature scale.

HEAT EXCHANGER: A device for transferring heat from one fluid to another. For example, to rapidly cool a patient during extracorporeal circulation, the blood is pumped through tubes sitting in a cold water bath and heat is dissipated to the water in the bath. The important principle of any heat exchanger is that the two substances exchanging heat do not come into direct contact with one another.

HEAT EXHAUSTION: See Heatstroke.

HEATING OR COOLING BLANKET: See Temperature blanket.

HEAT SINK: A device employed to dispose of unwanted heat, thereby preventing a damaging rise in temperature. Most often used in electronics, heat sinks are usually passive, multifinned metal mounts with a large surface area.

HEATSTROKE (HEAT HYPERPREXIA; SUNSTROKE): A condition marked by the cessation of sweating, extremely high body temperature, and collapse. A breakdown of the body's heat regulatory system occurs following prolonged exposure to excessive temperatures. Internal body temperatures higher than 43 degrees Celsius have been recorded. Clinical signs of heatstroke are an increased bounding pulse; hot, dry skin; and rapid, weak respirations. Heatstroke is a threat to life and immediate reduction of body temperature is necessary. An ice water bath and vigorous massage to increase circulation are indicated. Heatstroke should be differentiated from the less dramatic heat exhaustion, the symptoms of which are cold, sweaty skin; weak, rapid pulse; shallow respirations; and no discernable elevation in body temperature (in fact, it may be subnormal). These patients are treated with appropriate electrolyte and fluid administration.

HEAT TRANSFER: The movement of heat energy from one body to another. It can occur by any of the following methods: (1) conduction (heat energy is transferred directly from one molecule to another), (2) convection (heat energy in a fluid is transferred by the movement of the fluid itself), and (3) radiation (heat energy is transferred by means of electromagnetic waves in the infrared range emanating from the body).

HELIUM: A light, colorless, nonflammable gaseous element. It is difficult to liquefy even at temperatures of -195 degrees Celsius. It lowers the specific gravity of any gas(es) with which it is mixed. Therapeutically, a mixture of O_2 and helium can be beneficial in cases of partial respiratory obstruction. In this situation, the mixture decreases the work of breathing and oxygenation improves. However, the use of O_2/helium combinations has been nearly eliminated due to the current practice of tracheal intubation to manage respiratory obstruction.

HELIUM DILUTION TECHNIQUE: A technique for measuring functional residual capacity and/or residual volume using helium, a nearly blood-insoluble gas. A patient breathes in and out of the spirometer which contains a known volume of helium and air. After a few breaths (to reach equilibrium), the helium concentration is measured in the spirometer. From this concentration, the volume into which the helium has been diluted in the lung can be calculated.

HEMATOCRIT: The percent volume of erythrocytes (packed by centrifugation) in a given volume of whole blood. The normal hematocrit value differs from males to females and is extremely labile in the immediate postoperative period due to ongoing fluid shifts.

HEMATOMA: A mass of blood, usually clotted, in an organ, space, or tissue.

HEMICHOLINIUM: An experimental drug which blocks the synthesis of acetycholine by interfering with the transport of choline across the neuronal membrane.

HEMOCONCENTRATION: See Hemodilution.

HEMODIALYSIS (DIALYSIS): A procedure for removing certain unwanted products from the blood. These substances may include (1) natural metabolic end products which have accumulated due to renal disease, (2) ingested toxins, and (3) drug overdoses. The technique requires the creation of an artifical shunt between a large artery and vein. Blood is diverted from the artery into a long coil of semipermeable tubing which is bathed in a dialysate solution into which the undesirable blood constituents migrate. For anticoagulation purposes, heparin is added as the blood leaves the artery, and the heparin effect is reversed by protamine as the blood is returned. In peritoneal dialysis, the dialyzing solution is introduced either continuously or intermittently into the peritoneal cavity. After a period of time the dialysate containing the noxious products is withdrawn. Peritoneal dialysis is often the technique of choice in treating acute poisoning because it requires less time and technology.

HEMODILUTION: An increase in the volume of the blood plasma with a resulting decrease in red blood cell (RBC) concentration. Hemodilution is most frequently seen in clinical practice when non-RBC-containing volume expanders have been administered to counteract blood loss. Hemoconcentration, in contrast to hemodilution, is a decrease in plasma volume resulting in increased RBC concentration.

HEMOGLOBIN (Hb): The O_2-carrying pigment of the erythrocytes which is formed in the bone marrow. It is a conjugated protein: heme is an iron-porphyrin compound joined to the protein globin which consists of four polypeptide chains. Differences in the amino acid sequences of the polypeptide chains give rise to variations in human Hb. Normal adult Hb is called type A; fetal Hb is called type F, and is gradually replaced in the infant's first year by type A. In Hb type S (sickle), glutamic acid replaces valine in the polypeptide chains. With this rather minor change, the deoxygenated Hb form becomes poorly soluble and crystallizes within the red cell at low O_2 tension. This changes the cell shape from biconcave to crescent and greatly increases its fragility. Normal Hb A contains iron in its ferrous (Fe^{2+}) form. Drugs such as some local anesthetics (prilocaine and benzocaine), nitrates, and a number of the sulfonamides oxidize the Fe^{2+} of Hb to the ferric (Fe^{3+}) form. In this state, Hb cannot carry O_2 and is known as methemoglobin. Hemoglobin level in the blood is measured in grams per 100 milliliters. The normal range is 12-16 g/100 ml; women usually have lower Hb levels than men.

HEMOLYSIS: The destruction of red cells resulting in the liberation of hemoglobin into the surrounding fluid. It can be caused by changes in osmolarity and by numerous toxins and drugs.

HEMOLYTIC JAUNDICE: An inherited chronic disease characterized by a yellow appearance to the skin, increased fragility of red blood cells (leading to their destruction), absence of bile pigment in urine, and splenomegaly. Elements of this condition may also be seen following massive red blood cell destruction in a mismatched transfusion.

HEMOPHILIA: A bleeding disorder, almost invariably occurring in males, caused by an inherited (sex-linked recessive) deficiency of at least one blood-clotting factor. It is characterized by spontaneous or traumatic intramuscular and subcutaneous hemorrhages. Classic hemophilia is a deficiency of factor VIII. Christmas disease (pseudohemophilia), a deficiency of factor IX, resembles classic hemophilia in clinical features. See Blood coagulation.

HEMOPTYSIS: The expectoration of blood or blood-stained sputum from the bronchi, trachea, or lungs.

HEMORRHAGE: The heavy loss of blood.

HEMOSTASIS: The process by which bleeding is stopped. This may be accomplished by vasoconstriction, coagulation, or surgical methods. See Fig. See Blood coagulation.

HENDERSON-HASSELBALCH EQUATION: The formula for calculating the fundamental relationship of buffer systems such as bicarbonate-carbonic acid. The general equation for any buffer system is $HA \rightleftharpoons H^+ A^-$ (A^- represents any anion and HA the undissociated acid). For the bicarbonate-carbonic acid buffer system the equa-

Hemostasis: (I) Clotting factors and the minimal levels (percent of normal) required for surgical hemostasis, along with the in vivo half-life and therapeutic preparation used to supply a deficient factor to a patient.

Factor	Minimal Level for Surgical Hemostasis (Percent of Normal)	In Vivo Half-Life (Hr)	Therapeutic Agent
I	50-100	72-144	Cryoprecipitate
II	20-40	72-120	Plasma
V	5-20	12-36	Fresh or frozen plasma
VII	10-20	4-6	Plasma
VIII	30	10-18	Cryoprecipitate
von Willebrand	30	---	Plasma
IX	20-25	18-36	Plasma or II, VII, IX, X concentrate
X	10-20	24-60	Plasma
XI	20-30	40-80	Plasma
XII	0	?50-70	Plasma
XIII	1-3	?72-120	Plasma
Platelets	50,000-100,000/mm^3		Platelet concentrate

Hemostasis: (II) Common tests for the effectiveness of hemostasis and blood coagulation and some of the factors affecting them.

Test	Comment
1. Whole-blood coagulation time (WBCT)	Can be done in operating room; observe for clot retraction and lysis
2. Fibrinogen level	Depressed in DIC
3. Prothrombin time (PT)	Prolonged in hepatic disease, vitamin K deficiency, coumarin anticoagulation, DIC
4. Activated partial thromboplastin time (aPTT)	Prolonged in factor V and VIII deficiencies (massive transfusion), the hemophilias, or in the presence of heparin
5. Platelet count	
6. Bleeding time	Platelet function

tion is pH = pK + log (HCO_3^-/H_2CO_3). The pK for the bicarbonate-carbonate acid buffer system is 6.1. Thus, the equation becomes pH = 6.1 + log (HCO_3^-/H_2CO_3). In 1916, Hasselbalch changed the Henderson equation of 1909 into logarithmic form. The Henderson-Hasselbalch equation is used clinically when the pH and the $PaCO_2$ are determined. The equation can then be solved for bicarbonate and the value can be used to correct acid-base abnormalities. See Dissociation constant.

HENRY (H): The standard international unit of inductance. When a current variation of one ampere per second induces in a circuit an electromotive force of one volt, the inductance of that circuit is said to be one Henry. The milliHenry (mH — one one-thousandth of a Henry) is the sub-unit frequently used in electronics.

HEPA FILTER: An extremely efficient air filter often used in operating room heating and cooling systems. HEPA is an acronym for High-Efficiency Particulate Air. It actually increases in efficiency as it accumulates dirt. HEPA filters are used in laminar flow hoods. See Laminar flow hood.

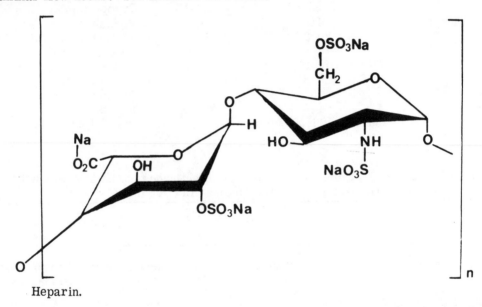

Heparin.

HEPARIN: A naturally occurring molecule produced by the mast cells which are found in connective tissue, especially around the lungs and liver, and in blood vessels. While the normal physiologic functions of heparin are in dispute, it is used in large, nonphysiologic doses to prevent clotting and platelet aggregation. (Heparin is the standard drug used to render blood nonclottable for extracorporeal circulation.) See Fig. See Anticoagulant, Protamine sulfate.

HEPATITIS: An inflammation of the liver usually caused by either viral or toxic agents. Subcategories of hepatitis are viral (type A, type B, and type non-A non-B), toxic (carbon tetrachloride poisoning), alcoholic, and halothane-induced. Viral hepatitis is often associated with either multiple transfusions (type B) or the ingestion of infected shellfish (type A). Populations at increased risk for hepatitis B include drug addicts, renal dialysis patients and personnel, dentists, and other health workers in general. Recently a vaccine has become available which provides a high level of protection against hepatitis B.

HEPATOJUGULAR REFLUX: See Cardiac tamponade.

HEPATOTOXICITY: The property of a substance to damage or destroy liver cells. Carbon tetrachloride is the classic example of a hepatotoxin. Exposure to this volatile chlorinated hydrocarbon in significant concentrations causes direct liver damage proportional to dose.

HERING-BREUER REFLEX: A mechanism which starts inspiration after lung deflation and then initiates deflation after inflation. The action is mediated by the vagus nerve in response to the stimuli of stretch receptors in the lungs. Of the two opposing effects, the one preventing overinflation is stronger. (In humans, the inherent rhythmicity of the respiratory center appears more important than these reflexes in controlling respiration.)

HEROIN (DIACETYLMORPHINE): A powerful narcotic which is physically and psychologically addictive. One of the most abused drugs of this century, it was originally synthesized for use as an antitussive. Produced by a simple chemical alteration of morphine, its relative potency is $2\frac{1}{2}$ times that of morphine. See Narcotic.

HERTZ (Hz): A unit of frequency measurement equal to 1 cycle/sec.

HETASTARCH; HYDROXYETHYL STARCH (HESPAN, VOLEX): A synthetic colloidal polymer used as a plasma expander to replace circulating volume following large blood loss. It is administered by infusion as a 6% solution in 0.9% sodium chloride. Hetastarch has been associated with bleeding difficulties, interfering with type and cross match, and a low incidence of anaphylactoid reaction. See Dextran.

HEXACHLOROPHENE: A phenol derivative that was extremely popular, e.g., Phisohex, as a skin antiseptic. Recently, however, toxicity studies have cast enough doubt on the long-term use of hexachlorophene that its clinical use has been curtailed.

HEXAFLUORENIUM (MYLAXEN): A skeletal muscle relaxant of the competitive (neuromuscular blocking) type which also inhibits plasma cholinesterase and prolongs the action of succinylcholine. It is given as an adjunct to succinylcholine to increase the duration of muscle paralysis and decrease the fasciculations. Its current use is limited.

HEXAMETHONIUM (DRUG C-6): A ganglionic blocking agent originally used to decrease sympathetic tone, thereby lowering blood pressure. The drug is now considered obsolete and is used for experimental purposes only.

HEXOBARBITAL (EVIPAL): An intravenous barbiturate anesthetic which is more potent than thiopental. It is used as an ultrashort-acting sedative and hypnotic. See Barbiturate.

HICCUP: An involuntary spasm of the diaphragm associated with closure of the glottis. Its etiology is obscure but it appears to occur frequently during light anesthesia. Many methods have been proposed for terminating hiccups since they can interfere with proper ventilation. The spasm can best be eradicated by deepening the anesthesia, less satisfactorily by increasing muscle relaxation.

HIGH-EFFICIENCY PARTICULATE AIR FILTER: See HEPA filter.

HIGH-FREQUENCY VENTILATION (HFV): The ventilation of the lungs at respiratory rates in excess of 60 times/min. Experimentally, respiratory rates upward of 600 times/min have been attempted. At such high rates tidal volume is dramatically decreased, almost invariably, to below dead space volume. Despite this, researchers have reported excellent gas exchange and maintenance of arterial blood O_2 and CO_2 concentrations. It is believed that HFV causes a negligible increase in airway pressures and therefore does not produce the circulatory depression which can occur with conventional techniques. It is claimed to be possible to impose HFV onto spontaneous respiration so that it can assist ventilation without having to paralyze the patient. The three subcategories of HFV (delineated by the mechanical means used for ventilation) are high-frequency positive pressure ventilation (HFPPV), high-frequency jet ventilation (HFJV), and high frequency oscillation (HFO). One proposed mechanism of action for HFV is that it works by oscillating the air column in the tracheobronchial tree, thus facilitating diffusion of O_2 downward and CO_2 upward without the actual mass movement of gas.

HIGH VOLTAGE: A term denoting voltage in excess of 650 V, usually used in reference to electric power generation or distribution.

HIPPOCAMPUS: A stratified, curved structure bulging into the inferior horn of the lateral ventricle of the brain. The hippocampus, one of the deep structures of the limbic system, plays a primary role in olfaction and feeding behavior.

HIS BUNDLE: See Heart, conduction system of.

HIS BUNDLE ELECTROCARDIOGRAPHY: See Electrocardiography, His bundle.

HISTAMINE: A naturally occurring substance widely distributed in the body. It can be found in high concentrations in blood (particularly within basophils and mast cells), skin, intestinal mucosa, and lungs. Although its functions are not well understood, it may act as a neurotransmitter. There appear to be at least two types of receptors for histamine, H_1 and H_2. The H_1-receptors are located in the smooth muscles of the intestine, bronchi, and blood vessels. The classic antihistamines bind with this receptor. The H_2-receptors are located in the smooth muscle of some blood vessels and in gastric parietal cells. Useful antagonists are cimetidine, metiamide, and burimamide. Stimulated H_1-receptors generally cause contraction of small muscles and an increase in vascular permeability, whereas stimulated H_2-receptors cause an increase in gastric acid secretion and some vasodilatation. See Fig. See Antihistamine.

Histamine: Structure of histamine and distribution of histamine receptors in the body.

Histamine Receptor	Tissue	Antagonist
H_1	Smooth muscle of intestine, bronchi, blood vessels.	Classic antihistamines (diphenhydramine).
H_2	Gastric parietal cell. Smooth muscle of some blood vessels. Guinea pig atria. Rat uterus.	Cimetidine Metiamide Burimamide

HISTIOCYTE: See Macrophage.

HISTOGRAM (FREQUENCY HISTOGRAM): A graphic representation using a set of rectangles on an X-Y axis to present a mass of data in a summarized and easily understandable form. Histograms are most often used to demonstrate the relative contribution of individual frequencies to a complex signal. See Fig.

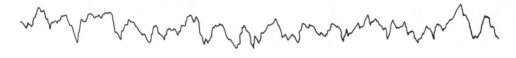

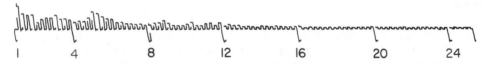

Histogram: Frequency histogram generated by fast Fourier analysis of an EEG signal.

HIVES: See Urticaria.

HOFMANN ELIMINATION: A major means of terminating the neuromuscular blockade of specific newer muscle relaxants. The quarternary ammonium rings, on which the blockade depends, spontaneously rupture as the pH and temperature of the drug molecules equilibrate with the body. (A muscle relaxant, such as atacurium, is at refrigerated temperatures when administered and undergoes nonenzymatic degradation when its pH and temperature are equilibrated with the body.)

HOLE, ELECTRIC: See Carrier, electric.

HOMOLOGOUS: See Autologous.

HORMONE: A chemical substance which has a specific regulatory body function. In general, rapid adaptation to stimuli is mediated by the nervous system whereas slower adaptation to stimuli is mediated by hormones. A hormone may stimulate changes in the "target" organ or may directly affect the activities of all cells in the body. The major endocrine glands and the hormones they produce are as follows. (1) The anterior lobe of the pituitary (adenohypophysis) secretes human growth hormone, adrenocorticotropic hormone, thyroid-stimulating hormone, follicle-stimulating hormone, luteinizing hormone, prolactin, and melanocyte-stimulating hormone. (2) The posterior lobe of the pituitary (neurohypophysis) secretes but does not synthesize antidiuretic hormone and oxytocin. (3) The adrenal cortex secretes glucocorticoids, mineralocorticoids, and, in insignificant amounts, estrogen and androgen, the female and male sex hormones. (4) The adrenal medulla secretes epinephrine and norepinephrine. (5) The thyroid secretes thyroxin, triiodothyronine, and thyrocalcitonin. (6) The pancreas secretes insulin and glucagon. (7) The parathyroid secretes parathormone. (8) The testes secrete testosterone and limited amounts of estrogen. (9) The ovaries secrete estrogen, progesterone, and androgen. (10) The placenta, considered a temporary endocrine gland, secretes human chorionic gonadotropin, estrogen, progesterone, and human placental lactogen. The adrenal medulla and the adenohypophysis differ from the other endocrine glands in that they appear to secrete their hormones under direct nervous system control. For example, the adrenal medulla can be said to function like a secretory ganglion of the central nervous system, as the actions of epinephrine and norepinephrine are quite broad and the duration of their action is quite short.

HORNER SYNDROME: The effects seen when the cervical sympathetic chain is successfully blocked by anesthetic injection (stellate ganglion block) or destroyed by disease (apical lung tumors). Miosis, ptosis, and exophthalmos are present on the affected side. These comprise the original triad of Horner syndrome. Other changes seen on the affected side are reduced sweating, blockage of the nose due to congestion of the nasal mucosa, and flushing of the skin.

HORSEPOWER (HP): A unit of power in the foot-pound-second system in which 1 HP is equal to moving 550 lb 1 ft vertically in 1 sec. One horsepower also equals 746 watts.

HOSPAL/MONAGHAN COMPANY: A manufacturer of anesthesia equipment, particularly ventilators. The company began in the 1940s when its founder, J. J. Monaghan, developed the cuirass ventilator (chest respirator) which permitted patients on iron lung ventilation to become semimobile. In 1977, the Hospal Corporation succeeded the Monaghan Company. The headquarters of the major segment of the company is located in Littleton, Colorado.

HOT VERUS COLD ELECTRIC CIRCUITS: A convention used in describing electric power circuits. The cold side of the circuit (connected to ground) is the conductor distal to the equipment using the electric power. The hot side is the conductor proximal to the equipment. The conductors are usually in a single cord separated by an insulator.

HOT WIRE RESPIROMETER: See Anemometer, hot wire.

HOWARD JONES SOLUTION (JONES SOLUTION): A proprietary solution of dibucaine that was commonly used for hypobaric spinal anesthesia.

HUFFMAN PRISM: A plastic lenslike device which attaches to the proximal end of the Macintosh laryngoscope blade, allowing greater vision of those structures near the tip of the blade.

HUM: An unwanted tone or series of tones heard in the output of an audio circuit. It is caused by extraneous alternating currents generated by the coupling of the audio circuit with nearby power lines. It is an example of incidental capacitance or inductance.

HUMIDIFIER: An apparatus that both supplies and maintains desired water vapor levels in the air. It is used in operating rooms to maintain a minimal relative humidity of 50-60% (a level which ensures the continuous discharge of built-up static charges). It is also used on anesthesia machines and ventilators to add water vapor to the dry fresh gas flow, keeping the respiratory tract moist and secretions loose and preventing the patient (particularly small children) from losing moisture from the respiratory tract. See Nebulizer, Vaporizer.

HUMIDITY: A measure of the degree of dampness in the form of water vapor found in room air or in a breathing circuit. Relative humidity is the ratio of the amount of water vapor present in the air to the maximum amount possible at the same temperature. Humidity is dependent on temperature, i.e., the warmer a gas mass the more water vapor it can hold. If the gas mass is saturated with water vapor and suddenly cooled, water droplets will form. Fully saturated air at 37 degrees Celsius contains 44 mg water vapor/L which exerts 47 torr partial pressure. Fully saturated air at room temperature contains approximately 24 mg water/L. This means that 20 mg of water must be added to each liter of inspired gas to fully saturate it.

HUNTING: The continuous attempts made by automatic control mechanisms to find and maintain a desired equilibrium.

HUSTEAD EPIDURAL NEEDLE: A needle with a rounded point used for epidural anesthesia. The point directs a catheter up or down the epidural space depending on needle position. See Epidural needle, Spinal needle.

HYALURONIDASE: A soluble enzyme found in some animal tissues (and in some malignant human tissues). Hyaluronidase for injection, prepared from mammalian testes, is reported to promote drug absorption and diffusion.

HYDRATE CRYSTAL THEORY OF ANESTHESIA (CLATHRATE THEORY): The theory which states that an anesthetic effect is produced by anesthetic molecules organizing water molecules to form hydrated microcrystals (clathrates) which interfere with the excitability of neurons. No experimental evidence exists to confirm this action of anesthetics and the theory remains unproven.

HYDROCEPHALUS: The excessive or abnormal accumulation of cerebrospinal fluid (CSF) in the ventricles of the brain. The skull may become enlarged and the brain may atrophy. Hydrocephalus, which may be congenital or acquired, can be classified as either communicating or noncommunicating depending on whether or not the CSF in the lateral ventricles is in communication with the lumbar subarachnoid space. In communicating hydrocephalus the ventricles are not obstructed and the CSF passes out of the brain into the spinal canal, but is not absorbed by the sub-

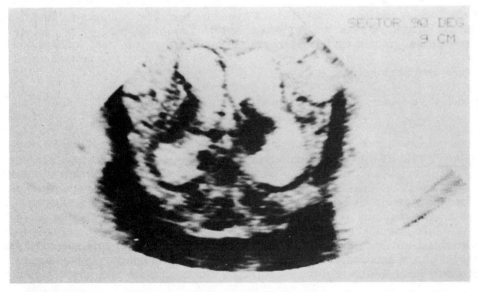

Hydrocephalus: Ultrasound demonstration of the enlarged ventricles of hydrocephalus.

arachnoid villi. In noncommunicating hydrocephalus there is an obstruction of the aqueduct of Sylvius to the fourth ventricle caused by scarring, malformation, or posterior fossa hemorrhage. It can also occur because of obstruction of the foramens of Magendie and Luschka (Dandy-Walker syndrome) blocking flow to the subarachnoid space. Hydrocephalus is treated in an attempt to prevent brain damage due to the progressive encroachment of the ventricles upon the brain mass. It requires the insertion of a Silastic shunt from the ventricles to the peritoneal cavity or, infrequently, to the right atrium. Prognosis is favorable for those infants without brain deformities who have shunts placed prior to brain damage. The shunt becomes a permanent part of the patient; it must be replaced if it becomes infected and lengthened as the patient grows. See Fig.

HYDROCORTISONE: See Corticosteroid.

HYDROGEN: A colorless, odorless, tasteless gas which is the lightest chemical element. It is flammable and explosive when combined with air. The hydrogen ion concentration is an index of the relative acidity of a solution. Hydrogen, which has an atomic number of 1, is a constituent of water and of nearly all organic compounds. The three isotopes of hydrogen — protium, deuterium, and tritium — are all naturally occurring. See Acid-base balance.

HYDROMETER: A flotation instrument for determining the relative density or specific gravity of a liquid.

HYDROMORPHONE (DILAUDID): A semisynthetic derivative of morphine used as a narcotic analgesic. It is approximately 10 times more potent than morphine.

HYDROXYDIONE (VIADRIL): A mildly potent steroid preparation used as a general anesthetic. It is not currently available for clinical practice in the United States.

5-HYDROXYTRYPTAMINE (5-HT): See Serotonin.

HYDROXYZINE (ATARAX, VISTARIL): A synthetic compound closely related to the antihistamine drugs. It is an antianxiety drug with antiemetic properties and produces drowsiness. It is a useful preanesthetic medication.

HYOSCINE: See Scopolamine.

HYPERALGESIA: An abnormal increase in sensitivity to pain.

HYPERALIMENTATION: See Amigen.

HYPERBARIC CHAMBER: See Hyperbaric oxygen therapy.

HYPERBARIC OXYGEN THERAPY: A treatment modality using high-pressure O_2. The patient is placed in a chamber of great structural strength within which O_2 pressure can be contained at 2-3 times atmospheric pressure. At high pressure more O_2 dissolves in blood and tissue so its content increases. The driving pressure differential for O_2 is raised allowing it to reach into areas of low PO_2. Current indications for hyperbaric O_2 therapy include gas gangrene, CO poisoning, and acute arterial insufficiency.

HYPERBARIC SOLUTION: A hypertonic solution used in spinal anesthesia. Its specific gravity is greater than that of cerebrospinal fluid. See Hypobaric solution.

HYPERBARIC TECHNIQUE: See Hyperbaric oxygen therapy.

HYPERBARISM: The deleterious condition resulting from exposure to atmospheric pressures which are higher than the pressures within the body.

HYPERCAPNIA (HYPERCARBIA): An excessive amount of CO_2 in the blood. It refers to an increase in CO_2 arterial tension above 44 torr.

HYPERESTHESIA: An abnormal increase in sensitivity to sensory stimuli.

HYPERINSULINEMIA: An excess of insulin in the blood. The condition can be caused by islet cell tumors, the injection of excess insulin, or the ingestion of sulfonylureas (which stimulate the islet tissue to secrete insulin). Hyperinsulinemia almost invariably leads to hypoglycemia.

HYPERPATHIA: An exaggerated subjective response to noxious or painful stimuli. The patient may incorrectly localize or identify a stimulus and perceive the pain as radiating from nonstimulated areas.

HYPERPNEA: A ventilatory increase which is proportional to an increase in CO_2 production. It is seen in moderate exercise states.

HYPERPOLARIZATION: A brief increase in electric charge across excitable membranes. This period of greater than normal polarization follows membrane depolarization which in turn is followed by the return to normal polarization. See Depolarization. See Action Potential.

HYPERPYREXIA: An extreme elevation of body temperature. See Malignant hyperthermia.

HYPERSTAT: See Diazoxide.

HYPERTENSION: A condition in which the arterial blood pressure (particularly diastolic pressure) is higher than the norm for the age of the patient. It may be idiopathic or may be associated with other diseases (such as pheochromocytoma or renal parenchymal disease). See Arterial blood pressure.

HYPERTENSION, ESSENTIAL: See Essential hypertension.

HYPERTONIC SOLUTION: In biologic terms, a fluid having an osmotic pressure which is greater than that of blood. When cells are surrounded by a hypertonic solution, a net flow of water out of the cells results.

HYPERVENTILATION: An augmented ventilation disproportionate to CO_2 production. An increased amount of air enters the alveoli resulting in a decrease of CO_2 tension and ultimately alkalosis. Prolonged voluntary hyperventilation is often used as a test for epilepsy or tetany. See Epilepsy.

HYPERVOLEMIA: An abnormally increased volume of body fluids.

HYPNOSIS: An altered state of consciousness in which an individual will accept suggestions. An alternate view states that the individual's power to criticize is either partially or fully suppressed during hypnosis. It is postulated that the power of criticism is largely a function of the conscious mind and is therefore bypassed in hypnosis. Hypnosis theoretically deals with the unconscious mind (that portion of the mind which constantly influences thought and behavior although an individual is normally unaware of its presence). In many ways, the state of clinical anesthesia and the state of hypnosis are similar in that both deal with the brain, can be easily demonstrated and described, and are poorly understood. It is a demonstrable fact, however, that in certain individuals deep hypnotic states can completely replace pharmacologic anesthesia for the suppression of noxious stimuli. In clinical terms, it is important to remember that practical hypnosis and pharmacologic anesthesia can be used as adjuncts to one another. For example, the induction of general anesthesia by inhalation can be made smoother in all patients if it is accompanied by a hypnotic state suggesting concentration on quiet, even respirations.

HYPNOTIC DRUG: A compound which produces central nervous system depression resembling normal sleep. See Fig.

HYPOBARIC SOLUTION: A hypotonic solution used in spinal anesthesia in which the specific gravity is less than that of cerebrospinal fluid. See Hyperbaric solution.

Hypnotic Drugs: Approximate serum half-lives of sedative hypnotic drugs.

Generic Name (Trade Name)*	Half-Life (hr)
Benzodiazepines	
Bromazepam (Lectopam)	8-19
Chlordiazepoxide (Librium)	7-28
Diazepam (Valium)	20-90
Flunitrazepam (Rohypnol)	10-20
Flurazepam-HCl (Dalmane)	24-100
Lorazepam (Ativan)	10-20
Nitrazepam (Mogadon)	18-34
Oxazepam (Serax)	3-21
Oxazolam (Serenal)	4.5
Prazepam (Verstran)	24-200
Temazepam (Cerepax, Levanxol)	
Triazolam (Halicon)	2.7-4.5
Barbiturates	
Amobarbital (Amytal)	8-42
Amobarbital Na (Amytal Sodium)	8-42
Aprobarbital (Alurate)	
Butabarbital Na (Butisol Sodium)	34-42
Butalibital (Sandoptal)	
Hexobarbital (Sombulex)	2.7-7
Pentobarbital (Nembutal)	15-48
Pentobarbital Na (Nembutal Sodium)	15-48
Phenobarbital (Various Trade Names)	24-140

* British names used when only available in England.

HYPOCAPNIA (HYPOCARBIA): A deficiency of CO_2 in the blood. It refers to a decrease in arterial CO_2 tension below 36 torr.

HYPOESTHESIA: A diminished sensitivity to stimulation of the skin or sense organ.

HYPOGLOSSAL NERVE: See Cranial nerves.

HYPOGLYCEMIA: A condition in which the glucose concentration in the blood is below normal. The patient may exhibit hyperactivity, sweating, skin pallor, confusion, bizarre behavior, or obtundation.

HYPOKALEMIC PERIODIC PARALYSIS: See Familial periodic paralysis.

HYPOPHYSECTOMY: The surgical removal of the pituitary gland. It is commonly performed through an oral incision, a procedure which causes mild chronic anxiety on the part of the anesthetist due to the proximity of the surgical site to the endotracheal tube.

HYPOTENSION: An arterial blood pressure which is lower than normal for the age and level of physical activity of the patient. It may be seen in shock. Hypotension per se is not a disease and is not considered harmful unless it leads to inadequate tissue perfusion, which can be demonstrated by the onset of metabolic acidosis or, more subtly, by derangement of central nervous system function. The conventional treatment includes position change to increase cardiac return, fluid administration to increase circulating volume, and administration of vasoconstrictors to decrease peripheral blood pooling.

HYPOTHALAMUS: The deep part of the brain forming the floor and part of the lateral wall of the third ventricle. It includes the mamillary bodies, tuber cinereum, infundibulum, and the optic chiasm. Through the autonomic nervous system, the hypothalamus appears to control or regulate visceral functions (mostly related to homeostasis) such as systemic temperature control, food and fluid intake, heart rate, movement of food through the digestive tract, and stimulation or inhibition of the anterior pituitary gland.

HYPOTHERMIA: A subnormal body temperature. This condition may be either deliberately induced or accidental, e.g., environmental. Hypothermia lowers metabolism and the need for O_2 (helpful during cardiac surgery). Under these circumstances the blood pressure is reduced and bleeding is minimal. At 28 degrees Celsius the basal metabolic rate is reduced by approximately 50%; at 18 degrees Celsius the basal metabolic rate is reduced by approximately 87%. However, below 30 degrees Celsius spontaneous ventricular fibrillation becomes an increased hazard. As the body cools, the electroencephalogram shows a less active pattern. At 30 degrees Celsius, the O_2 consumption of the brain is decreased by 50%; at 25 degrees Celsius the O_2 consumption is reduced by 75%. At 15 degrees Celsius the brain can go without circulation for approximately 45 min. Hypothermia can be accomplished by surface cooling (which is quite inefficient) or by extracorporeal circulation (heart-lung machine) of the blood volume through a heat exchanger). Anesthesia must be deep enough so that shivering is inhibited. Deliberate or inadvertent lowering of body temperature below 15 degrees Celsius is called supercooling (profound hypothermia). See Cardiopulmonary bypass, Heat exchanger.

HYPOTHERMIC SUBARACHNOID IRRIGATION: See Cold saline injection.

HYPOTONIC SOLUTION: In biologic terms, a fluid having an osmotic pressure which is less than that of blood. When cells are surrounded by a hypotonic solution, a net flow of water into the cells results. This can lead to cell bursting.

HYPOVENTILATION: A reduced ventilation which is insufficient in rate and/or total volume to maintain alveolar O_2 tension and eliminate CO_2 (PaO_2 falls and $PaCO_2$ rises).

HYPOVOLEMIA: An abnormally diminished volume of body fluids, particularly in the intravascular space.

HYPOVOLEMIC SHOCK: See Shock.

HYPOXIA: The relative lack of O_2 transported to or used by the tissues. There are four types of hypoxia. (1) Anemic hypoxia is a relative lack of O_2 in the tissues due to a reduction of the O_2-carrying capacity of the blood. This is usually caused by an insufficient amount of hemoglobin (Hb) in the red cells. (2) Anoxic hypoxia is a relative lack of O_2 delivered to the tissues due to insufficient oxygenation of Hb in the lungs. (3) Histotoxic hypoxia is a relative lack of O_2 due to impaired ability of the tissues to use O_2, e.g., cyanide toxicity. (4) Stagnant (ischemic) hypoxia is a relative lack of O_2 due to a too-slow delivery of oxygenated blood to the tissues which does not compensate for O_2 uptake and usage. See Fig.

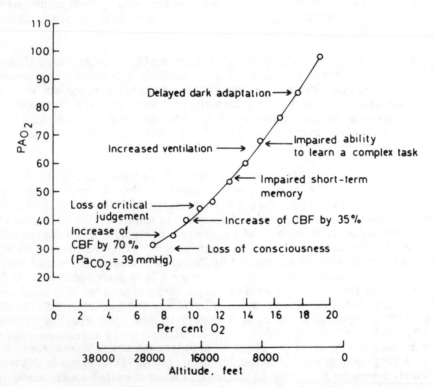

Hypoxia: Influence of inspired O_2 concentration on PAO_2 in humans as well as on some symptoms of and physiologic responses to hypoxia. From Siesjo, B. et al. 1974. Brain Dysfunction in Metabolic Disorder. p. 72. New York: Raven Press.

HYPOXIC SHUNT: A physiologic response of normal lung tissue triggered by a sharp decrease in inspired O_2 tension. This effect is best seen experimentally when a hypoxic gas mixture is administered to only one lung. The pulmonary vascular resistance of the hypoxic lung rises, thereby shunting blood to the normal lung. The effect may occur in small areas of the lung after regional airway obstruction. The shunted fraction of pulmonary blood flow may rise for many hours before peaking. The peak is reached faster in younger individuals with healthy lungs.

HYPOXIC VASOCONSTRICTION: A phenomenon which occurs in the lung when the PAO_2 is reduced. It is characterized by smooth muscle contraction in the walls of the arterioles in the hypoxic region. (It is the PAO_2, not the PaO_2, which causes this response.) A salutary effect of hypoxic vasoconstriction is that it directs blood flow away from the hypoxic regions of the lung. For example, in bronchial obstruction, the diversion of blood flow diminishes the deleterious effect on gas exchange by halting perfusion of poorly ventilated alveoli. Reversal of hypoxic vasoconstriction occurs at birth. Upon the infant's first breath, the vascular resistance falls dramatically and the pulmonary blood flow greatly increases. However, should the infant become hypoxic, the sudden rise in pulmonary vascular resistance caused by hypoxic vasoconstriction can overload the right side of the heart.

HYSTERESIS, LUNG: A demonstration of the effect of lung surfactant. It is a phenomenon seen in the laboratory in an isolated lung which is first degassed, then inflated with air to its maximum volume, and then deflated. The relationship between pressure and volume is different on the inflation curve from what it is on the deflation curve. For a given pressure, the volume of the lung is greater during deflation

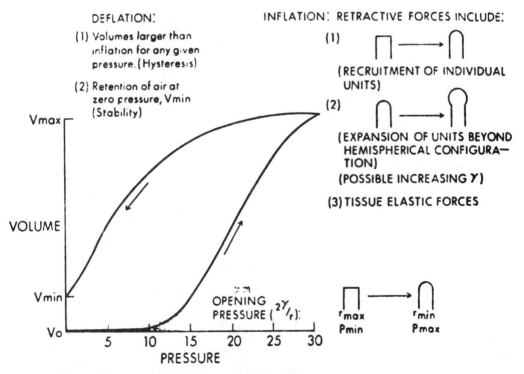

Hysteresis, Lung: Volume-pressure diagram of a degassed lung.

than inflation. This separation of the curves of inflation and deflation is termed hysteresis. Hysteresis is caused by surface forces at the air-liquid interface which exist in the air-filled lung. Evidence for this explanation is that when the degassed lung is filled and emptied with a liquid, hysteresis is negligible. See Fig. See Surfactant.

H ZONE: See Actomyosin.

I

IATROGENIC: A term applied to any adverse condition which occurs as the result of treatment by a health care worker. A sore throat after intubation of the trachea is an example of an iatrogenic complication.

IDEAL GAS: A theoretic entity which perfectly obeys Boyle law, Charles law, Joule law of internal energy, Dalton law of partial pressure, and Avogadro hypothesis. Actual gases only obey these laws as their pressure tends toward zero.

I/E RATIO: The ratio of the time for inspiration versus expiration. Because it is a slow passive process (particularly in the patient on a ventilator), expiration should be given as much of the breathing cycle time as possible. The minimum expiratory time should be equal to the inspiratory time. Many ventilators have an I/E ratio control which can be preset at 1:1, 1:2, or 1:3. As the respiratory rate increases, the time available per minute for expiration decreases. High ventilatory rates are often precluded by the requirement that expiration time be (at least) equal to inspiration time.

IGNITION TEMPERATURE: The temperature to which a fuel/air or fuel/O_2 mixture must be raised to start deflagration.

IMAGE INTENSIFIER: A device that combines the capabilities of x-rays and television to produce an image with minimal radiation exposure to the patient. In conventional x-ray techniques, a relatively large amount of radiation must be used to "expose" an x-ray plate. With an image intensifier only a low dose of radiation is necessary to penetrate the patient and then strike a fluorescent screen. This screen is scanned by a television camera, the signal output of which is amplified, increased in contrast, and displayed on a TV monitor. The key to the technique is the electronic amplification provided by the TV technology.

IMPEDANCE: See Bypass capacitor.

IMPEDANCE PLETHYSMOGRAPHY: The measurement of cardiac output or tissue volume changes of a body part based on the detected alterations in electric impedance between two surface electrodes. A constant difference in voltage is maintained between the electrodes. As the impedance of tissue varies, due to the ingress and egress of blood, current flow changes between the electrodes and is related to cardiac output or volume changes. See Ohm law.

IMPLANT TESTED (IT): See Z-79.

IMPLIED CONSENT: A legal term relating to the inferred approval by a patient for medical intervention during emergency situations. Although the patient is unable to communicate, it is assumed that he or she would agree to the necessary treatment. In addition, a patient may imply consent by his or her actions, e.g., by extending an arm, consent is given for palpating the pulse.

IMPLIED CONTRACT: See Contract.

IMPURITIES, ELECTRIC: A naturally occurring or deliberately implanted foreign atom found in semiconductors. Impurities fundamentally affect basic electric conductivity. The technique of implanting impurities is called doping. See Doping.

IN VITRO STUDY: A test or observation made "within a glass," such as a test tube or Petri dish, or outside the intact organism, e.g., withdrawing an arterial blood sample for gas analysis in a blood gas machine.

IN VIVO STUDY: A test or observation made within the intact organism, e.g., arterial pH measured by an appropriate electrode placed in an artery.

INAPPROPRIATE ANTIDIURETIC HORMONE (ADH) SECRETION SYNDROME: A disorder in which an abnormal amount of ADH is excreted, leading to water retention with respect to body fluid osmolality. It is frequently associated with small cell carcinoma (oat cell variant) of the lung, a variety of pulmonary and central nervous system disorders, or it may be idiopathic.

INAPSINE: See Droperidol.

INCANDESCENCE: The emission of visible radiation from a substance at high temperatures.

INDEPENDENT VARIABLE: A quantity the value of which bears no direct relationship to any other variables of concern. For example, the time of day is an independent variable in plotting a patient's pulse rate.

INDERAL: See Propranolol.

INDIFFERENT ELECTRODE: See Dispersive electrode.

INDIRECT MONITOR: See Noninvasive monitor.

INDOCYANINE GREEN (CARDIO-GREEN): A dye injected for the measurement of cardiac output by the dye dilution technique. See Cardiac output.

INDUCTANCE: The resistance a coil offers to an alternating current due to the creation of a magnetic field surrounding the coil. Capacitance, simple resistance, and inductance constitute electric impedance. See Capacitance, Impedance.

INDUCTION: The period in anesthetic administration which includes the time that the first drug is administered until the desired depth of the anesthetic state is reached. Various subcategories of induction exist. Inhalation induction refers to the steady increase of anesthetic vapor concentration delivered to a patient's airways. Intravenous (IV) induction is the IV administration of an anesthetic agent in

a stepwise or continuous infusion. Routine induction implies that the drug administration occurs in a controlled incremental manner. Crash induction (rapid sequence
induction) involves the administration (usually IV) of a single overwhelming dose of
anesthetic, commonly with a neuromuscular blocking agent, in order to gain control
of the patient's respiration and reflexes as rapidly as possible. Crash induction is
indicated in a patient with a full stomach in whom regurgitation and aspiration of
gastric contents would be a possibility with prolonged induction. However, it is important to remember that crash induction involves an increased risk since there is
a concurrent stepwise change in the vital signs. See Sellick maneuver.

INDUCTION HEATING: A method of producing heat in a conducting material by
passing a high current through it.

INFANT RESPIRATORY DISTRESS SYNDROME (IRDS; HYALINE MEMBRANE DIS-
EASE): A major cause of death in premature infants. The immature lung does not
manufacture sufficient quantities of surfactant to reduce alveolar fluid surface tension in order to stabilize the alveoli. The air sacs collapse on expiration producing
atelectasis, and the infant becomes cyanotic and hypoxic. Prediction of whether a
premature infant will develop IRDS is based on the ratio of lecithin, a major component of surfactant, to sphingomyelin in the amniotic fluid. If the ratio is greater
than 2:1, the probability that the fetus will have IRDS is less than 10%. Infants with
severe IRDS require long-term intensive care. See Adult respiratory distress syndrome, Surfactant.

INFARCT: An area of tissue necrosis caused by local obstruction of the arterial
blood supply. This obstruction is usually an embolus or thrombus, and the actual
cause of the tissue necrosis is insufficient oxygenation. See Myocardial infarction.

INFERIOR VENA CAVA SYNDROME: See Aortocaval syndrome.

INFLOW OCCLUSION: A technique used during myocardial surgery. A snare is
placed around the superior and inferior vena cavas and the pulmonary veins to prevent flow of blood into the heart. At normal body temperature, approximately 3 min
of surgical time is available before cardiac damage occurs; at 30 degrees Celsius
8 min is available. The technique has generally been abandoned in favor of extracorporeal circulation, which provides more surgical time and better operating conditions. See Cardiopulmonary bypass.

INFORMATION THEORY: A mathematic technique concerned with the analysis of
parameters involved in information acquisition and handling.

INFORMED CONSENT: The legal doctrine that every patient must understand the
potential complications of any procedure before it is performed. To give informed
consent for anesthesia, a patient must be aware that it is conceivable that the anesthetic process could result in debility, disfigurement, or death. See Consent form.

INFRARED ANALYZER: A device for measuring the content of a particular gas in
a gaseous mixture. It is most useful for the quantification of N_2O and CO_2 since
both of these gases absorb infrared light of a specific band proportional to their concentration with correctable overlap. See Halothane analyzer.

INFRARED RADIATION (IR): A part of the electromagnetic spectrum which trans-
fers heat energy from its source to its surroundings. See Electromagnetic spectrum.

INFRASOUND: An automated device for the determination of arterial blood pressure. The principle involves detection and amplification of sounds (in a frequency range below human hearing) created by turbulent blood flow past a deflating cuff. It is favored for pediatric and low arterial pressure situations. See Arterial blood pressure, Sound.

INHALATION ANESTHESIA: The administration of volatilized pharmacologic agents via the respiratory tract for the purpose of producing anesthesia. The outstanding advantage of administering drugs in this manner is that they can be retrieved by the same route as long as respiration is maintained. This, of course, presupposes that the drugs are neither metabolized nor excreted via another route by the body. Inhalation administration allows drugs to reach the central circulation rapidly and appear on the arterial side of the circulation faster than by intravenous injection. Significant disadvantages of inhalation anesthesia include the necessity of complex and sophisticated equipment to assure controlled administration. Inhalation anesthesia also requires manipulation of the upper airway. In addition, if the agent used is a liquid, it must have a vapor pressure at room temperature high enough to assure administration of a therapeutic dose. See Halothane.

INHALER: An apparatus for vaporizing liquids which will be inhaled. When used for analgesia it is a simple device which has a fixed upper limit of output and can therefore be safely used for self-administration. See Goldman vaporizer.

INHIBITION OF OXIDATION: A theory which attempts to explain the action of general anesthetics. It states that anesthetics primarily inhibit the utilization of O_2. (The theory is more an observation than an explanation of the anesthetic mechanism.)

INHIBITOR: An agent which slows or stops a chemical reaction or a biologic process.

INHIBITORY POSTSYNAPTIC POTENTIAL (IPSP): See Excitatory postsynaptic potential.

INITIAL SEGMENT: The nonmyelinated part of an axon hillock from which the axon arises. This is the area of a neuron in which the threshold for depolarization is lowest.

INK SPACE CUFF (DURAL SLEEVE) REGION: The thin area of the dura which may be the site for transdural anesthetic transfer from the peridural space to the perineural region. This area has been found to permit the passage of colloidal carbon particles and it is therefore presumed to permit passage of crystalloid particles and local anesthetic agents.

INNERVATION: The supply of nervous pathways (or the conveyance of nervous impulses) to or from a body part or organ.

INNOVAR: A proprietary combination of droperidol and fentanyl in a 50:1 ratio (by weight). It is useful as both a preoperative medication and as a supplement to N_2O/O_2 anesthesia. Innovar produces neuroleptanesthesia. See Neuroleptanesthesia.

INOTROPISM: The ability to influence muscular contraction either negatively or positively. Propranolol is a negative inotropic agent in relation to myocardial contractility whereas isoproterenol is a positive one.

INPUT-OUTPUT (I/O): A term that generally refers to the equipment used to communicate with a computer and to receive its results. For example, a cathode ray tube terminal is an I/O device.

INSENSIBLE WATER LOSS: The water loss directly from the skin (due to evaporation of sweat) and from the lungs (due to the exhalation of 100% water-saturated gas). In adults, insensible water loss is approximately 100-400 ml/day.

INSPIRATORY HOLD: A technique of respiratory therapy used to expand atelectatic areas of lung tissue. The lungs are maintained in the inflated state either by hand pressure on a breathing bag or by inhibition of the expiratory cycle on a ventilator.

INSTANTANEOUS PULMONARY BLOOD FLOW: A measurement of pulmonary blood flow taken while a patient is in a body plethysmograph (air-tight chamber). The patient breathes a mixture of N_2O and O_2 from a rubber bag inside the chamber. The N_2O is abosrbed into the pulmonary blood. This decreases the total amount of gas in the chamber and reduces its volume. The blood flow can be calculated by measuring (1) the small, stepwise drops in pressure and volume in the chamber, (2) the N_2O concentration in the alveoli, and (3) the solubility coefficient of N_2O in the blood. See Body plethysmograph.

INSTANTANEOUS SAMPLE (GRAB SAMPLE): A single sample of atmospheric gas taken in a leak-free and nonabsorbent container to spot-check for trace anesthetic gas contamination.

INSUFFLATION: The act of blowing a gas, powder, or vaporized drug into a body cavity. See Insufflation, intraperitoneal.

INSUFFLATION ANESTHESIA: A technique in which a high flow of anesthetic gas is delivered via an "ether" hook inserted at the corner of the mouth. The patient breathes spontaneously. Although insufflation anesthesia is simple to administer, it has been largely replaced by more sophisticated delivery systems which do not waste gas, dry the airways, or pollute the operating room environment.

INSUFFLATION, INTRAPERITONEAL: A technique in which CO_2 is introduced into the abdomen via a trocar through a small infraumbilical incision. Carbon dioxide is the gas of choice as N_2O may combine with bowel gas released by an inadvertant puncture of the intestines to form a flammable or explosive mixture. Insufflation with CO_2 enlarges the abdominal cavity thereby facilitating direct visual examination of the organs with a laparoscope. The technique is often used in electrosurgical tubal ligation and for investigation of possible abdominal or pelvic disease or trauma where a conventional laparotomy is contraindicated because of the patient's condition.

INSULIN: An essential hormone secreted by the islets of Langerhans in the pancreas. It is important for the proper control of plasma glucose levels. Interference with or nonproduction of insulin results in a constellation of abnormalities collectively referred to as diabetes mellitus. See Diabetes mellitus.

INSULT: An action or event that decreases the functional integrity of an organism or system.

INTENSIFYING SCREEN: A plate or screen, coated with a material such as calcium tungstate, which emits light when bombarded with x-rays. This light further exposes the x-ray film placed on it, making it possible to achieve a better x-ray picture while lowering the amount of radiation needed to produce it.

INTENSITY MODULATION: The process (or effect) of varying electron-beam current in a cathode ray tube. Since the brightness of a particular spot on the tube becomes proportional to the magnitude of the signal, modulation allows a two-dimensional display to provide three simultaneous pieces of information: the X coordinate, the Y coordinate, and brightness.

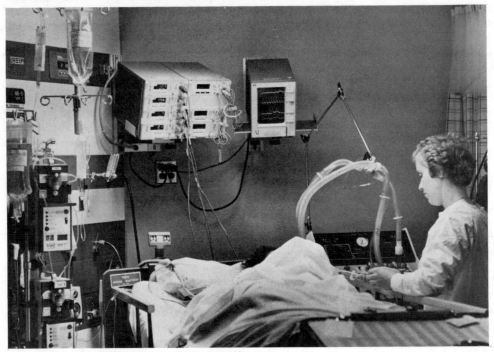

Intensive Care Unit: Typical unit.

INTENSIVE CARE UNIT (ICU): A specialized hospital unit in which seriously ill patients are given continual nursing care aided by enhanced monitoring techniques. Intensive care units are often separated into surgical and medical divisions. The care in these units is always extremely expensive but its effectiveness is demonstrated in treating diseases that may be devastating but potentially reversible.

INTERCOSTAL BLOCK: A regional nerve block in which a local anesthetic is injected into the intercostal space(s). The block (1) provides pain relief after rib fractures or abdominal surgery, (2) facilitates deep breathing and coughing after surgery, and (3) is useful for superficial surgery of the chest, back, or abdominal wall. The production of a pneumothorax is the potential major complication of an intercostal block. See Figs.

INTERMITTENT FLOW MACHINE (DEMAND FLOW MACHINE): A type of anesthesia delivery system used mainly for outpatient dental anesthesia. There is a single control that continuously varies the percentages of O_2 and N_2O delivered by the machine. (The dentist is able to perform the necessary dental work while operating the simple control mechanism on the machine.) There is no gas flow out of the com-

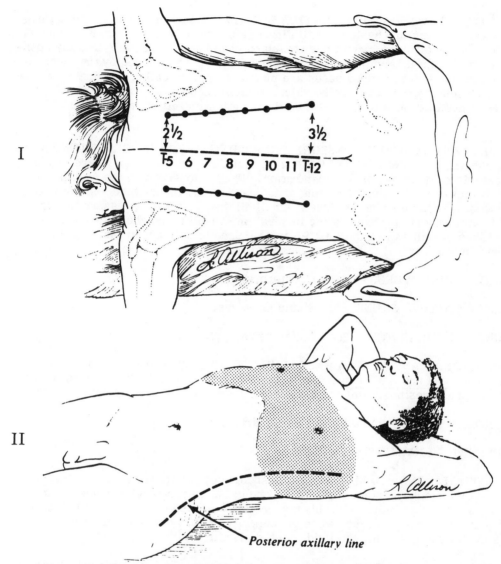

I

II

Posterior axillary line

Intercostal Block: (I) Superficial landmarks for block of the intercostal nerves on the posterior aspect of the body. The needles are inserted $2\frac{1}{2}$-$3\frac{1}{2}$ in from the midline. The arms are drawn upward and outward to move the scapulae away from the field. (II) Position of the patient for block of the intercostal nerves along the posterior axillary line. The light shaded area shows the sensory distribution of the nerves more easily blocked in this position.

mon outlet until a patient creates a negative pressure within the mask and the gas delivery hoses during inspiration. This negative pressure causes a valve to open and gas to be delivered in the proportion and pressure set by the adjustment controls. The intermittent flow system has some inherent disadvantages. Most commonly, the single mixture control can become blocked by dirt rendering it inaccurate. The flow control is also subject to wide variation in calibration, so that if a patient inspires deeply, it is often impossible for the machine to produce enough flow to supply all the patient's required gas without being diluted by room air.

INTERMITTENT MANDATORY VENTILATION (IMV): The process by which a patient is weaned from mechanical ventilation in a progressively decreasing manner.
A T-tube and respiratory circuit are combined enabling the patient to breathe spontaneously with a predetermined number of mandatory breaths aided by the mechanical ventilator. Arterial blood gases are measured periodically to evaluate the adequacy of alveolar ventilation. If the values remain acceptable, the rate of mechanical assistance continues to decrease until the patient is fully weaned. See Weaning.

INTERMITTENT POSITIVE PRESSURE BREATHING (IPPB); INTERMITTENT POS-
ITIVE PRESSURE VENTILATION (IPPV): A technique of respiratory care in which
the airway is pressurized during inspiration. Used extensively in the postoperative
period to improve pulmonary function, it is based on the theory that positive pressure encourages the opening of closed, small airways. Airway pressure is allowed
to fall to atmospheric pressure after inspiration, enabling the chest wall and lungs
to recoil and permit expiration. (IPPB is also used to deliver aerosol drugs to the
bronchopulmonary tree.) See Continuous positive airway pressure.

INTERNAL CARDIOVERSION: See Cardioversion.

INTERNAL CAROTID SHUNT: See Stump pressure.

INTERNAL JUGULAR VEIN: See Jugular veins.

INTERNATIONAL ANESTHESIA RESEARCH SOCIETY: The organization which pub-
lishes Anesthesia and Analgesia. Based in Cleveland, Ohio, it was founded in 1919
as the National Anesthesia Research Society and adopted its present name in 1925.

INTERNODAL ATRIAL PATHWAYS: See Heart, conduction system of.

INTERSPINOUS LIGAMENT: See Lumbar puncture.

INTERSTITIAL LUNG EDEMA: The earliest form of pulmonary edema. It is characterized by the engorgement of the peribronchial and perivascular spaces which
normally serve as conduits for fluids that might otherwise escape into the alveoli.
Frank pulmonary edema occurs when the capacity of the lymphatics to drain these
spaces is exceeded, forcing the fluid into the alveoli.

INTESTINAL OBSTRUCTION: A blockage to the normal flow of solids and fluids in
the intestine. It can be due to solid particles blocking the lumen, infection, inflammation, malignant tumor, extrinsic pressure, stricture, or twisted bowel. Any obstruction causes an increase in the anesthetic risk since the elevated pressure proximal to the obstruction makes the patient more susceptible to esophageal reflux and
possible aspiration.

INTESTINAL STERILIZATION SYNDROME: A condition in which there is a marked
decrease in the normal bacterial count in the intestine. It is seen in patients who
have received large doses of antibiotics. Since bacteria produce most of the vita-
amin K normally available to the body, an effect on the prothrombin time may be
evident within 7 days if vitamin K supplementation is not administered.

INTRA-AORTIC BALLOON PUMP (IABP): A device used to assist or improve circulation in patients with inadequate cardiac output. The IABP may be used in patients (1) with ischemic heart disease due to cardiogenic shock, acute myocardial

infarction, or refractory ventricular arrhythmias; (2) undergoing cardiac catheterization, cardiac surgery, or noncardiac surgery; or (3) with pediatric congenital heart disease. The IABP is inserted into the descending thoracic aorta; the tip of the balloon is inflated (with helium or CO_2) during diastole, thereby producing an increase in blood pressure and coronary blood flow. Ventricular afterload is decreased by balloon deflation just prior to systole. The actual inflation and deflation of the IABP is timed from the T wave (or dicrotic notch) and QRS complex of the electrocardiogram.

INTRACARDIAC ELECTROCARDIOGRAM: The graphic recording of electric currents generated by the heart by means of an electrode introduced into the heart via an intravenous catheter. The technique requires the precise placement of the catheter and monitoring of the movement of the catheter tip during introduction. Proper placement of the catheter is evidenced by an increasing amplitude of the P wave, which is upward deflecting as the catheter approaches the right atrium and downward deflecting as it traverses the right atrium and approaches the right ventricle.

INTRACEREBRAL STEAL SYNDROME: The unpredictable shifts in the distribution of cerebral blood flow in damaged or diseased areas of the brain. One region may be hyperperfused while another may be ischemic due to the breakdown of normal autoregulatory control of cerebral blood flow. In the hypothetical Robin Hood syndrome, deliberate hypocapnia causes constriction of normal cerebral blood flow areas and redirects it to maximally dilated ischemic areas. In the hypothetical Sheriff of Nottingham syndrome, hypercapnia dilates normal areas, directing the blood flow away from ischemic areas which are already maximally dilated.

Intracranial Hypertension.

Etiology	Treatment
Intracranial mass	Surgical removal

Cerebral edema	Fluid restriction
	Diuretics
	  Osmotic
	  Tubular
	Steroids
	Hyperventilation
	Hypothermia
	Barbiturates
	Controlled hypotension
	Surgical decompression

Increased intravascular blood volume	Position Hyperventilation Blood pressure stability Muscle relaxants Barbiturates
CSF retention	Osmotic agents Reduction of CSF formation CSF shunting procedure

INTRACRANIAL HYPERTENSION: A condition that exists when the measured intracranial pressure (ICP) is greater than 15 mmHg (normal range is between 5 and 15 mmHg). Elevated intracranial pressure, however, is not an absolute predictor of neurologic function. ICPs in the range of 80-100 mmHg associated with low cerebral perfusion pressures have been demonstrated to exist in patients with little or no neurologic deficit, but, as a generality, neurologically significant intracranial hypertension is associated with rapid increases in the ICP. The relevance of ICP measurement to patient care is compromised in cases where bony defects due to traumatic, congenital, or surgical causes exist. See Fig.

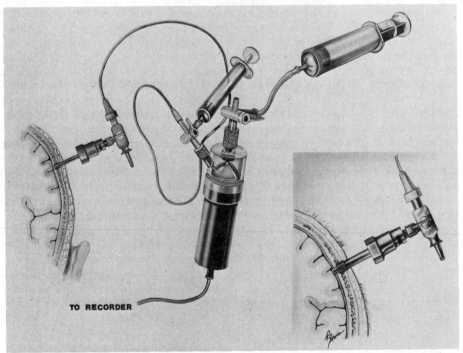

Intracranial Pressure Measurement: Typical setup for measurement.

INTRACRANIAL PRESSURE MEASUREMENT: A technique for determining the pressure within the cranium. Intracranial pressure (ICP) measurement is an invasive procedure and requires access through the skull. The measurement may be made via a fluid-filled catheter passing through the skull, brain, and into the cerebral ventricles, or it may be made via a small transducer resting on the dura or on the brain surface. The transducer technique, referred to as an intracranial screw or bolt, is less hazardous than the ventricular catheter but does not permit withdrawal of fluid. See Fig. See Subarachnoid screw.

INTRAGASTRIC PRESSURE: The pressure within the stomach which may vary with respiration. The pressure can increase dramatically during positive pressure ventilation performed with an inadequate airway because gas will be blown down the esophagus inflating the stomach. It is believed that intragastric pressure rises significantly during the fasciculations induced by succinylcholine. See Sellick maneuver.

INTRAMEDULLARY ANESTHESIA: See Intraosseous anesthesia.

INTRAOCULAR PRESSURE (IOP): The tension in the interior chamber of the eye produced mainly by the aqueous humor and, to a lesser extent, the vitreous humor. The aqueous humor is continually being formed and reabsorbed and the balance between the two processes regulates the total intraocular fluid volume and pressure. The normal IOP ranges from 10 to 30 mmHg (average is 15 mmHg) and is measured clinically by tonometry or estimated by palpation of the eye. The IOP is elevated in glaucoma. All anesthetic agents with the exception of ketamine tend to decrease IOP as do nondepolarizing muscle relaxants and intravenous barbiturates. Topical eye application of atropine, a mydriatic agent, increases IOP in eyes predisposed to closed-angle glaucoma. Succinylcholine can cause an elevated IOP but this effect may be inhibited by prior administration of a nondepolarizing muscle relaxant. Succinylcholine must not be used in patients with penetrating eye wounds because even a transient increase in IOP would lead to the loss of vitreous humor. See Glaucoma.

INTRAOSSEUS ANESTHESIA: A technique in which a local anesthetic solution is injected into the bone marrow of an extremity that is isolated from the systemic circulation by a tourniquet. Although quite similar in many respects to intravenous regional anesthesia, sterile technique is critical because of the possibility of directly introducing an infection into the bone. Intraosseus anesthesia may also be called intramedullary anesthesia. This latter term, however, is more frequently used to indicate spinal anesthesia.

INTERSCALENE BLOCK: See Brachial plexus block.

INTRATHECAL INJECTION: The injection of a pharmacologic agent through the sheath (theca) of the spinal cord into the subarachnoid space. Spinal anesthesia is accomplished with an intrathecal injection. An alcohol or phenol intrathecal injection is given to alleviate intractable pain. Since both of these agents are neurolytic on direct contact with nerves, the technique requires great skill on the part of the operator.

INTRAUTERINE PRESSURE: The pressure within the uterus measured near term by means of a catheter placed in the amniotic cavity. Normal baseline values are 8-20 torr. Contractions occur between 25 and 75 torr with peak values of 130 torr in conjunction with bearing down efforts. Uterine hypertonicity is a condition in which the baseline pressure is in excess of 20 torr.

INTRAVAL: A British trade name for thiopental sodium. See Barbiturate, Thiopental sodium.

INTRAVASCULAR ELECTROCARDIOGRAM: See Intracardiac electrocardiogram.

INTRAVENOUS ANESTHESIA: The introduction of pharmacologic agents into a vein to create a general anesthetic state. Intravenous anesthesia is useful for surgical procedures of short duration or for induction purposes prior to inhalation anesthesia. It may also supplement regional anesthesia. Short-acting barbiturates such as thiopental and methohexital are frequently used for intravenous anesthesia.

INTRINSICALLY SAFE DEVICE: An apparatus which is designed and built so that any internal spark which may occur or any point of high internal temperature will not ignite an explosive mixture within or around the device. "Explosion-proof" indicates a device or apparatus enclosed in a case which is capable of withstanding an explosion without touching off surrounding explosive mixtures.

INTRINSIC PATHWAY: A mechanism for activating blood coagulation by the formation of prothrombin activator. This pathway begins with trauma to the blood itself (or by contact with collagen in the vascular wall) which alters or damages factor XII and the platelets. The resulting activated factor XII and platelet factor III (platelet phospholipids) then activate factor XI, which in turn activates factor IX. Factor IX, with the aid of factor VIII and platelet factor III, then activates factor X. The last phase of the intrinsic pathway occurs when activated factor X combines with factor V and the platelet phospholipids to form the prothrombin activator complex which cleaves to form thrombin. Calcium ions are required for the promotion of most of these reactions (except for the activation of factors XII and XI); clotting will not occur in the absence of calcium ions. Various substances (citrate ions or oxalate compounds) that decrease the concentration of calcium ions or deionize the calcium in the blood are used to prevent blood coagulation. The partial thromboplastin time (PTT) laboratory test is performed to evaluate the intrinsic pathway functions. See Blood coagulation, Extrinsic pathway.

INTROPIN: See Dopamine.

INTUBATION: The process of passing a tube through the nose or the mouth so its tip rests below the vocal cords and above the division of the trachea into right and left mainstem bronchi. This procedure assures a patent airway if the tube remains mechanically intact. Intubation decreases the anatomic dead space. Intubation is not a benign procedure due to the need for instrumentation and to the introduction of a foreign body. It should be reserved for those patients who demonstrate difficulty in maintaining an airway or who will require long-term respiratory support. See Double-lumen tube, Endobronchial intubation.

INTUSSUSCEPTION: An acute condition, most often seen in children, in which one part of the intestine becomes pushed into the lumen of an adjoining segment of the intestine.

INULIN: A poorly metabolized polysaccharide (found in certain plants) used to measure the glomerular filtration rate to estimate kidney function. The test is known as inulin clearance. See Glomerular filtration rate.

INVERTER: An electronic or mechanical device that converts direct current (DC) into alternating current (AC). Inverters are often used in the operating room to provide standby AC service for emergency equipment. They allow a group of storage batteries with DC output to power AC equipment. An inverter also refers to an electronic device which inverts the polarity of a signal.

ION: An atom or molecule which is either positively (cation) or negatively (anion) charged as a result of having lost or gained one or more electrons.

IONIZATION: The dissociation of compounds into their constituent ions. The process can occur spontaneously (in chemical reactions) or as the result of the deliberate bombardment of material with ionizing radiation.

IONIZATION POTENTIAL: The minimum energy required to cause ionization of a particular atom or molecule.

IONIZING RADIATION: Any radiation of sufficient energy to cause ionization. Ionizing radiation can be either particulate (alpha and beta rays) or pure energy (gamma rays and x-rays).

I^2R LOSS: A form of power loss measured in watts and dissipated as heat due to the flow of current (I) through a conductor, e.g., machine or transformer. The amount of heat that will be generated within a machine may be calculated if the current and resistance (R) are known.

IRON LUNG (TANK VENTILATOR; CABINET RESPIRATOR): A rigid tank encasing the entire body which was the first successful long-term respirator for patients who were unable to ventilate themselves adequately. In current terminology it is classified as a negative pressure ventilator.

IRREVERSIBLE INHIBITION: See Noncompetitive antagonism.

ISMELIN: See Guanethidine.

ISOBAR: One of two or more nuclides which have the same atomic weight but different atomic numbers.

ISOBARIC SOLUTION: An isotonic solution used in spinal anesthesia in which the specific gravity equals that of cerebrospinal fluid.

$$F-\overset{\overset{\displaystyle F}{|}}{\underset{\underset{\displaystyle F}{|}}{C}}-\overset{\overset{\displaystyle H}{|}}{\underset{\underset{\displaystyle Cl}{|}}{C}}-O-\overset{\overset{\displaystyle F}{|}}{\underset{\underset{\displaystyle F}{|}}{C}}-H$$

Isoflurane.

ISOFLURANE (FORANE): A volatile anesthetic agent which is a stereoisomer of enflurane. Induction and recovery from anesthesia are somewhat shorter than with enflurane. Cardiovascular function is said to be less depressed with this agent than with earlier halogenated hydrocarbon anesthetics at comparable dosage levels. Isoflurane is only metabolized to a very limited extent in the body. It has vaporization characteristics very similar to halothane. See Enflurane.

ISOLATED INPUT: See Isolated output.

ISOLATED OUTPUT: An electronic design parameter in which the final (output) stage of a series of circuits has no direct connection with the previous circuits. Isolated input is an electronic design parameter in which the first of a series of circuits (input stage) has no direct connection with later circuits. Direct connection involves coupling the circuits by wiring or by bridging the two circuits with an active component such as a capacitor. Isolation, on the other hand, is accomplished by interposing a transformer so that a signal is transferred by interaction of electromagnetic fields or by optical isolation, in which the signal is transferred between circuits by a variable light beam. Modern electrocardiograph monitors have isolated inputs to protect them from a current surge caused by defibrillator discharge on top of an electrode. See Transformer.

ISOLATION TRANSFORMER: A transformer used to separate a device from its power supply so that no direct connection between them will normally occur. Current from the power supply flows through the primary coil of the transformer, causing current to be induced in the secondary windings of the transformer. It is this current that powers the device. Modern operating rooms are powered through isolation transformers.

ISOMER: Any compound which has the same molecular weight and chemical composition as another compound but which differs in some physical and chemical properties due to varied structural arrangements of atoms within its molecules.

ISOMETRIC CHANGE: A change in a gas which occurs while the gas remains at a constant volume.

ISOMETRIC CONTRACTION: A muscle contraction with no change in muscle fiber lengths and associated with increased muscle tension. During the isometric contraction phase of the ventricle, the ventricular pressure rises but there is no change in the ventricular volume.

ISONATREMIC: See Dehydration.

ISOPRENALINE: See Isoproterenol.

ISOPROPYL ALCOHOL (ISOPROPANOL): A volatile, flammable alcohol (C_3H_8O) used as a topical bactericidal preparation in concentrations of 70-100%. (The 70% strength is known as rubbing alcohol.) The germicidal action is inconstant, however.

ISOPROPYLNOREPINEPHRINE (ISOPROPYLNORADRENALIN): See Isoproterenol.

ISOPROTERENOL (ISUPREL; ISOPRENALINE): A synthetic drug closely related to the naturally occurring catecholamines: norepinephrine, epinephrine, and dopamine. (It is also known as isopropylnorepinephrine or isopropylnoradrenalin.) Isoproterenol is a very potent stimulator of beta receptors. It also has powerful positive inotropic and chronotropic effects on the heart and dilates bronchial smooth muscle and blood vessels. It is often used in aerosol form to treat bronchial asthma and related conditions. Overdosage of isoproterenol may cause tachycardia, angina, and headache. It increases cardiac O_2 consumption and stimulates cardiac output and, therefore, can actually increase the volume of infarcted tissue if administered during, or immediately after, a cardiac ischemic/infarct episode.

ISOTHERMAL PROCESS: A process which occurs at a constant temperature.

ISOTONIC SOLUTION: In biologic terms, a fluid having the same osmotic pressure as that of blood. Cells surrounded by an isotonic solution neither gain nor lose water.

ISOTOPE: A nuclide which has the same atomic number but a different atomic mass due to differences in the number of neutrons in the nucleus. Isotopes are nearly identical in chemical properties but vary in their physical properties. See Cesium-137, Gamma camera, Technetium, Xenon-133.

ISOVOLUMIC CONTRACTION TIME (ICT): See Systolic time intervals.

J

JACKSON, CHARLES: See Morton, William T. G.

JACKSON-REES APPARATUS: A modification of the Ayre T-piece system for pediatric anesthesia. The basic change is that a double-ended bag is fitted to the expiratory limb of the T-piece. This bag allows breathing to be assisted and/or controlled. See Fig.

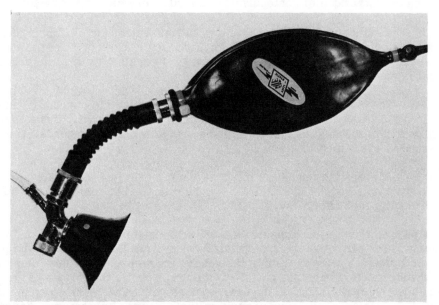

Jackson-Rees Apparatus: Jackson-Rees modification of an Ayre T-piece used for the administration of pediatric anesthesia.

JEHOVAH WITNESS: An international religious sect which originated in the United States at the end of the nineteenth century. Its members interpret the Old Testament literally. They believe that the soul resides in the blood, and therefore consider transfusion with blood or blood derivatives to be a sacrilege.

JITTER: A short-term, often recurring instability in either the phase or amplitude of a signal. This phenomenon is most often seen in a cathode ray tube display.

JOINT COMMISSION ON ACCREDITATION OF HOSPITALS (JCAH): A private, non-profit organization, formed in 1951, that fosters quality medical care by establishing optimal standards for American hospitals. Five major organizations are represented on the Board of Directors: American College of Physicians, American College of Surgeons, American Hospital Association, American Medical Association, and American Dental Association. The JCAH currently accredits approximately 5000 hospitals, 1200 psychiatric facilities, and 1100 related health care facilities. The JCAH stresses that accreditation is voluntary and that it surveys each institution only after the individual health care facility requests it. However, JCAH accreditation is mandatory in order for many institutions to receive funding from various public medical assistance programs. Accreditation is given for either a 1- or 2-year period. An institution does not have to comply with all JCAH standards but must substantially comply with most of them. JCAH headquarters are located in Chicago.

JORGENSEN TECHNIQUE: A method of sedation for dental procedures. Pentobarbital is injected slowly by the intravenous route until a predetermined point of patient relaxation is achieved. A fixed combination of meperidine and scopolamine is then injected slowly, followed by injections of appropriate intraoral anesthetic agents. Depending on the total dose of pentobarbital, the recovery can be prolonged.

JOULE (J): The standard international unit of measurement for all forms of energy. It is the energy equivalent to the work performed when a force of 1 newton moves a body a distance of 1 m. In electric equivalence, 1 J equals 1 watt-sec. In heat energy, 1 cal is equivalent to 4.1868 J.

JOULE LAW: The law stating that heat produced by an electric current (I) flowing through a resistance (R) for a fixed time (t) is determined by I^2Rt. If the current is expressed in amperes, the resistance in ohms, and the time in seconds, then the heat produced is expressed in joules.

JUGULAR BULB: A dilatation of the internal jugular vein just as it leaves the base of the skull. Blood removed from the jugular bulb is used to approximate mixed venous blood from the brain.

JUGULAR VEINS: The great veins of the neck composed of the external and internal jugular veins. The bilateral external jugular veins drain the blood from the parotid glands, facial muscles, and scalp into the subclavian veins. They run inferior and traverse the sternocleidomastoid muscle to a point opposite the middle of the clavicle, where they enter the subclavian veins. These veins are readily accessible in the patient who is in a Trendelenburg position (head down), but they are difficult to stabilize and therefore difficult to cannulate. This is due to several factors: the angle at which the external jugular veins enter the subclavian veins, the presence of valves in the external veins (impeding passage of the cannula), and the visibility of the external veins beneath the skin (which varies from individual to individual). The internal jugular veins begin in the base of the skull at the jugular fossas and are a continuation of the transverse sinuses of the brain. Coursing down through the neck, they accompany first the internal carotid arteries and then the common carotid artery. The internal jugular veins descend on either side of the neck and receive blood from the brain and superficial parts of the face and neck. They pass behind the clavicles and join with the right and left subclavian veins forming the brachiocephalic veins and the superior vena cava. The internal jugular veins are fairly easily cannulated and are often used for central venous pressure monitoring or placement of a Swan-Ganz catheter. A right-sided cannulation is preferred because

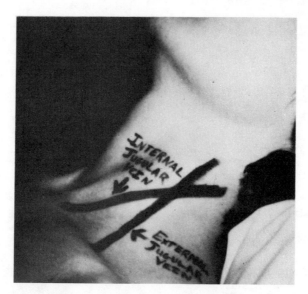

Jugular Veins: Internal and external jugular veins are outlined.

the right internal jugular vein leads directly into the superior vena cava. In addition, the apex of the right lung is lower than the left, thereby lessening the chances for inadvertent puncture of the lung. Furthermore, entry on the right side avoids possible injury to the thoracic duct, which is a left-sided structure. See Fig.

JUST NOTICEABLE DIFFERENCE (JND): The increase in the intensity of a painful stimulus that will just barely cause an appreciable difference in the perception of pain. It has been shown that an average individual can distinguish approximately 22 JNDs measured from a level of no pain to a level of intense pain.

KALLIDIN: See Kinins.

KALLIKREIN: See Bradykinin.

KEEPER: A magnetic conductor placed over the ends of a magnet to prevent the gradual loss of its magnetism.

KELVIN (K): The standard international unit of temperature equal to 1/273.16 of the thermodynamic temperature of the triple point of water. On the K scale, 1 K = 1 degree Celsius. Absolute zero on the K scale = -273 degrees Celsius, theoretically the lowest possible temperature. See Triple point of water.

KETAMINE: A nonbarbiturate intravenous general anesthetic. It is quite similar structurally to the veterinary anesthetic phencyclidine (Sernylan). Phencyclidine was abandoned for human use due to its propensity to cause severe and long-lasting hallucinations. Phencyclidine (angel dust) is popular for illicit drug use. Ketamine differs from the barbiturates because it tends to support, rather than depress, the cardiovascular system. With increased dosage, it causes epileptic-like electric activity of the brain and, in general, enhances muscle tone. The anesthesia is of short duration and may increase the blood pressure and induce dreams, hallucinations, and psychologic disturbances after recovery. These latter reactions are believed to occur less commonly in children. Ketamine produces "dissociative anesthesia," i.e., the patient becomes unresponsive to pain and to the environment. See Dissociative anesthesia, Neuroleptanesthesia.

KETONE BODY: See Anion gap.

KIDNEY: A prime organ of the urinary system. The paired kidneys are located in the retroperitoneum, the right slightly lower than the left. The main function of the kidneys is regulation of the composition and volume of body fluids. They play a critical role in the maintenance of acid-base balance, excretion of unwanted metabolic end products such as urea, uric acid, and creatinine, and elimination of drugs. The kidneys also have an endocrine function in that they elaborate erythropoietin (erythropoietic stimulating factor) and renin (a proteolytic enzyme which activates the angiotensin-dependent vasoconstrictor mechanism). The kidneys elaborate erythropoietin when they are hypoxic and renin when they are ischemic and arterial pressure decreases. The functional unit in the kidney is the nephron; each kidney con-

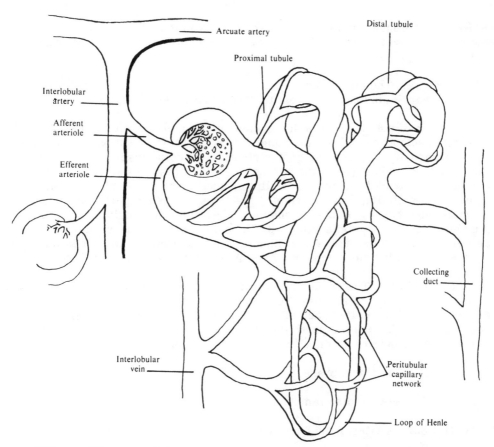

Kidney: Diagram of the nephron, the functional unit of the kidney.

tains approximately 1 million nephrons. The loss or destruction of nephrons results in an increase in size of the remaining nephrons. Life may still be maintained
with the loss of two-thirds of the nephrons. The components of the nephron include
the glomerulus, proximal convoluted tubule, loop of Henle, and distal convoluted tubule. The distal convoluted tubule terminates by merging with the collecting duct.
The circulation of the kidney is autoregulatory, i.e., the blood flow to the kidney
remains constant within a range of mean arterial pressure of approximately 60-180
mmHg. In general, inhalation anesthetics such as ether, cyclopropane, isoflurane,
enflurane, and methoxyflurane all cause depression of renal blood flow and glomerular filtration rate; the degree of depression appears to be dose-related. A similar
depression of renal blood flow is also seen with the use of the N_2O/O_2 muscle relaxant technique. Conversely, spinal anesthesia does not usually depress the glomerular filtration rate but may cause a decrease in the total renal blood flow. Epidural
anesthesia appears to have little or no effect on renal blood flow. Of all the anesthetic agents, only methoxyflurane seems to be directly nephrotoxic, depending on
dose and duration of administration. See Fig. See Glomerular filtration rate, Methoxyflurane.

KILO- (k): A prefix meaning 1000. In computer terminology it means 2^{10} (1024).

KILOGRAM (kg): The standard international unit of mass (1 kg = 2.204 lb).

KINESTHESIA: A sensation mediated by end organs in muscles, joints, and tendons. Movement is perceived by the individual who is then able to estimate the relative position of the body parts.

KINETIC ENERGY: The energy associated with motion. It is equal to the work that would be necessary to bring the system to rest. See Potential energy.

KININS: A group of polypeptides which causes dilation of the blood vessels in kidneys, vascular smooth muscles, and some glands. Bradykinin, a plasma kinin, constricts the bronchial, uterine, and gastrointestinal smooth muscles. It also causes release of catecholamines (from the adrenal medulla), histamine (from mast cells), and prostaglandin (from the kidney). Kallidin, another plasma kinin, has pharmacologic properties similar to bradykinin. The kinins increase permeability in the microcirculation, thereby producing edema. They also evoke pain by stimulating nerve endings. Edema in conjunction with the nerve stimulation results in the "wheal-flare" reaction to intradermal injections. The kinins take part in inflammatory responses and allergic symptoms. See Allergic response, Bradykinin.

KOROTKOFF SOUNDS: The sounds heard through the stethoscope during the auscultatory determination of arterial blood pressure. The blood pressure cuff is inflated to occlude the artery (usually brachial) and as the pressure is slowly released, the blood can then flow through the partially collapsed artery. The resulting turbulence in the vessels is thought to produce the Korotkoff sounds.

KUPFFER CELL: See Macrophage.

KUSSMAUL SIGN: See Cardiac tamponade.

KYPHOSCOLIOSIS: A lateral and backward curvature of the spinal column.

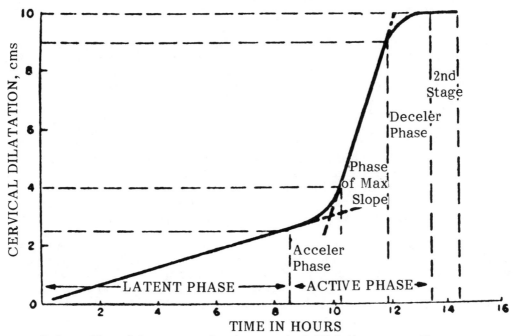

Labor: Mean labor curve showing cervical dilatation versus time, based on a study of 500 primigravidas at term.

LABOR: The process by which both fetus and placenta are expelled from the uterus through the vagina. Normal labor is divided into three stages. During stage 1, regular uterine contractions are accomplished by the complete dilation of the cervical os and effacement of the cervix. Stage 2, the stage of expulsion, begins when the os is fully dilated and ends with the delivery of the fetus. Stage 3 involves the expulsion of the placenta and membranes and ends with the final uterine contraction. False labor, common in late pregnancy, consists of brief, ineffective, irregular contractions not accompanied by cervical dilatation and effacement. See Fig.

LACTATE/PYRUVATE RATIO: A biochemical ratio measured in a blood sample which has been advocated as a possible indicator of tissue hypoxia. However, the lactate/pyruvate ratio has not been shown to add significantly to an understanding of patient status if other careful physiologic and metabolic monitoring has been performed.

LAERDAL VALVE: See Nonrebreathing valve.

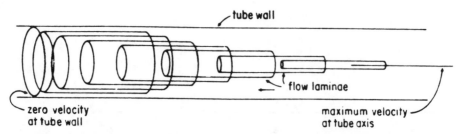

Laminar Flow: Laminar flow in a tube showing a few of the very large number of infinitely thin concentric flow laminae moving left to right. Each is at a different velocity, ranging from 0 at the tube wall to maximum at the tube center. The average velocity is half the maximum.

LAMINAR FLOW: The flow of an incompressible, viscous fluid in which the particles of the fluid move in distinct and separate layers (concentric laminae) parallel to each other and to the walls of a vessel or container. The velocity of the fluid particles is not uniform: there is little or no movement at the periphery of the flow and greatest movement in the center of the flow. This is different from turbulent flow in which there is no order and all molecules tend to flow at approximately the same velocity. More energy is necessary to produce turbulent flow and often this results in noise. See Fig. See Reynolds number, Turbulent flow.

LAMINAR FLOW HOOD: An enclosed work area (room, cabinet) which is protected from contamination by dust or microorganisms by HEPA filters. Air is continually moved in a single direction eliminating turbulence and backflow. Various units are available and are essential for use in laboratories for pharmaceutical research, tissue culture, biomedical research, and in hospital operating rooms. See HEPA filter.

LAPAROSCOPY: A method of visually examining the abdominal or pelvic organs by the insertion of a specially equipped endoscope through a small incision in the abdominal wall. This method, also known as peritoneoscopy, has both diagnostic and therapeutic value. Minor operative procedures, such as tubal ligation, ovarian or liver biopsy, and lysis of adhesions, may be performed through a laparoscope. See Insufflation, intraperitoneal.

LAPLACE LAW: A law of physics which has been applied to physiology. It defines the force which tends to stretch the muscle fibers in the vascular wall as proportional to the diameter (D) of the vessel times the pressure (P). The ventricular pressure depends on the tension produced by the contracted cardiac ventricular muscle and on the size and shape of the heart. This law helps explain the extra work load of the failing, dilated heart. As the D of the heart chamber is increased, more tension develops in the myocardium to produce any given P, thereby increasing the work of the dilated heart in maintaining the same arterial pressure as in the healthy heart. In the lung, the radii of the curvature of the alveoli become smaller during expiration. The surface tension-lowering substance, surfactant, prevents the alveoli from collapsing. If the surface tension does not remain low, the alveoli would collapse according to the law of Laplace. In spherical structures such as alveoli, the distending pressure (P) equals 2 times the wall tension (T) divided by the radius (R), $P = 2T/R$. Therefore, if T is not lowered as R is lowered, T overcomes P and collapse occurs. See Surfactant.

LARGE SAMPLES: A sample series large enough for the distribution of the individual observations to approach a normal distribution. See Normal distribution.

LARODOPA: See Levodopa, L-dopa.

LARYNGITIS: An inflammation of the larynx often caused by a respiratory infection or irritant. It is characterized by dryness and soreness of the throat, hoarseness, cough, and loss of voice. It is a relatively common sequela of endotracheal intubation and is dependent on cuff inflation pressure, tube position, length of procedure, type of endotracheal tubing, and the technical competence of the anesthetist.

LARYNGOSCOPY: The examination of the larynx either indirectly by means of a laryngeal mirror or directly by means of a lighted instrument, the laryngoscope.

LARYNGOSPASM: The sudden, forceful, and involuntary contraction (spasm) of the muscles of the larynx. Certain muscle groups normally act as sphincters to protect the airway, but during spasm they tend to close, obscuring the true vocal cords and the glottis. Closure of these sphincters separates the larynx and trachea. These sphincters include aryepiglottic folds, vestibular folds (false vocal cords), and true vocal cords. Laryngospasm can be a defensive reflex to prevent aspiration and is associated with a high-pitched squeak or whistle. (The complete absence of sound indicates that the vocal cords are in total apposition.) Laryngospasm is a serious potential complication during induction of anesthesia due to the seemingly innocuous manipulation of the upper airway. The administration of O_2 under pressure or the injection of a fast-acting neuromuscular blocking agent, such as succinylcholine, may be useful in treating laryngospasm; however, the condition is easier to prevent than to treat. See Larynx.

LARYNX (VOICE BOX): The short passageway that connects the pharynx with the trachea. The walls of this musculocartilaginous structure are supported by nine pieces of cartilage. The larynx lies in the midline of the neck anterior to the fourth-sixth cervical (C4-C6) vertebrae. It is lined with ciliated mucous membranes which trap particles not removed in the upper air passages. The vocal cords are usually thicker and longer in males and vibrate more slowly. See Fig.

LASER: An acronym for Light Amplification by Stimulated Emission of Radiation. It refers to a device which transforms energy of various frequencies into a narrow, extremely intense, and nearly nondivergent beam of monochromatic (single-frequency) radiation in the optical, ultraviolet, and infrared regions. Lasers are capable of producing a great deal of heat and power; however, the conversion efficiency of the change from one form of energy to laser energy is extremely inefficient. Laser techniques are being used with greater frequency in surgery.

LASIX: See Furosemide.

LATENT HEAT: The amount of heat absorbed or released by a unit mass of a substance during isothermal changes of state (such as fusion, sublimation, or vaporization) at a constant pressure. For example, a gently heated mixture of ice and water remains at 0 degrees Celsius as long as there is any ice in the mixture. Latent

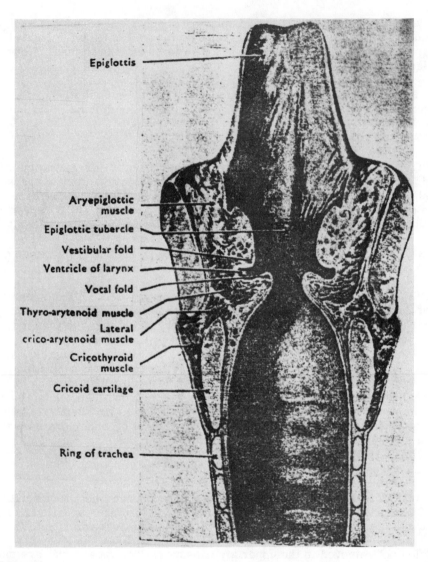

Larynx.

heat becomes an important consideration in the vaporization of liquids in anesthesia. In order for a liquid to vaporize at a constant rate, energy must be added to it to compensate for the heat loss and the resultant drop in temperature.

LAUGHING GAS: See Nitrous oxide.

LAVAGE: The therapeutic washing out or irrigating of an organ, such as the lung, bowel, or stomach. See Pulmonary lavage.

LD_{50} (LETHAL DOSE 50%): The dose of a pharmacologic substance which is fatal to 50% of test animals. As the difference between the LD_{50} and the ED_{50} (effective dose 50%) increases, so does the safety of the substance. See ED_{50}, Therapeutic index.

L-DOPA: See Levodopa.

LEAD (LEAD WIRE): A conductor, such as an electrocardiograph lead, used to connect two points in a circuit. See Electrocardiogram.

LEADING EDGE ANALYSIS (SPECTRAL EDGE ANALYSIS): An electroencephalograph (EEG) analysis technique. The EEG is displayed by compressed spectral array (CSA). The leading edge is the frequency below which a large percentage (90-98%) of the power in the EEG frequency band is contained. A shift in the leading edge from time interval to time interval on the CSA display is believed to indicate changes in depth of anesthesia. See Fourier analysis.

LEAKAGE: The undesirable flow of electric current in a path other than that intended, possibly due to imperfect insulation. See Fault current.

LEAST SQUARES, METHOD OF: A mathematic technique for finding the equation that best fits or describes the line or curve connecting points on a graph.

LECLANCHE CELL: The common dry cell, primary cell, or carbon-zinc battery in which the anode is made of carbon and the cathode is made of zinc. The least expensive of the common primary cells, it usually cannot be recharged. The voltage from a new cell is approximately 1.5 V, but it declines steadily with use.

LEFT VENTRICULAR EJECTION TIME (LVET): See Systolic time intervals.

LERITINE: See Anileridine, Narcotic.

LEU-ENKEPHALIN: See Enkephalins.

LEVALLORPHAN (LORFAN): A narcotic agonist/antagonist useful in the treatment of significant narcotic-induced respiratory depression. It is ineffective in alleviating respiratory depression due to other causes and, if used, may actually potentiate the problem. The use of levallorphan has diminished with the introduction of a newer antagonist, naloxone. See Naloxone.

LEVARTERENOL: See Norepinephrine.

LEVODOPA, L-DOPA (DOPAR; LARODOPA): A drug for treating Parkinson disease. Levodopa decarboxylates to dopamine, the neurotransmitter which is deficient in parkinsonian patients and must therefore by replenished. Relatively high doses of levodopa must be administered (orally) to produce the desired pharmacologic effects, e.g., reducing bradykinesia and rigidity. This enables a sufficient accumulation of the drug in the brain where the decarboxylation increases the dopamine concentration. (Dopamine itself does not readily penetrate the blood-brain barrier.) Side effects limit the usefulness of the drug, however.

LEVOPHED: See Norepinephrine.

LEVORPHANOL TARTRATE (LEVO-DROMORAN): A synthetic molecule closely related to morphine. See Narcotic.

LEWIS-LEIGH VALVE: See Nonrebreathing valve.

L-HYOSCINE: See Scopolamine.

LIBEL: A written unjust statement which defames an individual's reputation. It is a possible basis for countersuit in malpractice actions.

LIBRIUM: See Benzodiazepine.

LIDOCAINE (XYLOCAINE): See Local anesthetic.

LIFO: An acronym for "Last In First Out," referring to the ordering of machine tasks. The last task received is completed first.

LIGAMENTUM FLAVUM: See Lumbar puncture.

LIGHT: The electromagnetic radiation which is perceived by the eye. The visual spectrum is between wavelengths of 390 and 770 nm. The photon is the unit of light energy. The velocity of light in a free space, $2.997\ 925 \times 10^8$ m/sec, is considered one of the prime constants in the universe.

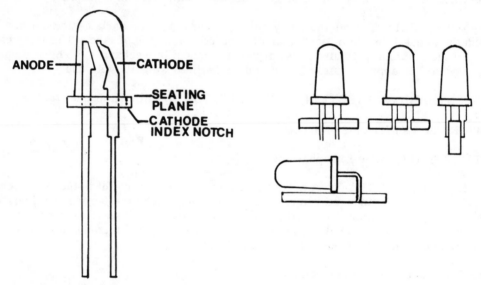

Light-Emitting Diode.

LIGHT-EMITTING DIODE (LED): A device which emits light at the junction of two semiconductor materials when the appropriate voltage difference is applied across the junction. Depending on the semiconductors used, the LED can be altered so as to emit different colors of visible light. The chief advantage that LEDs have over liquid-crystal displays (LCD) is that they can be seen in the dark because they generate light internally. To accomplish this, however, they use current and place higher demands on a circuit than does an LCD display. See Fig. See Liquid-crystal display.

LIGNOCAINE: The British term for lidocaine.

LIMBIC SYSTEM: The portion of the brain composed of the limbic lobe (subcallosal, cingulate, and parahippocampal gyri), hippocampal formation, amygdaloid nucleus, hypothalamus, and anterior nucleus of the thalamus. The limbic system appears to be involved in emotional behavior, particularly fear and anger, and sexual behavior. The hippocampus appears to be concerned with recent memory.

LIMITS OF EXPLOSIVENESS: See Detonability, limits of.

LIMIT OF FLAMMABILITY: The upper and lower end points of the concentration range at which a fuel/oxidizer mix will ignite. Generally, the upper and lower limits of flammability for a given fuel are much higher with O_2 than with air.

LINE ISOLATION MONITOR: A device which continually determines the actual electric separation of the input and output sides of an isolated power supply. It measures the potential for current flow (electric shock) if an individual simultaneously contacts a conductor located on the isolated side and a grounded conductor. See Ground, Isolation transformer.

LIPID SOLUBILITY THEORY OF ANESTHESIA (MEYER-OVERTON THEORY): A theory which correlates lipid solubility with the potency of an anesthetic agent. Anesthetics are lipophilic and therefore the greater the solubility, the lower the concentration needed to be effective. In actuality, however, the theory does not explain anesthesia but only describes the actions of anesthetics in the lipid areas of body tissues.

LIQUID-CRYSTAL DISPLAY (LCD): A technique for displaying numbers or letters which employs the physical characteristics of liquid crystals. These semiamorphous materials reorient themselves internally when a voltage difference is placed across them. This internal reorientation changes the percentage of light reflected by the crystal. This change in reflected light enables the liquid crystal element of the display to be seen. The LCDs have very low power requirements; however, they are not visible in darkness when no light exists for reflection. See Fig. See Light-emitting diode.

LIQUID OXYGEN: Oxygen cooled to -183 degrees Celsius at 1 atmosphere pressure. This is the most convenient form for bulk movement of O_2. One cubic foot of liquid O_2 yields over 24,000 L gaseous O_2 at room temperature.

LIQUID VENTILATION: An experimental technique in which gas exchange through the lungs is maintained by filling the lungs with a fluid. Liquid ventilation utilizes the properties of various silicone oils and fluorocarbons. Disadvantages of the technique include the viscosity of the fluid (which limits respiratory rate and tidal volume) and the long-term toxic effects on the cell linings of the alveoli. Theoretic advantages of the technique include the potential of delivering high O_2 concentrations while lowering O_2 toxicity and maintaining airway patency.

LITHIUM: A metallic element of the alkali group with an atomic weight of approximately 7. The carbonate salt of lithium is widely used in the treatment of the manic phase of manic-depressive psychiatric disease. Therapeutic doses of lithium carbonate have no discernible psychotropic effects in normal subjects. Its use is recommended only for medically healthy patients with acute mania or to prevent recurrences of manic-depressive states. Lithium toxicity is enhanced when sodium intake is lowered; this effect should be recognized if it is imperative to administer the drug to patients who are on intravenous therapy or have cardiac or renal disease. Toxic reactions and side effects include a benign, diffuse thyroid enlargement, vomiting, diarrhea, tremor, and polyuria.

LIVER FUNCTION TESTS: A series of blood tests that attempt to determine the functional integrity of the liver. Examples of such tests include prothrombin time, serum bilirubin, alkaline phosphatase, and serum glutamic oxaloacetic transaminase

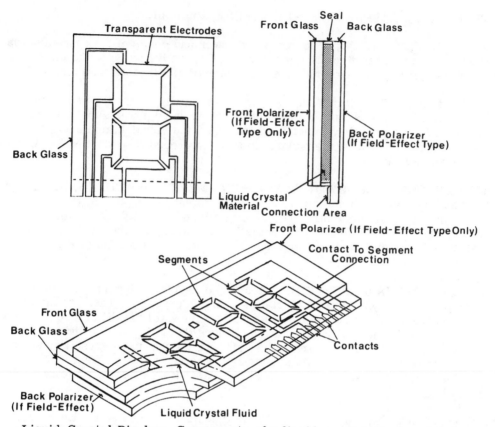

Liquid-Crystal Display: Components of a liquid-crystal display showing that each number is generated from seven transparent electrodes (segments) which are visible or not, depending on the figure generated.

(SGOT). Because of the tremendous capacity of the liver to function despite injury, much of the liver has to be damaged before the tests show any deviations from normal.

LOBAR ATELECTASIS: See Atelectasis.

LOBAR BRONCHI: See Conducting airways.

LOCAL ANESTHETIC (LA): An agent which produces a transient and reversible loss of sensation in a circumscribed portion of the body. This primary effect of LAs is due to the decreased permeability of the nerve membrane to sodium ions, thereby preventing an action potential. The nerve membrane remains in a polarized state, and the block produced by LAs is therefore known as a nondepolarizing nerve block. Modern LAs (all weak bases) are classified as either amides or esters depending on their chemical linkages. Most LAs are combined with an acid (usually hydrochloric) to form a salt which is stable and soluble in water. The specific method by which the amide or ester LA undergoes metabolic breakdown constitutes a major difference between the two classes. Esters such as procaine (Novocain) and tetracaine (Pontocaine) are mainly hydrolyzed in the plasma by pseudocholinesterase, whereas amides, such as lidocaine (Xylocaine), dibucaine (Nupercaine), bupivacaine (Marcaine), and mepivacaine (Carbocaine), are metabolized in the liver. The

Local Anesthetic: Some of the common local anesthetics and the molecular linkages which differentiate each.

Amide/Ester	Generic Name (Trade Name)
Amides	Lidocaine (Xylocaine)
	Dibucaine (Nupercaine)
	Mepivacaine (Carbocaine)
	Prilocaine (Citanest)
	Bupivacaine (Marcaine)
Esters of Benzoic Acid	Cocaine
	Tetracaine (Pontocaine)
	Piperocaine (Metycaine)
	Hexylcaine (Cyclaine)
	Ethyl Aminobenzoate (Benzocaine)
	Butacaine (Butyn)
Esters of Meta-Aminobenzoic Acid	Cyclomethycaine (Surfacaine)
	Metabutoxycaine (Primacaine)
Esters of p-Aminobenzoic Acid	Procaine (Novocain)
	Butethamine (Monocaine)
	Chloroprocaine (Nesacaine)
	Proparacaine (Ophthaine)

toxicity of an LA is dependent on the plasma level of the drug. This, in turn, is influenced by the rate of absorption into the bloodstream, degree of plasma binding, rate of distribution to the tissues, and rate of removal via tissue metabolism and/or excretory pathways. Most LAs (except cocaine) have vasodilating properties, the clinical effects of which are to increase the rate of absorption of the drug in the blood, thereby increasing the anesthetic level in the blood and the potential for overdose. Absorption of the LA is also dependent on the injection site, the degree of vasodilation, the dose, and the presence of a vasoconstrictor in the solution. Vasoconstrictors, such as epinephrine, are frequently added to the LA solution (used for nerve block or infiltration) to prevent absorption of the drug, prolong its local pain control activity, and reduce systemic reactions. Once the LAs are absorbed from the injection site, they can affect the cardiovascular system and central nervous system (CNS) (paradoxical excitation and then CNS depression or linear cardiac depression with increasing dose). Side effects, such as anxiety, tachycardia, and hypertension, may be related to the added epinephrine. In general, toxic reactions are related to overdosage or, rarely, to allergic manifestations. Lidocaine is also used intravenously for its antiarrhythmic effect. See Fig. See Dissociation constant, Sodium channel.

LOGARITHM: A system of notation in which every positive number is expressed as a power of 10. For example, 1000 can be expressed as 10^3, 10 X 10 X 10, or log 1000 = 3.

LONG, CRAWFORD: See Morton, William T. G.

LOOK-THROUGH PHENOMENON: An observation seen when radioisotopes are used to determine flow characteristics of particular organs. A local area of ischemia (which receives no isotope) is not detected because it is lost in the radiation picked up from surrounding normal tissue which "looks through" the ischemic area.

LOOP (LOOPING): A closed series of computer instructions which are repeated continuously until a terminal condition is satisfied. The loop may start at any point, but it must return to that point for completion.

LORAZEPAM (ATIVAN): See Benzodiazepine.

LORFAN: See Levallorphan.

LUDWIG ANGINA: A diffuse suppurative infection of the connective tissues, muscles, and glands of the submaxillary area. This cellulitis may become so extensive as to cause respiratory embarrassment.

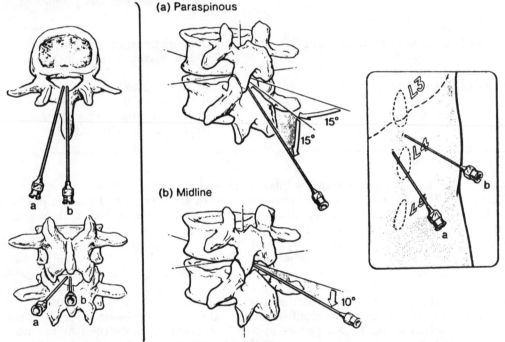

Lumbar Puncture: Two common techniques of lumbar puncture for spinal anesthesia. (a) Paraspinous, paramedian, or lateral approach. (b) Midline approach.

LUMBAR PUNCTURE: A technique used to administer local anesthetics or to sample cerebrospinal fluid. A long spinal needle is inserted into the subarachnoid space, penetrating the supraspinous and interspinous ligaments, ligamentum flavum, and dura. See Fig.

LUMEN (LM): The cavity of a tube or tubular organ. It is also the unit of measurement of light flux.

LUMINAL: See Phenobarbital.

LUMINESCENCE: The emission of electromagnetic radiation from a substance as the result of a nonthermal process. Luminescence also relates to visible radiation. If the luminescence terminates when the energy source is removed, it is known as fluorescence, whereas if it persists, it is phosphorescence. See Fluorescence, Phosphorescence.

LUNG, NONGAS EXCHANGE FUNCTIONS OF: The specific lung functions other than the oxygenation of blood. The lungs (1) act as a reservoir for blood and can increase their blood volume with only a slight increase in pulmonary and venous pressures; (2) act as a filter, removing thrombi and clots; (3) secrete the phospholipid dipalmitoyl lecithin, a major component of surfactant (necessary for lung expansion); and (4) inactivate circulating serotonin, bradykinin, and some prostaglandins.

LUNG VOLUMES AND CAPACITIES: The nomenclature useful in respiratory physiology to describe the air in the lung at maximum inspiration, maximum expiration, and at agreed upon points in between. There are four primary volumes. (1) The tidal volume (TV) is the volume of air inspired or expired with each normal breath. (2) The inspiratory reserve volume (IRV) is the maximal amount of gas which may be inspired in excess of the normal tidal volume. (3) The expiratory reserve volume (ERV) is the maximal volume of gas that can still be expired by active forceful expiration after normal tidal expiration. (4) Residual volume (RV) is the gas remaining in the lungs after a maximal expiratory effort. Pulmonary capacities are combinations of two or more lung volumes. Total lung capacity (TV + IRV + ERV + RV) is the maximal volume to which the lungs may be expanded with maximum inspiration. Vital capacity (IRV, TV, plus ERV) is the greatest volume of air that can be expelled from the lungs following maximum inspiration. Functional residual capacity (ERV plus RV) is the amount of air remaining in the lungs at the end of a normal tidal volume expiration (resting expiratory level). Inspiratory capacity (IRV plus TV) is the maximum amount of air that can be inspired at the end of a normal tidal volume expiration. See Figs.

LUTZ NEEDLE: See Epidural needle.

LUXURY PERFUSION: A localized excessive cerebral blood flow in relation to metabolic requirements. See Intracranial hypertension.

LYTIC COCKTAIL: The combination of chlorpromazine, promethazine, and meperidine which induces a state of lethargy, apathy, and tranquility from which a patient can be aroused. This mixture of drugs tends to decrease blood pressure as well. The lytic cocktail depresses the hypothalamic thermostat and the patient may be maintained under hypothermic conditions (artificial hibernation).

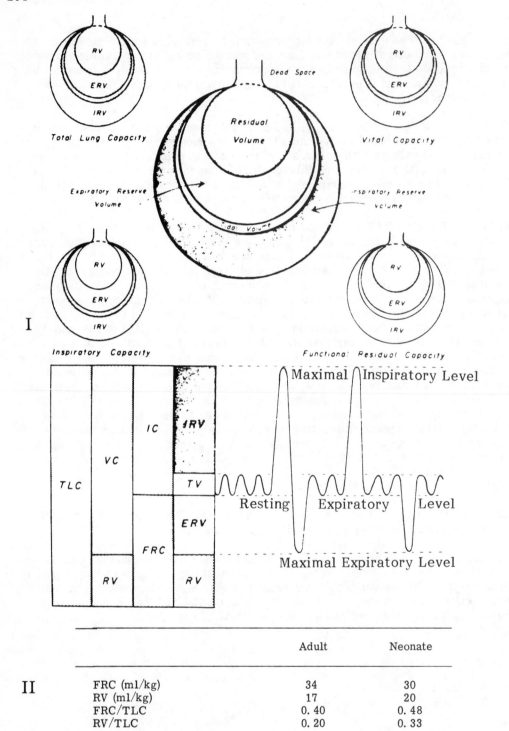

Lung Volumes and Capacities: (I) Static lung volumes and their relationship to the capacities of the lung. (II) Approximate volumes and capacities in neonates and adults.

	Adult	Neonate
FRC (ml/kg)	34	30
RV (ml/kg)	17	20
FRC/TLC	0.40	0.48
RV/TLC	0.20	0.33

MAC: See Minimum alveolar concentration.

MAC AWAKE: The minimum alveolar concentration of an inhalation anesthetic at which 50% of a patient population will respond to simple direct verbal commands.

MACROGLOSSIA: An enlargement of the tongue frequently seen in congenital disorders such as Down syndrome. Airway maintenance is a potential problem with this disorder. In patients with macroglossia, abnormal positioning of the head during general anesthesia may occlude the venous outflow of the tongue.

MACROPHAGE (HISTIOCYTE): A large phagocytic cell of the reticuloendothelial system. These cells are found in the loose connective tissue and are capable of engulfing bacteria and cellular debris, thereby providing a defense mechanism against foreign matter. Tissue macrophages include the Kupffer cells in the liver and alveolar macrophages (dust cells) in the lung. See Alveolar cell types.

MACROSHOCK: An electric current passing through the body which is strong enough to produce a physically perceptible response. This response can take the form of sensory stimulation, muscular contraction, or burns. The threshold of perception for 60-cycle alternating current is approximately 1 mA.

MAGILL SYSTEM: A modification of the basic Ayre T-piece for pediatric anesthesia purposes. It is useful with spontaneous, assisted, or controlled ventilation. In the Mapleson classification of breathing systems, the Magill system is known as the A system, based on the relative positions of the fresh gas flow, expiratory valve, and reservoir bag. See Ayre T-piece.

MAGNESIUM (Mg): A silvery, metallic element with an atomic number of 12 and atomic weight of 24.3. Its salts are essential in nutrition. Magnesium is necessary as a catalyst for many intracellular enzymatic reactions, especially those pertaining to carbohydrate, lipid, and protein metabolism. Normal extracellular Mg concentration is approximately 1.8-2.5 mEq/L. Hypomagnesemia (<1 mEq/L), seen in alcoholic cirrhosis, chronic nephritis, prolonged parenteral fluid therapy (without Mg supplementation), and cancer, is characterized by neuromuscular and central nervous system (CNS) hyperirritability, cardiac arrhythmia, convulsions, depression, and psychotic behavior. Hypermagnesemia (>3 mEq/L), associated with chronic renal disease and magnesium sulfate enemas, is characterized by drowsiness, CNS depression, and decreased skeletal muscle contraction (similar to hyper-kalemia). The body's normal Mg content is approximately 25 g, half of which is in the bone. See Ion.

MAGNESIUM HYDROXIDE (MILK OF MAGNESIA): A useful antacid and cathartic.

MAGNESIUM SULFATE (EPSOM SALT): A magnesium salt useful as a cathartic and antacid. It is also used to treat seizures associated with acute nephritis and eclampsia. Magnesium sulfate may accentuate the action of muscle relaxants.

MALIGNANT HYPERTENSION: A progressive elevation of blood pressure which ultimately produces degenerative changes in the walls of blood vessels; papilledema; retinal, cerebral, and renal hemorrhages; and left ventricular hypertrophy. A persistent diastolic blood pressure of < 120 mmHg associated with these clinical features is indicative of malignant hypertension. Approximately 1% of patients with essential hypertension develop malignant hypertension. Untreated patients usually live < 1 year and typically die of uremia, heart failure, or stroke. Diet and drug therapy are implemented to reduce the hypertension, and many of these patients may survive for several years without renal disease. See Hypertension.

MALIGNANT HYPERPYREXIA: See Malignant hyperthermia.

MALIGNANT HYPERTHERMIA (MH; MALIGNANT HYPERPYREXIA): A genetically determined (autosomal dominant) syndrome which becomes evident following an abnormal reaction to various anesthetic agents. Although any potent inhalation anesthetic agent or skeletal muscle relaxant may precipitate an acute crisis of MH in susceptible individuals, most frequently implicated are halothane and succinylcholine. Malignant hyperthermia can also occur following the use of a monoamine oxidase inhibitor or psychotropic agent. Malignant hyperthermia is characterized by a markedly elevated body temperature, tachycardia, unstable blood pressure, arrhythmias, cyanosis, skin mottling, and profuse diaphoresis. Muscle rigidity may or may not be present. (Temperature levels as high as 44 degrees Celsius have been recorded.) Laboratory findings include respiratory and metabolic acidosis; hyperkalemia; hypercalcemia; and elevated levels of serum creatine phosphokinase (CPK), lactic dehydrogenase, and myoglobin. The overall incidence of MH in anesthetic administrations is approximately 1/15,000 in children and 1/50,000 in adults. Mortality rate is approximately 60% if treated late or inadequately. The ability to determine susceptibility to MH preoperatively would aid in decreasing this rate. Evaluation of patients should include a complete medical history and physical examination to detect subclinical muscle weakness or abnormality. Specific information about anesthetic exposures in family members should be obtained as well. Measurement of CPK levels, although not completely reliable, may be used as a screening test. Muscle biopsies may be taken for halothane-caffeine contraction tests and for light and electron microscopic studies to determine certain myopathies in patients susceptible to MH. Awareness of MH susceptibility should alert the anesthetist to use neuroleptanesthesia (fentanyl and droperidol), pancuronium, or a barbiturate/N2O/ narcotic combination and to avoid succinylcholine and other depolarizing relaxants, local anesthetics of the amide type, and halogenated anesthetic agents. The classic presentation of MH (in a previously unsuspected case) is muscle rigidity (frequently jaw muscles) following intravenous (IV) succinylcholine administration. Anesthesia should be terminated immediately and, if the surgery is of an emergency nature, neuroleptanesthesia should be administered. Dantrolene, a muscle relaxant which acts directly on skeletal muscle, should be given intravenously as soon as the syndrome of MH is recognized. It decreases the amount of calcium released from the sarcoplasmic reticulum, thereby reversing the probable defect found in MH, i.e., an inability to control calcium levels within the muscle fibers which leads to an elevated intracellular calcium concentration. See Caffeine test, Creatine phosphokinase.

MALPRACTICE: A treatment rendered by a health practitioner which is improper, unskillful, and possibly injurious to the patient. An acceptable level of professional skill, "the standard of care," is not rendered. This "standard" varies with the amount and type of training the individual practitioner possesses and is determined by expert testimony.

MANDATORY MINUTE VOLUME (MMV): A technique of ventilatory support in which the overall minute volume is maintained at a preset level. The patient's responses regulate the volume supplied by spontaneous respiration and the remainder is supplied by intermittent positive pressure breathing.

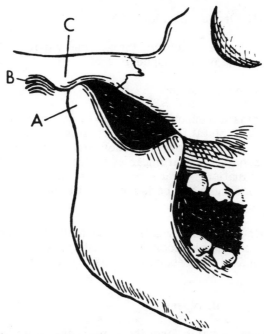

Mandible: Dislocated mandible, a potential mishap of anesthesia which can occur with muscle paralysis and manipulation of the mandible. The condyle (A) is out of the fossa (B) in the base of the skull and has jumped anterior to the articular eminence (C). Direct movement posteriorly is impossible. The condyle must descend before it can move posteriorly to regain normal position.

MANDIBLE: The lower jaw. It is the largest and strongest facial bone and the only movable bone in the skull. It consists of the body, ramus, angle, coronoid process, and condylar process. (The condylar process forms part of the articulation of the temporomandibular joint.) The mental nerve and vessels pass through the mental foramen and the inferior alveolar nerve and vessels pass through the mandibular foramen. These are frequently the sites for dental local anesthetic injections. See Fig.

MANNITOL: A naturally occurring sugar alcohol which is useful as a diuretic when administered intravenously. It rapidly decreases brain mass and cerebrospinal fluid pressure prior to neurosurgery and intraocular tension during an acute attack of congestive glaucoma or prior to ophthalmic surgery. Mannitol is known as an osmotic diuretic because it filters at the glomerulus, is not reabsorbed by the tubules, and is resistant to metabolic changes. In large amounts it adds to the osmolality of the plasma, the glomerular filtrate, and the tubular fluid. The extracellular fluid volume increases following administration of mannitol.

MANOMETER: An instrument for measuring the pressure of liquids and gases. A sphygmomanometer, for example, measures blood pressure.

MAO INHIBITOR: See Monoamine oxidase inhibitor.

MAPLESON SYSTEM: See Magill system.

MARCAINE (BUPIVACAINE): See Local anesthetic.

MASK, ANESTHESIA: A device for delivering gas and vapor to the nose and mouth simultaneously, while sealing out atmospheric air.

MASS NUMBER: See Nucleus, atomic.

MASS REFLEX: An automatic response exhibited by an area which is innervated by a segment of the spinal cord distal to a cord disruption. It may be evident in paraplegic individuals. A mild stimulus to the denervated area causes uncontrolled massive sympathetic discharge, resulting in sweating, pallor, blood pressure shifts, defecation, and urination. There may be a withdrawal response of the limbs. The fluctuation in blood pressure can be harmful to the patient since it may potentially overload the circulatory system.

MASS SPECTROMETER: An analytic instrument which identifies a substance by separating and quantifying its ions according to their mass. A mass spectrometer may be used for rapid analysis of respiratory gases accurate to a few parts per million.

MAST CELL: See Alveolar cell types.

MAXILLA: The paired bones which form the upper jaw. It articulates with every facial bone except the mandible and forms the floor of the nasal cavities and part of the floor of the orbit and palate. The infraorbital nerve and artery pass through the infraorbital foramen, an opening in the maxilla inferior to the orbit. The incisive foramen and greater and lesser palatine foramens are other canals through which nerves and vessels travel. These are common sites for dental local anesthetic injections.

MAXIMUM BREATHING CAPACITY (MBC): See Maximum voluntary ventilation.

MAXIMUM VOLUNTARY VENTILATION (MVV): The volume of air that can be breathed per minute by the greatest voluntary effort. To test the MVV, a patient is asked to breathe as deeply and rapidly as possible for 15 sec. The MVV is reduced in patients with such conditions as airway obstruction and emphysema. The MVV is also known as maximum breathing capacity (MBC).

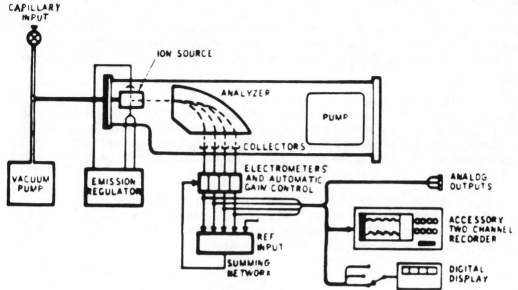

CAPILLARY INPUT

ION SOURCE

ANALYZER

PUMP

COLLECTORS

VACUUM PUMP

EMISSION REGULATOR

ELECTROMETERS AND AUTOMATIC GAIN CONTROL

ANALOG OUTPUTS

ACCESSORY TWO CHANNEL RECORDER

REF INPUT

SUMMING NETWORK

DIGITAL DISPLAY

Mass Spectrometer: Simplified schematic.

MEAN ARTERIAL PRESSURE (MAP): The average blood pressure throughout the cardiac cycle. The formula used to approximate this pressure is: MAP = diastolic pressure + 1/3 pulse pressure (systolic pressure - diastolic pressure). See Arterial blood pressure.

MECHANICAL NEBULIZER: See Nebulizer.

MEDIAN: The middle number of a set of numbers arranged in order of magnitude. For example, the median of the set of serum sodium values 135, 138, 139, 140, 142, 142, and 145 is 140. Note that this is not the same as the arithmetic mean.

MEDIAN POWER FREQUENCY (MPF): A means of analysis of an electroencephalograph (EEG) signal along with the peak power frequency (PPF). The MPF and PPF are determined after the EEG signal is broken down by Fourier analysis. Shifts in the MPF and PPF have been used to monitor changes in depth of anesthesia. The MPF is the median frequency of the set of frequencies determined by the Fourier equation. The PPF is the component frequency with the highest amplitude in the same set. See Fourier analysis, Leading edge analysis.

MEDIASTINAL FLAP: The movement of the heart and great vessels in the mediastinum toward the unaffected lung during ventilation when the other lung has collapsed. This may be a dangerous occurrence, especially if the patient is in a lateral position, because the entire weight of the mediastinal contents compresses the normal lung.

MEDIASTINAL SHIFT: The abnormal position of the mediastinum, which can be visualized by x-ray. It occurs in patients with atelectasis.

MEDIASTINOSCOPY: An examination of the mediastinum using a lighted endoscope which is inserted through a cervical incision at the suprasternal notch. The instrument is passed along the anterior surface of the trachea to the bifurcation of the trachea. Direct visualization allows the surgeon to perform a biopsy of a suspicious area, e.g., lymph nodes or bronchi. This procedure, which requires general anesthesia, is used in the evaluation of hilar adenopathy and metastatic bronchogenic cancer. It is a potentially hazardous procedure, however, because of the possibility of injury to the great vessels present in the area due to improper scope manipulation.

MEDIASTINUM: The tissues and organs between the pleuras of the lungs that extend from the sternum to the vertebral column. It is subdivided into the superior mediastinum (containing many large vessels), anterior mediastinum (containing the thymus gland), middle mediastinum (containing the pericardium and heart), and posterior mediastinum (containing the esophagus, trachea, and many large lymphatic and blood vessels).

MEDLARS: An acronym for MEDical Literature Analysis and Retrieval System. It is a computerized service of the National Library of Medicine (available to most medical and dental school libraries) which organizes published material into key words and topics to aid a complete literature search.

MEGA-: See SI unit.

MEMBRANE OXYGENATOR: A method to facilitate gas exchange in extracorporeal circulation. The blood and the gases are separated by a membrane which allows diffusion of O_2 and CO_2. This attempts to simulate the physiologic state (no gas-blood contact). This type of oxygenator, however, is expensive and difficult to use, and its capacity is limited. Because of its theoretic advantages it is still being improved and may in the future replace other oxygenators, particularly in long-term cases.

MEMORY, COMPUTER: A mechanism (human or mechanical) used for the storage of information within a designated system. Many categories of machine memory exist: (1) volatile, a temporary type, in which power loss causes a loss of the information; (2) nonvolatile, a permanent type, in which loss of electric power leaves the information intact; (3) random access memory (RAM), in which all stored information is available in the same amount of time; (4) read-only memory (ROM), in which information can only be read out and not added to by the user; and (5) programmable read-only memory (PROM), which is a ROM that can be changed or added to in toto. Reprogramming this type deletes all earlier information. (In the changing world of microelectronics, these definitions are subject to alteration at least every 18 months.)

MENDELSON SYNDROME: See Aspiration.

MEPERIDINE (DEMEROL): A synthetic analgesic drug which is useful as a supplement to N_2O/O_2 anesthesia. See Narcotic.

MEPHENTERMINE (WYAMINE): A drug related to ephedrine which has both direct and indirect vasoactive properties. It causes the release of endogenous norepinephrine and it has a positive inotropic effect on the heart.

MEPIVACAINE (CARBOCAINE): See Local anesthetic.

MEPROBAMATE (EQUANIL; MILTOWN): A drug with mild sedative and tranquilizing properties. Side effects tend to be dose-related; high doses cause drowsiness and may induce allergic reactions (skin rash and itching). Meprobamate has an additive effect with alcohol and other central nervous system depressants.

MERCURY SWITCH: A device in which electric contact can be established between a pair of electrodes by a drop of mercury enclosed in a glass cylinder. Depending on the tilt of the cylinder, the mercury will move either toward or away from the contacts to make or break a circuit.

MESH: A network or screen composed of small openings which allow various sized particles to pass through or to be retained. Mesh size is designated according to the number of openings per linear inch and is used to grade soda lime granules.

MESTINON: See Pyridostigmine.

METABOLIC ACIDOSIS: A condition in which there is a decrease in the pH of the body fluids not caused by an excess of CO_2. Metabolic acidosis may result from severe diarrhea (which would eliminate excessive amounts of sodium bicarbonate), kidney malfunction (which would interfere with normal excretion of metabolic acids), excessive amounts of metabolic acids in the body (from exogenous or endogenous sources), or a loss of alkali from body fluids. It depresses the central nervous system to such a level that it may lead to coma. The acid pH also leads to an increased rate and depth of respiration (compensatory respiratory alkalosis).

METABOLIC ALKALOSIS: A condition in which there is an increase in the pH of the body fluids not caused by reduction in CO_2. This may result from excess ingestion of alkaline substances, excessive vomiting of gastric contents (and a subsequent decrease in acid content), or excessive secretion of aldosterone by the adrenal gland. Metabolic alkalosis tends to overexcite the nervous system and leads to tetany.

METABOLIC COMPENSATION: See Acid-base compensation.

METABOLITE: A substance produced by metabolism. Metabolites are classified pharmacologically as active or inactive. Active metabolites can produce further changes in physiologic function; inactive metabolites are breakdown products which cause little or no change in physiologic function. Halothane is a general anesthetic with active metabolites undergoing metabolic breakdown in the body. Up to 30% of inhaled halothane is transformed into nonvolatile metabolites. It is now postulated that bromine (a known sedative), which is a metabolite of the halothane molecule, may account for prolonged awakening after a long halothane anesthetic.

METARAMINOL (ARAMINE): An antihypotensive drug that causes profound peripheral vasoconstriction by acting directly on alpha receptors. See Receptor/receptor site.

METARTERIOLE: See Microcirculation.

MET-ENKEPHALIN: See Enkephalins.

METER (m): The standard international unit of length (approximately equal to 39.37 in), which is defined in terms of the wavelength of the orange light emitted during the electric excitation of krypton.

METHADONE (AMIDONE; DOLOPHINE): A synthetic narcotic related to meperidine. Although it has an analgesic potency approximately equal to that of morphine, it has a much longer duration of action. It produces respiratory depression, but causes less sedation, nausea, and constipation than morphine. Methadone is useful in the treatment of narcotic addiction. Subsequent withdrawal symptoms are less severe but may be more prolonged. See Narcotic.

METHAMPHETAMINE: See Amphetamine.

METHEMOGLOBIN: See Hemoglobin.

METHOHEXITAL (BREVITAL): See Barbiturate.

METHOXAMINE (VASOXYL): A sympathomimetic drug which acts directly on alpha receptors. It tends to increase blood pressure by causing vasoconstriction and is therefore used primarily to treat hypotensive states. It has no significant stimulant effect on the heart. See Receptor/receptor site.

Methoxyflurane.

METHOXYFLURANE (PENTHRANE; 2,2-DICHLORO-1,1-DIFLUOROETHYL METHYL ETHER): A halogenated hydrocarbon, liquid, general anesthetic. It is lipid-soluble and has a very low vapor pressure at room temperature. It produces analgesia and relaxation of skeletal muscles. Its use is limited to short-term intermittent administration to lessen the accumulation of the agent in the body. (It may be used during the first stage of labor for its analgesic properties.) Methoxyflurane is nephrotoxic as the drug is metabolized to free fluoride ions and other toxic derivatives which may cause permanent renal damage. See Fig.

METHYLDOPA (ALDOMET): An antihypertensive agent that decreases both blood pressure and total peripheral resistance. It has been reported to both maintain cardiac output and decrease cardiac output. Its precise mechanism of action is unknown but it is currently believed to act primarily on the central nervous system. Methyldopa, given orally or parenterally, tends to produce sedation and some depression. This drug and its metabolites interfere with laboratory tests for catecholamines and their presence in blood and urine produces false positive results for pheochromocytoma.

METHYLENE BLUE: A dark green crystalline powder, producing a distinct blue color in solution, which is a useful histologic-biologic stain. Since it can be reduced to a colorless form and oxidized to its blue form, methylene blue may be used as an indicator in reversible oxidation-reduction reactions. The dye has weak bactericidal properties but is no longer used for this purpose. Currently, methylene blue in low doses is relied on as a treatment for methemoglobinemia. It hastens the conversion of methemoglobin to hemoglobin. Conversely, high concentrations of methylene blue oxidize the ferrous ion of reduced hemoglobin to the ferric form, thereby inducing methemoglobinemia.

METHYL METHACRYLATE: A volatile flammable liquid which is easily polymer-ized and is useful as a monomer for resins and as a bone cement. To form the ce-ment, a powder (polymer which contains short chains of methyl methacrylate) and a liquid (monomer which contains single molecules) are rapidly mixed to form a semiviscous mass which hardens as molecular chains lengthen and cross-link (poly-merization). There is controversy as to what effect this semisolid material has on the circulation when placed onto raw bone surfaces, i.e., both hypertension and hy-potension are seen.

METHYLMORPHINE (CODEINE): See Narcotic.

METHYLPARABEN: See Preservative.

METICORTELONE: See Corticosteroid, Prednisolone.

METICORTEN: See Corticosteroid, Prednisone.

METRAZOL: See Pentylenetetrazol.

METUBINE: See Dimethyl tubocurarine iodide, Neuromuscular blocking agent, Tu-bocurarine chloride.

METYCAINE: See Local anesthetic, Piperocaine.

MEYER-OVERTON THEORY: See Lipid solubility theory of anesthesia.

MICROCIRCULATION: The part of the vascular network comprising the arterioles, capillaries, and venules, and their smaller branches. The arterioles divide into metarterioles (precapillaries), which are lined with discontinuous muscle cells. Blood flows from the metarterioles into the venules via a capillary thoroughfare ves-sel. True capillaries are connecting side branches of this thoroughfare vessel or channel and are lined with a single layer of endothelial cells. The openings of the true capillaries are surrounded by smooth muscle precapillary sphincters, which regulate the surface area of the capillary-venule network. Venules merge to form collecting venules, which drain the entire microcirculatory unit. Arteriovenous anas-tomoses provide extensive collateral circulation. (Many capillaries originate from single metarterioles and branch and anastomose repeatedly to provide an increased surface area, which effectively lowers the velocity of blood flow.) Sympathetic block-ade causes the musculature of the metarterioles and precapillary sphincters to re-lax, making the entire capillary bed available for blood passage. If this occurs over a large enough portion of the microcirculatory bed, it can cause a profound drop in blood pressure as the resultant intravascular volume is enlarged 3-4 times that of circulating blood. Sympathetic blockade does not cause a maximal increase in intra-vascular volume because the capillary beds have an intrinsic vasomotor tone affected by the sympathetic nervous system. This vasomotor tone can be disturbed by hista-mine or local acid-base derangements. See Acid-base balance; Histamine; Micro-sphere, biologic.

MICROFUEL CELL: See Oxygen analyzer.

MICROGNATHIA: A congenital or acquired condition in which the jaws are abnor-mally small. This disorder is significant in anesthesia because a satisfactory fit of the mask is difficult to achieve and maintenance of the airway is therefore not op-timal. See Pierre Robin syndrome.

MICROHEMATOCRIT: The rapid determination of erythrocyte volume in an extremely small quantity of blood. This measurement is accomplished using a capillary tube of blood in a high-speed centrifuge.

MICROSHOCK: An electric shock of very small magnitude which is hazardous to patients with pacemakers, cardiac catheters, or other direct-current paths to the heart.

MICROSPHERE, BIOLOGIC: A minutely sized sphere (5-50 μm) composed of an inert material (cannot be broken down in circulation) or albumin (can be broken down). Microspheres are used to determine the extent and size of the microcirculation in an organ or part of an organ. They can be prepared to contain at least eight different radioisotopes. The spheres function by flowing distally with the blood and then lodging, according to size, in the capillaries. They can be identified microscopically (tissue sections) or radiographically (if they are tagged with a radiotracer).

MICROWAVE: An electromagnetic wave of high frequency (1-300 GHz) and short wavelength (0.1-100 cm) that is not sharply distinguishable from either infrared or radio waves. Microwaves are used in radar surveillance and cooking.

MIDAZOLAM: A new water-soluble benzodiazepine derivative that is virtually painless on injection and lessens the incidence of venous thrombosis. It is apparently 3 times as potent as diazepam, has a much shorter half-life, and may find significant use as an anesthetic induction agent. See Antianxiety.

MILLIHENRY: See Henry.

MILLIMETERS OF MERCURY (mmHg): A unit of pressure which is measured by the height, in millimeters, of a column of mercury at standard gravity. One standard atmosphere equals 760 mmHg.

MILLIOSMOLE: See Osmole.

MILL WHEEL MURMUR: An aberrant cardiac sound associated with venous air embolism. It is a relatively insensitive indicator of this condition and is often misinterpreted. (Having listened to a mill wheel on many occasions, the author does not find it very similar to the murmur of venous air embolism. The mill wheel was courtesy of the Mt. Vernon Historical Society, Alexandria, Virginia.) See Embolism.

MILTOWN: See Meprobamate.

MINIMUM ALVEOLAR CONCENTRATION (MAC): The anesthetic concentration at 1 atmosphere (after the alveolar gas has equilibrated with the inhaled gas mixture) which is necessary to produce a lack of response to a standard skin incision in 50% of subjects tested. MAC is the best available method for comparing the potencies of inhaled anesthetics. See MAC awake.

MINIMUM BLOCKING CONCENTRATION (C_m): The lowest level of local anesthetic that will block nerve impulse conduction. Each anesthetic has its own C_m, and the smaller the C_m, the more effective the agent. The thicker nerve filbers require a higher concentration of local anesthetic. See Duality of pain transmission; Nerve fiber, anatomy and physiology of.

MINUTE VOLUME: The total volume of air leaving the lung each minute, calculated by multiplying the tidal volume by the respiratory rate. The volume of air which enters the lung is slightly greater than the volume of air which leaves the lung because more O_2 is inhaled than CO_2 is exhaled. See Lung volumes and capacities.

MIOSIS: The contraction of the pupil of the eye.

MIOTIC: An agent that produces miosis.

MITRAL REGURGITATION (MITRAL INSUFFICIENCY): A condition in which the mitral (bicuspid; left atrioventricular) valve fails to close completely, thereby allowing reflux from the left ventricle into the left atrium. Chronic mitral regurgitation is usually the result of rheumatic heart disease and can remain stable for many years. Acute mitral regurgitation can occur due to papillary muscle dysfunction or rupture of chorda tendineae cordis. (The cusps of the mitral valve are attached by means of the chorda tendineae cordis to papillary muscles which are located on the inner surface of the ventricles. Functioning chorda tendineae cordis and the papillary muscles keep the valve flaps pointing in the direction of the blood flow. Contraction of these muscles prevents the valve from swinging upward into the atrium.) Mitral regurgitation is poorly tolerated and may result in death. As the left atrium becomes a low-pressure shunt for left ventricular ejection, the total stroke volume of the left ventricle consists of backflow into the atrium and forward flow into the aorta. This causes left atrial hypertrophy. Symptoms of mitral insufficiency include easy fatigability, exertional and nocturnal dyspnea, and, ultimately, congestive heart failure. Deliberate peripheral vascular dilatation (nitroprusside) significantly decreases backflow into the atrium and enhances forward flow.

MITRAL STENOSIS: A narrowing of the orifice of the mitral valve which causes obstruction of blood flow from the left atrium to the left ventricle. It is the most common form of rheumatic valvular heart disease in adults. The area of the adult mitral valve is 4-6 cm. When progressive narrowing of the valve reduces this area to 1 cm^2 or less, a mean left atrial pressure (LAP) of 25 mmHg (normal LAP is 8-12 mmHg) is required to maintain a minimally adequate left ventricular filling and cardiac output. This elevated LAP eventually causes an increase in pulmonary arterial and right ventricular pressures, which produces symptoms such as dyspnea on exertion and paroxysmal nocturnal dyspnea. As the disease progresses, orthopnea and fatigue become prominent and acute pulmonary edema may occur. Adequate control of the cardiac rate is an anesthetic consideration for a patient with this condition. Drugs which may induce tachycardia should be avoided. Mitral valve prostheses are employed to replace the diseased valve surgically.

MODE: The value which occurs most frequently in a set of variables.

MODEM: An acronym for MOdulator/DEModulator. This is a device which transforms or converts signals from one type of equipment into a form for use in another type. It is typically used to modulate and demodulate signals transmitted over communication networks.

MODULATION: The controlled variation of frequency, phase, and/or amplitude of a wave to transmit a message.

MOGADON (NITRAZEPAM): See Benzodiazepine.

MOISTURE EXCHANGER (ARTIFICIAL NOSE): A device, composed of a condenser or filter, which allows efficient humidification for a patient who is breathing through a tracheostomy or endotracheal tube. Since the temperature of the exchanger is lower than the body, some water vapor from expiration condenses on its inner surface and is thereby able to humidify the inspired air. This apparatus lessens fluid loss seen when the upper airways are bypassed. It also helps prevent excessive drying of the lower air passageways.

MOLAL SOLUTION: A solution which contains 1 mol solute dissolved in 1 kg solvent.

MOLAR PREGNANCY (HYDATIDIFORM MOLE): An abnormal pregnancy resulting from a pathologic ovum. The chorionic villi become hydropic and trophoblastic tissue proliferates. This condition is more common in older women. The majority of hydatidiform moles are benign. Urinary human chorionic gonadotropin (HCG) hormone levels are markedly elevated.

MOLAR SOLUTION: A solution in which each liter contains 1 gram-molecule of the dissolved substance.

MOLE: See Gram-molecular weight.

MOLECULE: The smallest quantity into which a substance may be divided while still retaining all its chemical properties.

MONITOR: An instrument used to measure, display, and/or record (continuously or intermittently) certain physiologic variables such as pulse, blood pressure, and respiration.

MONOAMINE OXIDASE (MAO) INHIBITOR: A drug which blocks MAO, an enzyme important in catecholamine degradation. When this enzyme is inhibited, a resultant increase in the concentration of norepinephrine, dopamine, and serotonin occurs, producing side effects such as orthostatic hypotension, nervousness, and insomnia. Severe adverse reactions (hypertension, headache, heart palpitations) occur in patients who have ingested tyramine-rich foods and beverages (e.g., aged cheese, Chianti wine) or certain drugs (e.g., meperidine, barbiturates, sympathomimetic amines). MAO inhibitors were originally introduced to treat depression. Due to the pronounced side effects they can produce, however, their use has decreased.

MONTANDO TUBE: A U-shaped endotracheal tube previously used to deliver anesthetic gases through a tracheostomy.

MONTEVIDEO UNIT: A system for determining the relative force of uterine contractions using the intrauterine pressure (in torr) times the frequency of contractions in a 10-min period.

MORBIDITY: The condition of being ill. In common usage, morbidity describes the possibility and type of untoward effects following a specific procedure. For example, morbidity associated with endotracheal anesthesia includes sore throat or damaged teeth. In statistics, morbidity indicates the relative incidence of disease.

MORPHINE: A naturally occurring narcotic analgesic obtained from opium. It is the standard of comparison of potency for all narcotics. See Narcotic.

MORTALITY: The condition of being subject to dying. In common usage, mortality describes the possibility of dying from a given procedure or technique. In statistics, mortality rate indicates the proportion of deaths in a population.

MORTON, WILLIAM T. G.: A dentist and medical student who gave the first successful demonstration of general anesthesia, employing diethyl ether, at the Massachusetts General Hospital, October 16, 1846. (The operating room, known as the Etherdome, still exists as a memorial.) Diethyl ether was brought to the attention of Morton by Charles Jackson, his chemistry professor. Crawford Long, a Georgia surgeon, used diethyl ether as a general anesthetic on his own patients at least 4 years earlier (but without publishing). Gardner Quincy Colton demonstrated the use of N_2O as an anesthetic in Connecticut in 1844. Horace Wells, a dentist in the audience, was so impressed with the agent that he offered to test it on himself. Wells demonstrated N_2O the next year at Harvard, but the results were unfavorable and the technique was thought to be useless. Controversy developed as to who should receive recognition for inventing anesthesia. The four men involved never profited from the discovery and spent the rest of their lives in litigation.

MOUTH-TO-MOUTH RESUSCITATION: A method of artificial ventilation in which the rescuer's mouth is placed over the victim's mouth (mouth and nose in an infant) and air is blown forcefully into the lungs at a rate of 12 times/min in an adult or 30 times/min in an infant. It provides adequate O_2 for life support even though exhaled breath contains only 14-18% O_2. This technique is combined with external cardiac massage in cardiopulmonary resuscitation (CPR) to resuscitate patients with cardiac arrest.

MUCOCILIARY TRANSPORT: The cleansing action of the cilia in the trachea and respiratory passageways. Cilia are fine, hairlike structures approximately 7 μm long and 0.3 μm thick, projecting from specialized columnar cells of the mucous membrane. Ciliary movement occurs at a rate of 10-15 times/sec to move mucus and trapped foreign material upward toward the hypopharynx for swallowing. Ciliary activity is optimal at 28-33 degrees Celsius, stops at 7-10 degrees Celsius, and decreases above 35 degrees Celsius. In actuality, however, ciliary activity is directly influenced by the quantity of mucus secreted rather than by temperature changes. Low concentrations of volatile general anesthetics stimulate ciliary activity whereas high concentrations depress it. (N_2O has no effect on ciliary transport.) Nonhumidified gases dry the mucous membranes and hinder ciliary movement. This effect is even more pronounced following concomitant use of atropine as a premedicant.

MUCOMYST: See Respiratory care.

MUCUS: A viscous fluid suspension secreted by the mucous membranes and composed of mucin (a complex polysaccharide), water, desquamated cells, leukocytes, and inorganic salts. Mucus moistens and protects the respiratory tract and is essential for ciliary activity. See Mucociliary transport.

MULTIBREATH TEST: A test used to determine the rate of washout of pulmonary N_2 when 100% O_2 is administered starting at the end of a normal expiration. The N_2 concentration, continuously measured at expiration by a N_2 analyzer, is nearly linear (on semilogarithmic paper) when plotted against the number of breaths in normal patients. This is explained by the fact that the remaining N_2 in the lung is successfully diluted by each breath of pure O_2, thereby causing an exponential decay in N_2 concentration. When ventilation is uneven, as in a diseased lung, the line becomes successively curved because different regions of the lung eliminate N_2 at different rates. At the very end of the test only the N_2 left in the least ventilated spaces is being washed out. The test can be modified to determine the functional residual capacity (FRC). The FRC = the volume of N_2 washed out X 100/78 (since 78% of the gas in the lungs is N_2). See Infrared analyzer, Single-breath test.

MULTIPLEX: The simultaneous transmission of two or more signals via a common carrier wave by means of time, frequency, or phase divisions. See Modulation.

MUSCARINE: A naturally occurring alkaloid which acts like acetylcholine on receptors of smooth muscles and glandular cells. These receptors are blocked by atropine. Muscarine is not used clinically at the present time. See Neuromuscular blocking agent, Pilocarpine.

MUSCARINIC DRUG: A drug which produces effects similar to those of muscarine. These effects include marked diaphoresis, salivation, noticeable drop in blood pressure, and temporary slowing or cessation of the heart rate. Examples of muscarinic agents are acetylcholine, methacholine, bethanechol, and carbachol.

MUSCLE ACTION POTENTIAL (MAP): See Neuromuscular blocking agent.

MUSCLE CONTRACTION/RELAXATION: See Actomyosin.

MUSCLE RELAXANT: See Neuromuscular blocking agent.

MUSCLE TWITCH: A sudden solitary muscle contraction of extremely short duration (approximately 7.5-100 msec). The twitch can be elicited by exciting the motor nerve or by passing an electric current through the muscle itself.

MUSCULAR DYSTROPHY: A group of hereditary diseases characterized by progressive atrophy of the muscles and by the absence of central nervous system (CNS) involvement. Many types of muscular dystrophy have been described. Duchenne, the most common type, is sex-linked and, therefore, confined to young boys. Serum enzyme studies reveal markedly elevated levels of creatine phosphokinase (CPK). Female carriers may be identified with moderate increases in the serum CPK levels. Pseudohypertrophy of the calf muscles is evident; this is due to replacement of muscle cells by fatty and fibrous tissues. Cardiac abnormalities occur in many of these patients. Most Duchenne patients die within a decade from respiratory infection or cardiac failure. In other forms of muscular dystrophy, symptoms tend to appear later in life and localized areas of the body become affected.

MUTAGENICITY: The ability of a substance (mutagen) to produce a permanent alteration in the genetic material. Mutagens include radioactive substances and some chemotherapeutic agents.

MYASTHENIA GRAVIS (MG): A chronic disease characterized by muscle weakness and easy fatigability. Typically, there are alternating periods of remission and exacerbation of symptoms. Ptosis and diplopia are common early signs. Myasthenia gravis appears to be caused by an abnormality at the neuromuscular junction that prevents the muscle from contracting normally in response to nerve impulses. Functionally, it appears that the neurons fail to release enough acetylcholine, or excessive cholinesterase present in the neuromuscular junction destroys acetylcholine (ACh), or there is a decrease in acetylcholine receptors. (Motor neurons stimulate contraction of muscle fibers by releasing ACh.) Although the exact etiology of MG is unknown at the present time, it is thought to be an autoimmune disorder based on the following. (1) Evidence exists that thymectomy may produce clinical improvement. (Organ-specific autoimmunity has been established to have a pathogenic role.) (2) Autoantibodies to ACh receptors have been demonstrated in the sera of patients with MG. Myasthenia gravis results from this autoimmune damage to the ACh receptors, which in turn results in a failure of neuromuscular transmission. (3) Malignant thymomas may occur in patients with MG. Confirmation of an MG diagnosis may be accomplished by the "edrophonium test." An intravenous injection of edrophonium chloride, a short-acting anticholinesterase agent, produces a brief increase in muscle strength in the extremities. A nondepolarizing muscle relaxant may also be administered for diagnostic purposes; however, adequate means for patient resuscitation must be available. Patients with MG are extremely sensitive to drugs that produce respiratory depression (sedative-hypnotics and opiates) and to drugs that produce muscle weakness, e.g., neuromuscular blocking agents. These effects are potentiated with certain antibiotics (kanamycin, streptomycin, and neomycin) and some general anesthetics (ether, halothane, methoxyflurane, and cyclopropane). See Neuromuscular blocking agent.

MYASTHENIC SYNDROME: A weakness of the peripheral musculature usually seen in association with bronchial carcinoma. Patients with myasthenic syndrome are extremely sensitive to muscle relaxant agents. It differs from myasthenia gravis (MG) in that it first attacks limb muscles rather than ocular muscles, and has a poor response to anticholinesterases. See Myasthenia gravis.

MYCIFRADIN: See Neomycin.

MYDRIASIS: The excessive or extreme dilatation of the pupil. Unless induced by drugs or trauma, pupil dilatation is considered to be a sign of significant central nervous system damage.

MYELIN SHEATH: The lipid-ladened material which surrounds the axon of large nerve fibers. Its presence is critical for the rapid conduction of nerve impulses. It acts as an electric insulator by preventing the flow of ions between the axon and the extracellular fluid and as a pharmacologic insulator by protecting a nerve fiber from the actions of local anesthetics. It is possible for a local anesthetic to reach the nerve membrane only at the nodes of Ranvier, where the myelin thins out or is absent. Furthermore, these nodes act as circuits for electric impulses, i.e., impulses can actually jump from node to node faster than they can travel down the nerve membrane. This jumpwise conduction is called saltatory conduction. As a consequence of saltatory conduction, local anesthetics must cover a distance of at least two or three nodes (which in practical terms is a span of approximately 8-10 mm) to block myelinated fibers. See Fig. See Nerve fiber, anatomy and physiology of.

MYELOGRAPHY: The roentgenographic visualization of the spinal subarachnoid space following a lumbar or cisternal puncture and injection of air or an opaque medium.

MYELOMENINGOCELE: A congenital defect of the spinal canal through which the cord and its meninges protrude. Myelomeningoceles most frequently occur in the lumbosacral region. The abnormality is either exposed or covered by atrophic skin and infection is therefore a frequent complication. Paraplegia, absence of bowel and bladder control, and sensory disturbances below the level of the lesion are common. Surgical repair is aimed at preventing infection and correction of spinal abnormalities.

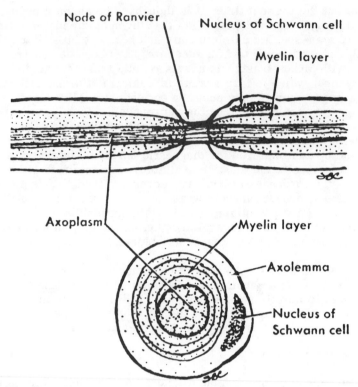

Myelin Sheath: Structure of a myelinated nerve fiber.

MYLAXEN: See Hexafluorenium.

MYOCARDIAL INFARCTION (MI): A syndrome resulting from sudden and persistent curtailment of myocardial blood supply due to a thrombus, embolus, or spasm (?) in a coronary artery. It is characterized by severe and prolonged chest pain (described as crushing or compressing) and electrocardiographic and laboratory evidence of myocardial necrosis. There is a rise in noncardiac-specific serum glutamic-oxaloacetic transaminase (SGOT) and in the serum levels of cardiac-specific isoenzymes of creatinine phosphokinase (CK) and lactic dehydrogenase (LDH). SGOT and CK rise and fall rapidly. While LDH rises slowly, the rise is sustained. The size of the infarct can be correlated with the amount of enzyme released. The electrocardiographic irregularities, if present, are usually abnormal Q waves and ST segment changes. Pulmonary edema and shock frequently accompany MI and pulmonary embolism and cardiac arrest are common complications. Paroxysmal atrial or ventricular arrhythmias may occur after MI. See QRS complex.

MYOCARDIAL IRRITABILITY: The tendency of the myocardium toward arrhythmia. Irritability is enhanced by circulating catecholamines, lowered body temperature, myocardial ischemia, acid-base imbalance, electrolyte abnormalities (particularly potassium), and certain drugs, e.g., halothane.

MYOCARDIUM: The specialized muscle tissue of the heart. Cardiac muscle fibers are involuntary and striated, and are responsible for the contraction of the heart. The myocardial tissue layer lies between the epicardial and endocardial layers. Cardiac muscle tissue contracts rhythmically about 70-80 times/min. Specialized conducting tissue of the heart transmits electric impulses that stimulate cardiac contraction. Two networks of cardiac muscle fibers exist: the muscle walls and septum of the ventricles. Each fiber is separated from the next by an intercalated disc. When a single fiber is stimulated, all the fibers in that network become stimulated. Each network therefore contracts as a functional unit. See Heart, conduction system of.

MYOFASCIAL SYNDROME (Myofascial Pain Syndrome, Myofasciitis): An entity characterized by pain and at times autonomic phenomena generated by compression at a hyperirritable location called a trigger point. The pain or dysfunction usually is located over a particular muscle, group of muscles, or fascial plane and need not obey dermatomal distribution. Treatment is usually aimed at eliminating the trigger points by physiotherapy or local anesthesia.

MYOGLOBIN: An O_2 transport and storage protein complex found in muscle fibers.

MYONEURAL JUNCTION: See Neuromuscular blocking agent.

MYOTONIA: An increased irritability and contractility of a muscle or group of muscles. It is temporary when brought about by excessive exercise. Myotonia is identical with tonic muscle spasm and is also seen in various disease states.

MYOTONIA ATROPHICA (MYOTONIC DYSTROPHY; STEINERT DISEASE): A rare, hereditary (autosomal dominant) disease characterized by a slowly degenerative myotonia and subsequent atrophy of the muscles (especially of the face and neck). Ptosis, cataracts, testicular atrophy, endocrine dysfunction, and mental retardation are associated with this disorder. Some patients develop diabetes mellitus. Cardiac musculature is frequently affected. These patients are particularly prone to cardiorespiratory abnormalities and therefore pose problems for anesthetic management. When continued muscle contraction occurs in this disease, neuromuscular blocking agents do not relax the affected muscles because the motor nerves are uninvolved.

MYOTONIA CONGENITA (THOMSEN DISEASE): A rare, inherited (autosomal dominant) disease characterized by rigidity and the tonic spasm of muscles upon movement after a period of rest. (The stiffness disappears following continual use of the muscles.) The disease is manifested clinically in the entire somatic and branchiomeric muscular system. Patients complain of difficulty in chewing, swallowing, talking, and walking, and show evidence of muscle cell hypertrophy. Although myotonia congenita is not often debilitating, patients with the disease present anesthetic problems similar to those of patients with muscular dystrophy. See Muscular dystrophy.

MYOTONIC DYSTROPHY: See Myotonia atrophica.

MYTOLON: See Benzoquinonium.

NALLINE: See Nalorphine.

NALORPHINE (NALLINE): A drug with both narcotic agonist and antagonist effects. It has been replaced by the pure antagonist naloxone.

Naloxone.

NALOXONE (NARCAN): A derivative of oxymorphone (Numorphan) and a popular narcotic antagonist which is neither analgesic nor addicting. It reverses the respiratory depressant action of drugs such as morphine, meperidine, and methadone. Naloxone administered alone does not cause respiratory depression, pupillary constriction, sedation, or analgesia. See Fig.

NALTREXONE: A derivative of Naloxone with longer-lasting narcotic antagonist properties.

NANO-: See SI unit.

NARCAN: See Naloxone.

NARCOTIC: See Fig.

NARKOTEST METER: A device for indicating the percentage of halogenated hydrocarbon anesthetics in the gas mixture of an anesthetic circuit. Values are registered by changes in the length of Silastic bands attached to a lever which moves in proportion to the concentration of anesthetic absorbed. The Narkotest meter is not very accurate, requires a large gas sample, is affected by water vapor, and has a very slow response time. See Halothane analyzer.

Narcotics.

Generic Name (Trade Name)	Duration of Action* (hr)	Dose (mg)**
Alphaprodine (Nisentil)	1-2	25-35
Anileridine (Leritine)	2-4	23-30
Butorphanol (Stadol)	3-4	2-3
Codeine	4-6 (oral)	120
Dihydrocodeine (Paracodin)	4-5	60
Fentanyl (Sublimaze)	0.5-1.5	0.1
Heroin	3-4	3
Hydrocodone (Hycodan)	4-8 (oral)	5-10
Hydromorphone (Dilaudid)	4-5	1.5
Levorphanol (Levo-Dromoran)	4-5	2-3
Meperidine (Demerol)	2-4	80-100
Methadone (Dolophine)	3-5	7.5-10
Morphine	4-5	10
Nalbuphine (Nubain)	4-5	10
Oxycodone (Percodan)	4-5	10-15
Oxymorphone (Numorphan)	4-5	1.0-1.5
Pentazocine (Talwin)	1-3	30-50 (parenteral) 60-100 (oral)

* Duration of action after subcutaneous administration, except codeine and hydrocodone which are administered orally. IV administration speeds onset and decreases duration. Narcotic depression of respiration usually outlasts analgesic effect.

** Doses listed are rough analgesic equivalents to 10 mg morphine.

NASAL CATHETER (NASAL CANNULA): A device which is inserted into the nose to supply O_2 enrichment to the inspired breath or to maintain an airway. Nosebleed is a fairly common consequence of its use. Nasal cannulas only augment inspired O_2 up to 50%; the high volumes of fresh gas flow required for this level of augmentation dry out the nasal mucosa, causing the patient extreme discomfort.

NASOTRACHEAL TUBE: An endotracheal tube which is introduced into the trachea via the nose. It has a smaller diameter than an orotracheal tube and less curvature, so that it passes easily along the posterior pharyngeal wall. Nasotracheal intubation is usually used in oral and maxillofacial operations and in patients with jaw fractures or trismus.

NATIONAL FIRE PROTECTION ASSOCIATION (NFPA): A voluntary nonprofit organization which writes codes and standards for fire prevention and safety for both the public and private sectors. It was founded in 1896 and its headquarters are in Boston. The NFPA has developed and continues to update approximately 240 codes and standards which cover such diverse areas as smoke detectors, firefighter clothing, stairway fire door standards, transportation of hazardous materials, electric wiring, and qualifications to be a firefighter. The single most popular code is the National Electric Code (NEC).

NAUSEA: A distinctly unpleasant sensation in the epigastrium or abdomen described as "bloating," "fullness," or "need to vomit."

NEBCIN: See Tobramycin.

NEBULIZER: A device which disperses water into a fine droplet spray. It is used to produce humidification of the respiratory airways. Two types exist: the high-pressure gas nebulizer and the ultrasonic nebulizer. The high-pressure gas type produces droplets of a large diameter (5-20 μm). The ultrasound type produces droplets of approximately 1 μm in diameter which easily penetrate the terminal bronchioles.

NEEDLE VALVE: See Flow control valve.

NFPA: See National Fire Protection Association.

NEGATIVE WATER BALANCE: A condition in which total water loss (sweat, urine, feces, lungs) exceeds water intake. Positive water balance exists when water loss is less than water intake. Negative water balance leads to dehydration; positive water balance leads to overhydration and water intoxication. See Water Balance.

NEGLIGENCE: The failure to administer ordinary care to an individual resulting in harm to that person.

NEGLIGENCE, GROSS: A legal term indicating willful behavior compounding neglect. This may be grounds for a malpractice suit.

NEMBUTAL: See Barbiturate, Pentobarbital.

NEOMYCIN (MYCIFRADIN): A broad-spectrum antibiotic of the aminoglycoside series. It is used topically against infections from burns, wounds, or ulcers and orally to reduce the microbial content in the intestines prior to bowel surgery. Intestinal malabsorption syndrome and yeast infection may result, however. Toxic effects such as renal damage and nerve deafness may occur with parenteral use. See Antibiotic.

NEOPRENE: See Elastomer.

NEOSTIGMINE (PROSTIGMIN): A reversible anticholinesterase drug used to improve neuromuscular transmission in diseases such as myasthenia gravis (alleviating muscle fatigue) and to reverse nondepolarizing muscle relaxants. It is also used to treat glaucoma and urinary retention and to enhance gastrointestinal smooth muscle tone. Intramuscular injections of neostigmine produce elevation of skin temperature, diaphoresis, salivation, constriction of the intestines, bradycardia, and fasciculations. Atropine will antagonize the muscarinic effects of neostigmine but will not antagonize the general fasciculations.

NEO-SYNEPHRINE: See Phenylephrine.

NERVE ACTION POTENTIAL (NAP): See Action potential, Depolarization.

NERVE CONDUCTION: See Action potential, Depolarization.

NERVE CONDUCTOR VELOCITY: See Nerve fiber, anatomy and physiology of.

NERVE FIBER, ANATOMY AND PHYSIOLOGY OF: The axons constituting a peripheral nerve and composed of both motor and sensory fibers. These fibers vary in size and are myelinated or unmyelinated. (Generally, large peripheral nerves are myelinated and small ones are unmyelinated.) These nerve fibers are classified as either A, B, or C based on anatomic and functional differences. The A and B fibers are both myelinated whereas the C fibers are not. The A fibers are divided into alpha, beta, gamma, and delta types. The A-alpha fibers, which range in size from 6 to 22 μm, are concerned with proprioception, motor function, and reflex activity. The A-beta fibers, 5-22 μm in size, are responsible for touch and pressure sensations. The A-gamma fibers are 2-8 μm in diameter and serve muscle tone. The A-delta fibers, only 1-5 μm in diameter, are concerned with pain, temperature, and touch. The B fibers are preganglionic sympathetic (autonomic) fibers <3 μm in diameter. The C fibers (postganglionic sympathetic fibers) measure only 0.1-1.3 μm in diameter and are important in temperature, pain, and reflex responses. The diameter of an axon is important in determining its ability to carry impulses and its sensitivity to local anesthetics. The larger (myelinated) nerve fibers can conduct impulses at an approximate rate of 100 m/sec, whereas the smaller (unmyelinated) fibers conduct impulses at an approximate rate of 0.1 m/sec. The A-delta fibers and C fibers are similarly sensitive to local anesthetics and are blocked by nearly the same concentration. The enhanced resistance of unmyelinated C fibers to local anesthetics is explained by the fact that the C fibers tend to group together and are then called fibers of Remak. The cells surrounding these groups tend to hamper drug access to the C fibers. The B fibers are more readily blocked than any other fiber and are therefore important during spinal or peridural anesthesia. When anesthetizing a peripheral nerve, pain sensation is often totally obtunded (A-delta fibers and C fibers are blocked) but motor function and touch (A-alpha and beta fibers) remain unaffected. This differential blockade indicates that only the thin fibers are blocked. At a nerve trunk, the local anesthetic effect progresses from the outer layer of axons (the mantle fibers) toward the inner layer of axons (the core fibers) and spreads in a proximal to distal direction. As the anesthesia wears off, this direction of diffusion reverses so that sensation is restored first to the proximal and then to the distal areas. With intravenous regional anesthesia (the Bier block), the anesthetic effect progresses from the core to the mantle fibers.

See Duality of pain transmission, Local anesthetic, Minimum blocking concentration, Myelin sheath.

NERVE GAS: An organophosphorus compound which had been used as a war gas. It interferes with nerve transmission and induces severe bronchospasm, which leads to respiratory depression. Nerve gases are now used as insecticides. Treatment of nerve gas poisoning includes administration of atropine or pralidoxime. See Organophosphorus compounds, Phosgene, Pralidoxime.

NERVE MEMBRANE: See Action potential; Myelin sheath; Nerve fiber, anatomy and physiology of.

NERVE PALSY: The paralysis of a peripheral nerve. Inadvertent compression or stretching of the nerve or poor positioning of the limbs during injection may lead to nerve palsy. In addition, the injection of an irritating solution into or near the nerve trunk may produce the same effect. Postoperative assessment of nerve damage is possible if knowledge of the preoperative condition exists. Diseased nerves are more susceptible to trauma, and certain illnesses such as diabetes mellitus, periarteritis nodosa, and alcoholism predispose the nerves to injury as well.

NESACAINE: See Chloroprocaine, Local anesthetic.

NEURALGIA: An acute paroxysmal pain radiating along peripheral nerves.

NEURITIS: The inflammation of a nerve or group of nerves which causes pain, sensory disturbances, or impaired reflexes.

NEURITIS, ALCOHOL: See Alcohol neuritis.

NEUROLEPTANALGESIA: See Neuroleptanesthesia.

NEUROLEPTANESTHESIA: A state of altered awareness, restfulness, and unconsciousness produced by the combined administration of (usually) intravenous Innovar (droperidol and fentanyl, a butyrophenone and opioid, respectively) with N_2O/O_2. The use of Innovar alone causes neuroleptanalgesia during which the patient remains conscious and minor surgical procedures such as bronchoscopy and cystoscopy may be performed. A neuroleptic agent has antipsychotic activity and typically belongs to either the butyrophenone or phenothiazine group. See Fentanyl, Innovar.

NEUROLYSIS: The destruction of nerve fibers. Substances which can cause this destruction are called neurolytic agents and include solutions of alcohol or phenol. They are used to treat intractable pain. See Neurotoxin.

NEUROMETRICS: A three-dimensional display technique for electroencephalographic data which shows the variables of time, frequency, and amplitude.

NEUROMUSCULAR BLOCKADE, ASSESSMENT OF: The technique by which the adequacy of muscular relaxation is determined. (1) Twitch response: after a single shock to a large motor nerve, the strength of the subsequent contraction of the muscles which the nerve supplies is evaluated. When the twitch is completely or nearly gone, the neuromuscular blockade is suitable for even the most severe retraction during surgery. (When curare is used, at least 75% of the receptors must be blocked in order to obtain a significant decrease in twitch response.) (2) Tetanic response: normally following administration of rapid, repeated shocks to a large motor nerve, no relaxation occurs between shocks and continuous contraction is seen. Frequent shocks deplete acetylcholine levels in the nerve endings and, when this is combined with endplate blockade, the tetanic response fades with continued stimulation. Commonly used frequencies to demonstrate tetany are 30, 50, 100 and 200 Hz. The higher the frequency of the stimulus, the more demand put on the neuromuscular junction. The rate of fade is related to the profoundness of the neuromuscular blockade. (3) "Train of Four": four supramaximal (above the current required to get a maximal response) shocks are given a half-second apart and the ratio of the height of the fourth twitch to the first twitch is used to determine the degree of block. (4) Physical diagnosis: these include hand squeeze on command, ability to raise the head from a pillow and hold for 5 sec on command, and respiratory measurements, such as vital capacity and inspiratory and expiratory force. See Blockade monitor.

NEUROMUSCULAR BLOCKING AGENT: A drug which produces skeletal muscle relaxation by altering the ability of the neurotransmitter acetylcholine (ACh) to activate the postsynaptic cholinergic receptor of the muscle fiber. Neuromuscular blocking agents are classified as nondepolarizing (competitive) or depolarizing (noncompetitive). Nondepolarizing drugs compete with ACh for the cholinergic receptor sites. If enough nondepolarizer is present, it prevents ACh from interacting with these receptors. Therefore, depolarization and contraction of the muscle cannot occur. (This is competitive inhibition.) These effects may be reversed if a cholinesterase inhibitor (e.g., neostigmine) is administered which would increase available ACh. Examples of nondepolarizers are tubocurarine chloride (Tubarine), gallamine (Flaxedil), dimethyl tubocurarine iodide (Metubine), and pancuronium (Pavulon). Depolarizing drugs, such as succinylcholine, structurally resemble ACh and have a shorter duration of action than nondepolarizing agents. They cause an initial depolarization and muscle contraction (fasciculation) followed by a block. The serum enzyme pseudocholinesterase quickly inactivates the succinylcholine. Depolarizing blockers are noncompetitive, i.e., they will not be displaced from the cholinergic receptor by any increase in ACh. Currently, there is no reliable antagonist to depolarizing agents. Their action is terminated by redistribution and metabolism. All neuromuscular blocking agents impair respiration and produce apnea. Ventilation must therefore be controlled until spontaneous respiration occurs. Neuromuscular blocking agents are useful during general anesthesia to aid in muscle relaxation and endotracheal intubation. Since patient response to neuromuscular blockers differs, it is recommended that a monitoring device, e.g., peripheral nerve stimulator, be used to determine the effectiveness of the drug. See Action potential; Neuromuscular blockade, assessment of.

NEUROMUSCULAR JUNCTION: The specialized synapse between a nerve fiber and a muscle membrane. See Fig. See Neuromuscular blocking agent.

NEUROMUSCULAR RELAXANT: See Neuromuscular blocking agent.

NEUROMUSCULAR TRANSMITTER, QUANTAL RELEASE OF: The unit of release of acetylcholine from the presynaptic membrane of a nerve terminal. Acetylcholine is stored in the nerve terminal as separate quanta. A nerve action potential appears to release many quanta. In the absence of an action potential, intermittent spontaneous release of single quanta occur from the presynaptic membrane. The release of quanta increases exponentially with each stepwise increase in depolarization caused by the action potential. For every 15-mV difference during depolarization there is a 10-fold increase in quanta release. See Acetylcholine; Neuromuscular blockade, assessment of.

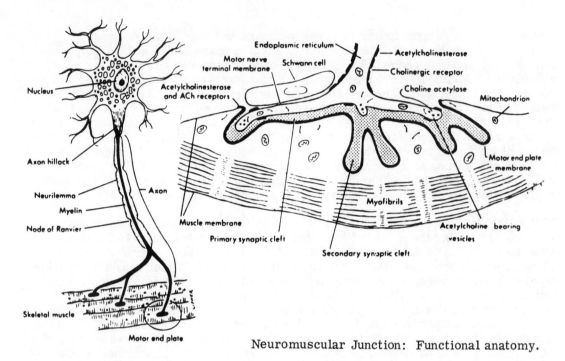

Nucleus

Axon hillock

Neurilemma

Myelin

Node of Ranvier

Axon

Skeletal muscle

Motor end plate

Endoplasmic reticulum

Motor nerve terminal membrane

Schwann cell

Acetylcholinesterase and ACh receptors

Acetylcholinesterase

Cholinergic receptor

Choline acetylase

Mitochondrion

Motor end plate membrane

Myofibrils

Muscle membrane

Primary synaptic cleft

Secondary synaptic cleft

Acetylcholine bearing vesicles

Neuromuscular Junction: Functional anatomy.

NEUROPATHY: A functional or pathologic disturbance of degeneration affecting the peripheral nerves. Neuropathy refers to noninflammatory lesions of the peripheral nervous system, whereas neuritis refers to inflammatory lesions. Possible causes of neuropathy include diabetes, alcoholism, trauma, nutritional deficiencies, and, indirectly, cancer. Less commonly, there are a few inherited neuropathies. Occasionally, no specific etiology is discovered. One nerve, several nerves, or bilaterally symmetric nerves may be affected.

NEUROTOXIN: A substance which is injurious or destructive to nerve tissue. See Intrathecal injection.

NEUROTRANSMITTER: A substance that transmits nerve impulses across a synapse. See Acetylcholine, Norepinephrine, Receptor.

NEUTRON: An uncharged elementary particle found in all known atomic nuclei except hydrogen.

NEWTON: The force which gives a mass of 1 kg an acceleration of 1 m/sec.

NICKEL: A metallic element (atomic number 28, atomic weight 58.7) used in the manufacture of alloys and as a catalyst. It adds strength to other metals and is resistant to chemical attack.

NICOTINE: A natural poisonous, colorless, soluble liquid alkaloid obtained from the tobacco leaf. It is used as an agricultural insecticide and veterinary external parasiticide. In humans, nicotine in small doses causes ganglionic stimulation and peripheral constriction. With larger doses, stimulation is quickly followed by neuromuscular blockade, decreased blood pressure, and diminished peripheral resistance. Nicotine also causes the release of catecholamines in some organs. It stimulates the central nervous system, producing tremors and, with large doses, convulsions. Toxic effects of nicotine are observed in children who ingest tobacco products. Nicotine poisoning may also result from the ingestion of insecticide-laden substances. Symptoms of acute nicotine poisoning include nausea, salivation, abdominal pain, vomiting, diarrhea, cold sweat, headache, dizziness, mental confusion, and weakness. A decrease in blood pressure, dyspnea, and a weak, rapid, irregular pulse follow. Death due to respiratory failure may result.

NIPRIDE: See Sodium nitroprusside.

NISENTIL: See Alphaprodine, Narcotic.

NITRAZEPAM (MOGADON): See Benzodiazepine.

NITROGEN (N_2): A gaseous, soluble element that is colorless, odorless, and tasteless. Its atomic number is 7 and atomic weight is 14. It constitutes 78% of the atmosphere by volume and is a constituent of all proteins. At pressures > 5 atmospheres, N_2 may be a general anesthetic agent (in combination with O_2). This anesthetic ability of N_2 parallels its lipid solubility. Liquid N_2 (at -196 degrees Celsius) is useful as a coolant in the laboratory. See Nitrogen narcosis, Nitrous oxide.

NITROGEN ANALYZER: See Infrared analyzer.

NITROGEN DIOXIDE (NO_2): A reddish brown, poisonous, irritant gas prepared from nitric oxide and air. Under pressure, it becomes nitrogen tetroxide (N_2O_4). NO_2 is an intermediate in the production of nitric and sulfuric acids. Inhalation of NO_2 at >100 ppm leads to pulmonary edema and possibly death. It was a significant contaminant in early nitrous oxide production.

NITROGEN NARCOSIS: A condition due to excessive exposure to high N_2 pressure (e.g., hyperbaric chamber, deep-sea diving) characterized by stupor and central nervous system depression. These symptoms usually begin with pressures >5 atmospheres for at least 1 hr. See Caisson disease.

NITROGEN TETROXIDE: See Nitrogen dioxide.

NITROGLYCERIN (NITROL; NITROSTAT): A yellowish, volatile liquid, also known as glyceryl trinitrate, formed by the action of nitric and sulfuric acids on glycerin. It is useful as a vasodilator in the management of angina pectoris. Nitroglycerin administered sublingually produces almost immediate pain relief from an acute anginal attack. (Given prior to exercise or stressful situations, nitroglycerin may be used to reduce the patient's susceptibility to an attack.) The mechanism of action appears to be that the drug reduces the work load of the cardiac muscles by decreasing afterload and producing coronary artery vasodilation and a decrease in the venous return to the heart. Nitroglycerin may also be administered topically since it is absorbed by the skin. This latter method has a much slower onset of action although its effectiveness is longer lasting.

NITROPRUSSIDE: See Sodium nitroprusside.

NITROUS OXIDE (N_2O; LAUGHING GAS): A colorless gas with a slight sweetish odor and taste that is used as an inhalation anesthetic and analgesic. It is the only inorganic gas useful as a general anesthetic agent. Although N_2O is neither flammable nor explosive, it will support combustion. It is both rapidly absorbed and eliminated from the body. The maximum concentration of N_2O that can be given safely is approximately 75% and it must be administered with at least 20% O_2 to prevent hypoxia. To provide complete anesthesia, supplementation with a barbiturate (such as thiopental sodium) and a neuromuscular blocking agent is advocated. When 70% N_2O in O_2 is used in conjunction with a halogenated hydrocarbon anesthetic, lower levels of the hydrocarbon may be used and a reduction in respiratory and circulatory depression occurs. In hyperbaric chambers, N_2O becomes a total general anesthetic, i.e., supplementation is no longer required. In concentrations below 50%, N_2O is often used as an analgesic during dental procedures. Chronic exposure to N_2O has been implicated in occupational disease among anesthesia and operating room personnel.

NITROUS OXIDE ANALYZER: See Infrared analyzer.

NOCICEPTOR: A nerve receptor that perceives pain. Nociceptors are end organs for A-delta fibers and C fibers. They have a high threshold to their specific stimulus but once activated do not show adaptation (rising threshold in response to a constant stimulus). In fact, reverse adaptation can take place when the threshold is lowered following prolonged stimulation. Subclasses exist which are determined by the initial stimulus causing the response. Such stimuli include temperature extremes, mechanical deformation, and locally released chemicals such as histamine and acetylcholine.

NOISE: An extraneous, unwanted disturbance in a communications or electronic system.

NOMOGRAM: A graphic representation of interrelated variables. The Radford nomogram, for example, was designed to show the relationship between body weight in pounds, the respiratory rate, and the basal tidal volume. When the first two are known, the third can be determined from the nomogram. Corrections for fever, altitude, etc., must always be taken into consideration. See Fig.

NONCOMPETITIVE ANTAGONISM (IRREVERSIBLE INHIBITION): A pharmacologic phenomenon seen when an agonist is prevented from acting at a specific receptor site by an antagonist, irrespective of the concentration of either. See Competitive antagonism, Receptor/receptor site.

NONDESTRUCTIVE MONITOR: See Noninvasive monitor.

NONFADE: See Oscilloscope, Shift register.

NONINVASIVE MONITOR: An instrument used to observe physiologic functions that does not invade or puncture tissues. It is also called a nondestructive, indirect, external, or transcutaneous monitor. Conversely, invasive monitoring techniques enter, puncture, or penetrate intact tissues.

NONREBREATHING VALVE: A type of valve found in respiratory apparatus which directs fresh gas to the patient and allows the release of exhaled gas into the atmosphere. These valves are useful in pediatric anesthesia and in portable resuscitators. Three functional types of nonrebreathing valves exist: (1) spontaneous ventilation (Stephen-Slater valve), (2) controlled ventilation (Ambu valve), and (3) spontaneous and controlled ventilation (Ambu E, Ambu Hesse, Ambu E2, Fink, Frumin, Laerdal, Lewis-Leigh, and Ruben valves).

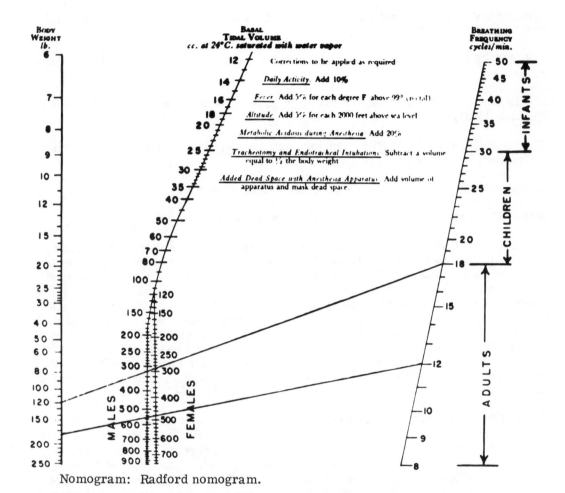

Nomogram: Radford nomogram.

NOREPINEPHRINE (LEVOPHED): A naturally occurring catecholamine produced by the adrenal medulla. It acts mainly on the alpha receptors and is a potent vaso-constrictor. Norepinephrine (also known as levarterenol or noradrenalin) in-creases systolic and diastolic pressures, mean arterial pressure, and peripheral resistance. Adverse effects of norepinephrine associated with high doses include severe hypertension, diaphoresis, vomiting, and chest pain. Arrhythmias may oc-cur if the drug is given with some general anesthetic agents. The sympathetic ner-vous system stimulates production of norepinephrine and epinephrine during physio-logic "fight-or-flight" responses. See Catecholamine, Dopamine, Epinephrine.

NORMAL CURVE: See Frequency curve.

NORMAL DISTRIBUTION: A display of many data points that are symmetric to either side of the mean (the center of the distribution). The standard deviation (SD) measures the variation of each measurement. A normal curve, which displays a normal distribution, depends on the two parameters, mean and SD, and is illustrated by a symmetric, bell-shaped curve. See Frequency curve, Standard deviation.

NORMALITY: The number of gram-equivalent weights of a solute per liter of solu-tion.

NORMOCAPNIA: A normal concentration of CO_2 in the arterial blood in young healthy individuals ($PaCO_2$ = 36-44 torr).

NORMOTHERMIA: An oral temperature of 37 degrees Celsius (98.6 degrees Fahrenheit).

NORMOXIA: A normal concentration of O_2 in the arterial blood of young healthy individuals (PaO_2 = 96-104 torr).

NORTH AMERICAN DRAGER: A major company which manufactures anesthesia equipment and is located in Telford, Pennsylvania.

NOVOCAIN: See Local anesthetic, Procaine hydrochloride.

NOXIOUS: A substance that is harmful and destructive.

NUCLEUS, ATOMIC: The central, positively charged, dense portion of an atom. Constituting nearly the entire mass of the atom, the nucleus is composed of protons and neutrons (nucleons). The atomic number (Z) is equal to the number (constant) of protons in each element, whereas the mass number (A) is equal to the number of neutrons. The mass number may vary depending on the various isotopes of each element. Most naturally occurring atoms have stable nuclei, whereas naturally occurring radioactive atoms do not. This instability gives rise to nuclear transmutations involving atomic and chemical alterations. Artificial nuclei are produced by bombarding a stable nucleus with charged particles of high energy. This bombardment leads to the creation of a new nucleus and the possible ejection of one or more particles.

NUCLEUS, CELL: The membrane-bound organelle which controls cellular structure and activity. The nucleus contains the genetic (chromatin) material deoxyribonucleic acid (DNA). (A mature red blood cell does not contain a nucleus and is therefore unable to reproduce.) The nucleolus, a protein structure containing ribonucleic acid (RNA), is also present within the nucleus. Multiple nucleoli may be present. The nucleolus is important in protein synthesis and becomes enlarged when active (during growth, repair, tumor formation). Microscopic abnormalities in the size and characteristics of the nucleus and nucleolus are evident in malignant cells.

NULL HYPOTHESIS: A statistical theory to be tested and accepted or rejected in favor of an alternative. A null hypothesis is used to aid in the design of appropriate experiments which prove or disprove a set of related statements. Any hypothesis which differs from a null hypothesis is known as an alternate hypothesis. See Type I error, Type II error.

NUPERCAINE: See Local anesthetic.

OBESITY: A condition characterized by excessive accumulation of body fat. Obesity may be due to exogenous (overeating) or endogenous (endocrine, metabolic, or hypothalamic abnormality) causes. See Pickwickian syndrome.

OBSTRUCTION: A blockage of vessels, ducts, or organs. For example, respiratory obstruction may occur if the upper airways are blocked by foreign material, tissue swelling, or the tongue falling backward in the unconscious patient.

OBSTRUCTIVE PULMONARY DISEASE: See Chronic obstructive pulmonary disease.

OCCUPATIONAL EXPOSURE: The unavoidable contact with a potentially harmful substance due to its presence in the work environment. Individuals working in operating rooms have an inevitable exposure to N_2 and other gaseous agents. Studies have shown that, at least at high concentrations, chronic exposure to N_2 is deleterious to health. The Occupational Safety and Health Administration (OSHA) determines the maximum safety levels for various toxic agents.

OHIO MEDICAL PRODUCTS: A company that manufactures anesthesia equipment. Its headquarters are located in Madison, Wisconsin.

OHM: The unit of electric resistance in the meter-kilogram-second (MKS) system of measurement equal to the resistance of a circuit in which a potential difference of 1 V produces a current of 1 amp.

OHM LAW: An expression of the relationship between the current, potential difference (voltage), and resistance. The current in a conductor is proportional to the potential difference between its ends. A voltage (E) across a direct current circuit equals current (I) in amperes through the element times resistance (R) of the element (E = IR). See Impedance.

OMPHALOCELE: A congenital condition characterized by the protrusion of part of the intestine through a defect in the abdominal wall at the umbilicus. This results from the failure of the intestine to return to the abdominal cavity during fetal development. A translucent amniotic sac covers the exposed intestine. The umbilical cord is generally located at the apex of the sac. If the amniotic sac ruptures in utero, a chronic peritonitis will result. If it ruptures at birth, emergency treatment to cover the viscera is necessary. Silastic sheets may be used to cover an intact omphalocele after birth. This allows for a slow, progressive reduction of the intestine into the growing abdominal cavity. Total parenteral feeding is necessary to provide adequate nutrition for the infant, who at this stage is unable to tolerate oral feedings. See Gastroschisis.

ONCOTIC PRESSURE: The osmotic pressure at the capillary membrane due to the plasma colloids. Normal oncotic pressure is approximately 28 mmHg. See Osmotic pressure.

ONE-LUNG ANESTHESIA: See Double-lumen tube, Pulmonary alveolar proteinosis.

ONE-TAILED TEST: See Two-tailed test.

ON-LINE: A term describing a device or process that is directly connected to and/or controlled by a central processing unit or computer.

OPEN CIRCUIT: An incomplete path for current flow.

OPEN CIRCUIT, ANESTHESIA: See Anesthesia system, open; Nonrebreathing valve.

OPEN CIRCUIT, ELECTRIC: A circuit in which either the input or output side (source-load-source connection) is cut (opened), stopping current flow.

OPEN DROP TECHNIQUE: A method for administering inhaled anesthetics introduced in 1847 for use with chloroform. The technique involved the dropping of a volatile liquid anesthetic onto a gauze-covered mask made of wire mesh. When used with diethyl ether, mask temperature could reach 0 degrees Celsius. Aside from use in emergencies or adverse field conditions, the technique is currently rarely employed.

OPERATING ROOM AIR CIRCULATION SYSTEMS (AIR HANDLERS): There are two basic types of air circulation systems in operating rooms: nonrecirculating and partial recirculating. The nonrecirculating or one-path system takes in fresh air, heats or cools it as appropriate, filters it, then circulates it through the operating room, and exhausts it outside the building. The partial recirculating or two-path system does not vent all air to the outside, but filters and places back in the room some previously circulated air. The former is quite costly as each new batch of air has to be modified to bring it to temperature and humidity standards. The latter system, on the other hand, while cheaper to operate, only slowly reduces room concentrations of anesthetics. Two methods of air handling are turbulent and laminar. Turbulent flow systems put in a very high velocity of air through a small grill, whereas laminar systems put in low velocity air via a very large grill which can typically comprise an entire wall or most of the ceiling (Allander air curtain). National Fire Protection Association codes require at least five complete air changes per hour in operating rooms; partial recirculating systems which balance expense versus dilution of contaminants have five to six complete changes per hour with 80% recirculation, meaning that air is completely filtered at least 25 times/hour. (It is to be remembered that with modern air conditioning systems, the older consideration that anesthetics were heavier than air and could therefore be safely assumed to settle to the floor is no longer operative.) The modern systems, to a large but variable degree, stir waste anesthetics throughout the entire room. See Allander air curtain, HEPA filter.

OPERATING ROOM ELECTRIC CONCEPTS: See Grounding, Isolation transformer.

OPERATIONAL AMPLIFIER: A type of amplifier that uses voltage feedback between output and input. Operational amplifiers are used to perform functions such as integrating, adding, and differentiating. Combinations of operational amplifiers can carry out complex mathematic manipulations on a signal. See Amplifier.

OPIATE: A group of chemical compounds extracted or derived from the opium poppy (Papaver somniferum). Opiates are used mainly for relief of moderate to severe pain. They depress respiration and may produce bronchoconstriction. Opiates induce a feeling of euphoria and tranquillity in combination with analgesia. Adverse effects include nausea, vomiting, orthostatic hypotension, constipation, and urinary retention. Opiates have significant abuse potential. Overdose or opiate poisoning renders the patient comatose and cyanotic; pinpoint pupils are common; respiratory failure is a prime cause of death. See Narcotic.

OPIUM: See Opiate.

OPTICAL CHARACTER READER (OCR): A light-sensitive photoelectric device used in data processing that scans printed material and produces electric signals proportional to the shades of light and dark it views.

OPTICAL ISOLATION: See Isolated output.

OPTIC NERVE: See Cranial nerves.

ORGANOPHOSPHORUS COMPOUNDS: The highly toxic alkyl phosphate compounds that irreversibly bind with and inactivate cholinesterase. They were developed as chemical warfare agents and are now used in insecticides (Malathion; Diazinon). Poisoning by these agents may result in paralysis and respiratory depression leading to death. Pralidoxime may be administered intravenously to counteract these anticholinesterase effects. Organophosphorus compounds may be used to treat glaucoma. See Nerve gas, Pralidoxime.

ORINASE: See Tolbutamide.

ORTHOSTATIC HYPOTENSION: A drop in blood pressure which is evident after changing from a supine or prone position to a standing or sitting position. The transient decrease in venous return and cardiac output causes a reduction of the blood pressure. Orthostatic hypotension may be due to drugs that impair autonomic reflexes or to excessive doses of antihypertensive agents.

OSCILLATION: A periodic variation between minimal and maximal values or a single swing of an object between the two extremes of its arc.

OSCILLATOR: An electronic device which converts energy from a direct current source to a periodically varying electric output. An oscillator is also a mechanical or electric device that, in the absence of external forces, regularly and repeatedly changes position, e.g., a pendulum.

OSCILLOMETRY METHOD OF TAKING BLOOD PRESSURE: See Arterial blood pressure.

OSCILLOSCOPE: An instrument that displays the instantaneous values and wave-forms of electric currents on the fluorescent screen of a cathode-ray tube. Most commonly, electrocardiographic (ECG) recordings are visualized on an oscilloscope. The bouncing ball and nonfade display techniques are two common methods used to display the information on an oscilloscope. The bouncing ball display shows a bright spot that moves along the screen from left to right. The light is nonpersistent and disappears within seconds. In contrast, the nonfade display remains on the screen until a blanking area clears the screen. Combinations of these two methods are possible; each half of the screen may use a different method. See Cathode-ray tube.

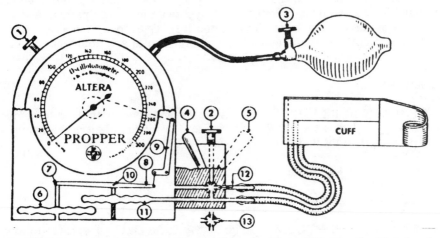

Oscillotonometer: Working elements. 1. Zero adjust. 2. Bleed valve adjustment screw. 3. Bulb pressure release valve. 4. Control valve lever: normal position, read pressure. 5. Control valve lever: position to bleed, observe oscillometry. 6. Pressure wafer. 7., 10., 8. Pivot points on internal lever. 9. Bell crank. 11. Sensitive oscillometric wafer. 12. Connection port to valve rotor shown in pressure or normal position (control lever in position 4). 13. Position of valve rotor to bleed, observe oscillometry.

OSCILLOTONOMETER: An instrument used for the indirect measurement of blood pressure. It is most accurate during hypotensive states. See Fig. See Arterial blood pressure.

OSMOLALITY: The osmotic concentration of a solution expressed as the number of osmoles of the dissolved substance per kilogram of solvent.

OSMOLARITY: The osmotic concentration of a solution expressed as the number of osmoles of the dissolved substance per liter of solution.

OSMOLE (Osm): The unit of measurement of osmotic activity based on the actual number of particles in solution, regardless of their charge. In physiologic practice, this is usually designated in milliosmoles (mOsm). One osmole is the number of particles in 1 gram-molecular weight of an undissolved solute; however, if that solute dissociates into two ions, then 1 gram-molecular weight will equal 2 Osm.

OSMOMETER: An instrument which measures osmotic pressure.

OSMOTIC PRESSURE: The amount of force necessary to prevent osmosis across a semipermeable membrane. The actual osmotic pressure is dependent on the number of particles in solution per unit volume of solution. Serum osmotic pressure is the osmotic pressure exerted by the serum and is primarily the result of concentrations of sodium, chloride, and bicarbonate, although sodium plays the dominant role. Serum protein and metabolites play a lesser role, although high levels of urea or glucose can increase the serum osmotic pressure. Urea can penetrate membranes and therefore does not produce long-term marked osmotic shifts. In contrast, glucose does not equilibrate well without sufficient insulin and can be responsible for maintaining osmotic differences across membranes. Normal serum osmotic pressure is 290 ± 5. The body, exquisitely sensitive to changes in serum osmolarity. expends great effort to maintain serum osmolarity in a narrow normal range.

OSTWALD SOLUBILITY COEFFICIENT (LAMBDA): A means for describing the equilibrium distribution between a gas and a solvent. The Ostwald solubility coefficient equals the volume of gas absorbed per unit volume of the solvent when the partial pressure of the gas is 760 torr. This coefficient is numerically equivalent to the partition coefficient. The Bunsen solubility coefficient (alpha) is the Ostwald solubility corrected to standard temperature (273 degrees absolute). See Partition coefficient.

OUABAIN: The most rapid and shortest acting of all the cardiac glycosides. See Digitalis.

OUTPATIENT ANESTHESIA: A technique in which general anesthesia is administered to individuals undergoing surgery who plan to leave the hospital, clinic, or office the same day.

OUTPUT: An electronics term relating to the current, power, voltage, driving force, or information that a device or circuit delivers. It is also an automatic data processing term indicating the data that have been processed.

OUTPUT IMPEDANCE: See Impedance.

OUTPUT TRANSFORMER: A coupling transformer between an output (e.g., amplifier) circuit and a load. See Transformer.

OVERCURRENT PROTECTION DEVICE: An instrument that prevents excessive electric current flow. Two types exist: (1) a fuse that melts if too much current passes through it, thereby opening the circuit, and (2) a circuit breaker that uses the current to create a magnetic field of sufficent strength to open a movable contact, thereby breaking the circuit.

OVERHYDRATION: See Dehydration, Water balance.

OXALOSIS (PRIMARY HYPEROXALURIA): A pathologic accumulation of calcium oxalate crystals, usually occurring in the kidneys, although it may also occur in the bones, arteries, or heart. The inhalation anesthetic methoxyflurane is metabolized, in part, to oxalate. Oxalosis is considered one of the possible causes of the nephrotoxicity of methoxyflurane.

OXAZEPAM (SERAX): An antianxiety drug of the benzodiazepine class. It is recommended for elderly patients or those with impaired liver function. See Benzodiazepine.

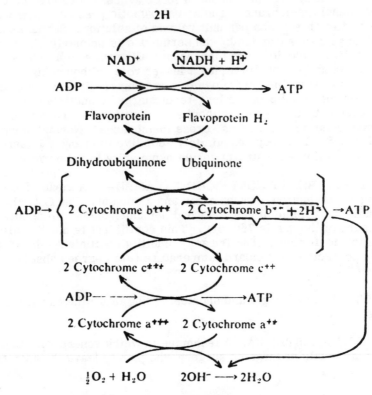

2H

NAD⁺ → NADH + H⁺

ADP → ATP

Flavoprotein / Flavoprotein H₂

Dihydroubiquinone / Ubiquinone

ADP→ { 2 Cytochrome b⁺⁺⁺ / 2 Cytochrome b⁺⁺ + 2H⁺ } →ATP

2 Cytochrome c⁺⁺⁺ / 2 Cytochrome c⁺⁺

ADP → ATP

2 Cytochrome a⁺⁺⁺ / 2 Cytochrome a⁺⁺

½O₂ + H₂O   2OH⁻ → 2H₂O

Net reaction:

$$2H + \tfrac{1}{2}O_2 + 3ADP \longrightarrow H_2O + 3ATP$$

Oxidative Phosphorylation: Chemical processes of oxidative phosphorylation showing the ionization of H_2 and O_2 and the formation of H_2O and adenosine triphosphate.

OXIDATIVE PHOSPHORYLATION: A process of obtaining adenosine triphosphate (ATP) from adenosine diphosphate (ADP) and phosphate by utilizing the energy produced when hydrogen molecules are oxidized to water. This process is performed by a complicated system of enzymes known as the cytochrome chain. See Fig. See Adenosine triphosphate.

OXIMETER: A photoelectric instrument designed to measure the amount of O_2 in whole blood. The instrument operates on the principle that the optical density of hemoglobin at the red and infrared wavelengths is linearly related to the percentage of O_2 saturation.

OXYGEN (O_2): An element present freely in the atmosphere as a colorless, odorless, tasteless gas (comprising approximately 21% of air volume.) It is frequently found in combination with many solids, liquids, and gases. It has an atomic number of 8 and an atomic weight of 16. Oxygen has a critical temperature of -183 degrees Celsius below which it becomes a liquid. It is often supplied commercially in bulk in the liquid state and stored in vacuum containers to remain cold. Smaller supplies of O_2 are delivered in standard colored cylinders (American color for O_2 is green; international color is white). Oxygen is an essential component in cellular respiration and combustion processes. See Atmosphere; Cylinder, gas; Liquid oxygen; Paramagnetism.

OXYGEN ANALYZER: A device which measures the percentage of O_2 in a mixture of gases. Two basic modes of operation exist: the discrete sampler and the continuous sampler. The discrete sampler (Pauling) has been in use since the early 1940s. It operates on the principle that O_2 molecules, unlike all other commonly encountered gases, exhibit magnetic properties. Samples of unknown gas are drawn into a test chamber spanned by a permanent magnetic field. The O_2 molecules migrate to one side and displace any other gas present. This unbalance in the magnetic field changes the position of a mirror reflecting a light beam along a calibrated scale dependent on the percentage of O_2. Continuous O_2 analyzers place a sensor in the gas volume to be tested and a reading is constantly displayed (except for a lag in time as the sensor responds to changes in O_2 content). Two types of sensors are commonly in use today: the galvanic cell (often wrongly called microfuel cell) and the polarographic cell. The galvanic cell is made up of a lead anode and a gold cathode sealed in a membrane (filled with a potassium hydroxide electrolyte bath) which allows for easy diffusion of gases but not of large molecules (proteins). When O_2 crosses the membrane and comes in contact with the gold, it is reduced to hydroxide ions (OH^-). These migrate to the lead anode and form lead oxide, releasing electrons which flow from the anode back to the cathode through a resistor which is external to the sensor. A sensitive meter measures the voltage across the external resistor and registers on a scale calibrated in O_2 concentrations. The cell life of the galvanic sensor is proportional to the O_2 concentration to which it is exposed because the electrodes are consumed in the process. The galvanic sensor is slow to respond and is quite expensive due to its gold content. However, it is rugged, easy to use, and requires no power input to the sensor. The galvanic sensor is rated in percent hours: $100\% \ O_2$ will last X hr, $50\% \ O_2$ will last X/2 hr. The polarographic O_2 sensor is a two-electrode system: a silver anode and a gold or platinum cathode, which are surrounded by an electrolyte solution of potassium chloride. The cathode is insulated from the electrolyte solution (except at its tip, which is covered by a membrane through which gas can permeate) and is kept negative in respect to the anode by an external battery. Oxygen crosses the membrane, is broken down at the cathode, and alters the conductivity of the electrolyte solution. Current flow be-

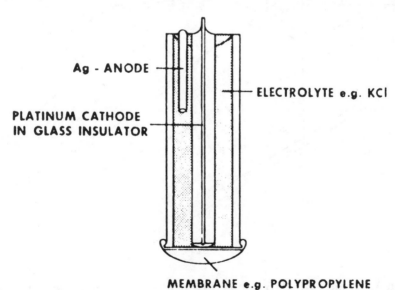

Ag - ANODE

ELECTROLYTE e.g. KCl

PLATINUM CATHODE
IN GLASS INSULATOR

MEMBRANE e.g. POLYPROPYLENE
(PERMEABLE TO O_2) OR TEFLON

I

Oxygen Analyzer: (I) Polarographic cell or sensor.

300

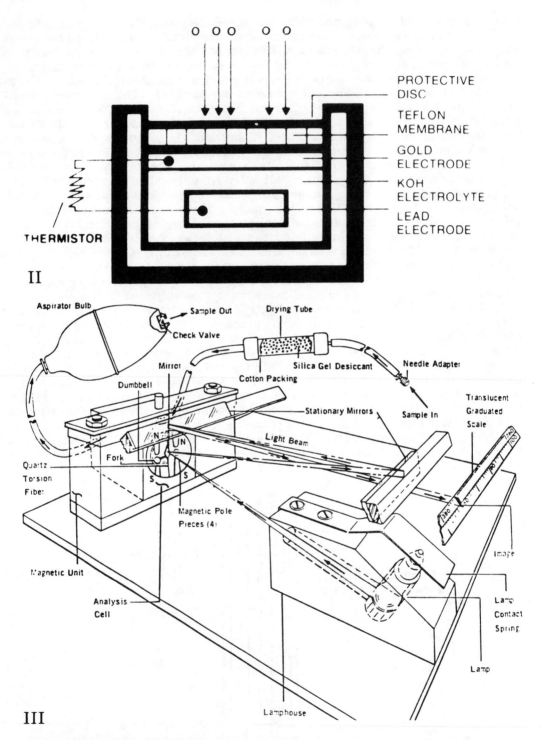

Oxygen Analyzer: (II) Galvanic cell or sensor. (III) Schematic diagram of the Beckman Model D2 Oxygen Analyzer which depends on the magnetic properties of O_2 to quantitate O_2 concentration.

tween the electrodes is proportional to the O_2 concentration. Polarographic sensors are less expensive than galvanic sensors but require frequent electrolyte changes and careful maintenance. They respond faster than galvanic sensors but require an external power source. See Figs.

OXYGENATOR: A mechanical device which oxygenates venous blood extracorporeally. In combination with one or more pumps, an oxygenator can maintain circulation during open heart surgery. (CO_2 is passively eliminated by diffusing from venous blood into the O_2 in contact with the blood.) Types of oxygenators include bubble, membrane, rotating disc, and screen. See Bubble oxygenator, Membrane oxygenator, Rotating disc oxygenator, Screen oxygenator.

OXYGEN CAPACITY: The maximum amount of O_2 that can be combined with hemoglobin (Hb) when the blood is fully saturated with 100% O_2 at a PO_2 of 760 mmHg. One gram of Hb can bind with 1.34-1.39 ml O_2; the O_2 capacity of normal blood is therefore approximately 21 ml O_2/100 ml blood. (Normal blood contains 15 g Hb/100 ml.) At a PO_2 of 760 mmHg the amount of dissolved O_2 is 0.3 ml/100 ml blood.

OXYGEN CONTENT: The amount of O_2 that can be extracted from 100 ml blood. This includes both the amount which is physically dissolved in plasma plus the amount bound to hemoglobin. The O_2 content of partially desaturated blood will be below the theoretic maximum. See Oxygen capacity.

OXYGEN DISSOCIATION CURVE: See Oxygen-hemoglobin dissociation curve.

OXYGEN ELECTRODE (CLARK ELECTRODE): One of three standard electrodes which make up a blood-gas analyzer. It is a device for determining PO_2 in solution. Oxygen molecules cross a plastic membrane and are ionized by a platinum cathode which is kept negative with respect to a silver/silver chloride anode. By various corrections the ionic current of O_2 between cathode and anode is converted to a reading of PO_2. See Fig.

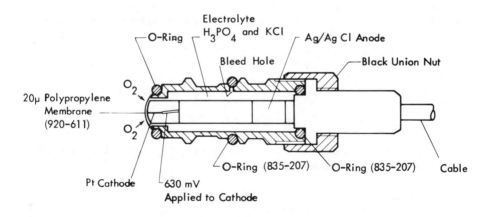

E5049 Po_2 Electrode

Oxygen Electrode: Standard O_2 electrode. (Courtesy Radiometer Corporation.)

OXYGEN FLUSH VALVE: A valve which directs high-flow O2 (at least 35-75 L/min) through an anesthesia machine outlet. Standards require that the O2 flush valve be spring-loaded so that when pressure on the valve button or handle is removed the flow shuts off. On some machines activation of the O2 flush valve eliminates all O2 flow through integral vaporizers. This flow must be restored manually when O2 flushing ceases. Modifications of O2 flush valves exist which vary the effect on other gases that may be flowing when the valve is activated, i.e., the flow may stop or be vented into the atmosphere. See Continuous flow anesthesia machine.

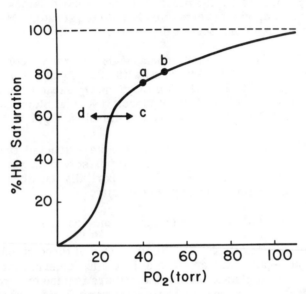

Oxygen-Hemoglobin Dissociation Curve: Oxygen-hemoglobin dissociation curve and the parameters which determine left or right shift of the curve.
   a. Point indicating normal mixed venous blood that has P_VO_2 40 torr and Hb 75 percent saturated
   b. Cyanosis not normally apparent until PaO_2 drops to approximately 50 torr (80 percent saturation) or less. Also, below this level a drop in PO_2 is related to a large drop in percent Hb saturation. (The neonate with fetal Hb will have a much lower than 50 torr PaO_2 level at 80 percent saturation.)
   c. Right shift of curve with increased H^+, PCO_2, temperature and 2.3 DPG
   d. Left shift of curve with decreased H^+, PCO_2, temperature and 2.3 DPG
   Also, left shift with Hb F. (Hb F, therefore, holds onto O2 "tighter" and gives up O2 at tissue level less readily.)

OXYGEN-HEMOGLOBIN DISSOCIATION CURVE: A graphic representation of the increased amount of hemoglobin that is bound to O2 as the PO_2 is increased. Three major conditions affect the curve: pH, temperature, and concentration of 2,3-diphosphoglycerate (2-3-DPG) in the red blood cell. A decrease in temperature or 2,3-DPG or an increase in pH, i.e., decreased CO_2, of the blood shifts the curve to the left. Conversely, an increase in temperature or 2,3-DPG or a decrease in pH, i.e., increased CO_2, of the blood shifts the curve to the right. (The concentration of 2,3-DPG is elevated in chronic hypoxia or in high altitudes.) P_{50} indicates the PO_2 at which hemoglobin is half-saturated with O2. The decrease in the affinity of hemoglobin for O2 when the pH of blood falls is known as the Bohr effect. See Fig.

OXYGEN HOOD: See Oxygen tent.

OXYGEN POINT: The temperature at which gaseous and liquid O_2 are in equilibrium at 1 standard atmosphere (-183 degrees Celsius).

OXYGEN SATURATION: The proportion of oxyhemoglobin to the total hemoglobin in a given blood sample expressed as a percentage. Normally, blood leaving the lungs via the pulmonary vein is approximately 97% saturated. See Oyxgen capacity, Oxygen content, Oxygen-hemoglobin dissociation curve.

OXYGEN TENT (OXYGEN HOOD): A light, portable, transparent, tentlike structure that is placed around a patient's head (hood) or bed (tent) and used for the administration of O_2. The concentration of O_2 within the tent may be increased by higher flow rates, elimination of leaks, or use of a smaller tent. This concentration rarely exceeds 50% and may be as low as 25%. In contrast, the O_2 concentration of a head hood may reach 90-100%. The low O_2 concentration of the tent and the restricted patient accessibility of the hood limit the usefulness of these methods for O_2 administration.

OXYGEN THERAPY: A treatment which involves the administration of O_2 by means of inhalation via an O_2 tent or hood, nasal cannula, or face mask. Such therapy is employed in the treatment of hypoxia.

OXYGEN TOXICITY: The injurious prolonged exposure to excessive concentrations of inhaled O_2. Rapid O_2 toxicity occurs only under hyperbaric conditions. Chronic O_2 toxicity, occurring when O_2 concentrations over 70% are inhaled at atmospheric pressure for a long period of time, may be due to the deactivation of surfactant and damage to the alveolar epithelium. (Clinically, exposure to 100% O_2 for 24 hr may be considered injurious, to some extent, to all patients whereas it may take more than a week for 70% O_2 to cause damage.) In the first stage of toxicity (exudative), the lungs become edematous and there is evidence of hemorrhage and capillary damage. In the second stage (proliferative), there is marked scarring and fibrosis. Some degree of tolerance to high concentrations of O_2 may occur in some patients. No patient, however, should be denied high O_2 concentrations because of a potential for O_2 toxicity if it is the only means to prevent hypoxia.

OXYMORPHONE (NUMORPHAN): See Naloxone, Narcotic.

OXYTOCIN: A hormone which is formed in the hypothalamus and stored in the posterior lobe of the pituitary gland (neurohypophysis). It has weak but noticeable contractile effects on smooth muscle, a characteristic it shares with vasopressin (antidiuretic hormone, ADH), the other major hormone released by the posterior pituitary. Oxytocin's primary use is to increase the strength of uterine contractions. See Antidiuretic hormone.

$\mathscr{P}$

PAIN: An unpleasant sensation, either conscious or unconscious, which signals the body that some tissue damage is occurring. In one system, pain sensation is classified into three major types: pricking, burning, and aching. Pricking pain and burning pain are felt at the skin surface, whereas aching pain is felt below the surface. In a second system, pain is described in terms of (1) onset, (2) severity, (3) quality, (4) duration, and (5) etiology. In a third system, pain is classified according to origin: (1) peripheral, (2) cerebral, and (3) psychogenic. See Nerve fiber, anatomy and physiology of; Nociceptor.

PAIN, GATE THEORY OF: See Gate theory of pain.

PAIN, LOCAL MECHANISM OF: See Pain signal transmission.

PAIN SIGNAL TRANSMISSION: The sensation of two types of pain due to the presence of two pain pathways, slow and fast. The first half of the double sensation is a pricking pain sensation which is carried rapidly by the small A-delta fibers at velocities of approximately 5-25 m/sec. The second part of the sensation is a burning sensation which is transmitted more slowly by type C fibers at velocities between 0.1 and 2 m/sec. See Gate theory of pain.

PAIN THRESHOLD: The lowest intensity of a pain stimulus which will elicit the sensation of pain. Implicit in the concept of pain threshold is the idea that the more intense the stimulus, the less time it has to be applied before it elicits a response.

PAIN TOLERANCE LEVEL: The greatest intensity of pain that a subject will tolerate, usually as part of an experiment.

PALLADIUM: A rare metal often found in conjunction with platinum. It is used in electric components because of its resistance to oxidation and corrosion and in jewelry because of its beautiful silver color.

PALSY: See Paralysis.

PANCURONIUM BROMIDE (PAVULON): A competitive neuromuscular blocking agent which is approximately 5 times as potent as d-tubocurarine. Since it does not appear to cause ganglionic blockage or histamine release, Pavulon does not (especially upon rapid intravenous injection) precipitate a rapid drop in blood pressure.

Rather, depending on dose and administration, it is more likely to cause tachycardia (by some degree of vagus nerve blockage) and an increase in cardiac output. See Neuromuscular blockade, assessment of.

PAPAVERETUM (OMNOPON; OPOIDINE): A mixture of all the water-soluble alkaloids of opium in their natural proportions (available in Great Britain).

PAPAVERINE: A naturally occurring alkaloid of opium. It is neither a narcotic nor an analgesic and is nonaddictive. Its major effect is smooth muscle relaxation. It has been used to treat peripheral vascular disease and has been advocated on occasion as a treatment for the inadvertent intra-arterial injection of irritants such as thiopental and diazepam.

PAPER TAPE: An information storage medium which consists of a strip of paper on which information can be stored as punched holes or chemical changes in discrete areas on the paper surface.

PARA-AMINOBENZOIC ACID (PABA): An acid associated with the vitamin B complex. Often used in topical preparations as a sunscreen, it has been reported to have some cross-sensitivity with the ester group of local anesthetics. PABA is a breakdown product of procaine and also a potent inhibitor of the bacteriostatic effects of the sulfonamides.

PARACERVICAL BLOCK (UTEROSACRAL BLOCK): An anesthetic nerve block of the inferior hypogastric plexus. The block interrupts uterine and cervical sensation and is therefore performed to ease pain during labor. The procedure has fallen into disfavor due to the possible inadvertent injection of local anesthetic into the placental circulation which delivers a high concentration of local anesthetic to the fetus, causing bradycardia. See Fig.

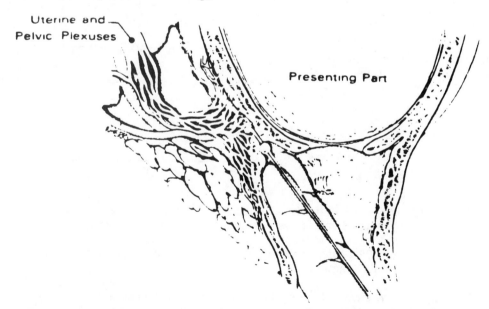

Paracervical Block: Schematic representation of paracervical block. The tip of the needle just penetrates the mucosa and points away from the myometrium and the fetal presenting part.

PARADOXICAL OXYGEN DEATH: A clinical circumstance which occurs when the respiratory center no longer responds normally directly to elevated arterial blood-CO_2 tension but is, in fact, being driven by the carotid bodies responding to low O_2. Arterial CO_2 rises so high that it acts as a depressant. The administration of high O_2 concentrations to the patient will be detected first by the carotid bodies. They will cease stimulating the central respiratory center, which will shut down completely, and the patient will die paradoxically from hypoxia and hypercapnia in the presence of adequate O_2. Paradoxical O_2 death is seen in respiratory cripples, e.g., end stage emphysema. Avoiding this iatrogenic catastrophe requires controlled administration of mildly elevated O_2 concentrations and mechanical ventilation with adjustment of acid-base balance as necessary. See Carotid body.

PARADOXICAL RESPIRATION: A phenomenon seen following a crush injury to the chest wall (flail chest) or surgical removal of part of the rib cage. On normal inspiration, the chest rises up and out. In paradoxical respiration, the normal side behaves as noted, while the damaged side is sucked inward. Similarly, on expiration, the unaffected side falls inward, while the affected side balloons outward. This reversal of normal movement of the chest wall is deleterious to normal respiratory function. See Flail chest.

PARALDEHYDE: A cyclic ether which is an effective hypnotic. It was formerly administered in the treatment of delirium tremens, psychiatric disorders characterized by excitement, convulsions from tetanus or eclampsia, and for basal and obstetric anesthesia. Paraldehyde has been implicated in both chronic intoxication (despite its unpleasant odor and taste) and fatal toxic reactions. It is damaging to tissues at the site of injection and has been replaced by other sedatives which do not have the offensive taste and odor and are not irritating on injection.

Parallel Circuit: Simple parallel circuit made up of three resistors connected across the same voltage source.

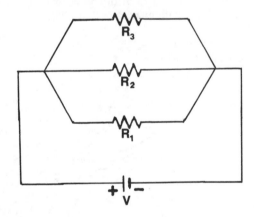

PARALLEL CIRCUIT: A circuit with elements that connect across the same pair of terminals, ensuring that the voltage is constant across each element. See Fig.

PARALYSIS (PALSY): The loss of motor function. Paralysis has also been used to mean loss of any organic function.

PARAMAGNETISM: A physical property of certain substances, such as O_2, in which the molecules behave as if they carry a magnetic charge.

PARAMEDIAN APPROACH: A spinal anesthetic technique in which the needle is placed offset from the midline below and to the side of the interspace and aimed cephalad. This technique is used when the usual midline perpendicular approach is not easily accomplished. See Spinal anesthesia.

PARAPLEGIA: The paralysis of the lower part of the body and of both legs.

PARASYMPATHETIC DIVISION (CRANIOSACRAL DIVISION): The craniosacral portion of the autonomic nervous system. There are two divisions of this system: the cranial outflow and the sacral outflow. The cranial outflow supplies the visceral structures of the head, thorax, and upper abdomen via the oculomotor, facial, glossopharyngeal, and vagus nerves. The sacral portion varies with each individual but most frequently consists of the second, third, and fourth sacral segments. Parasympathetic preganglionic fibers go to discrete ganglia nearest the organ they innervate. The parasympathetic ganglia include the ciliary, pterygopalatine, submandibular, and otic ganglia. Within the chest and abdomen, parasympathetic ganglia are diffuse and are therefore referred to as plexuses. These include the superficial cardiac, deep cardiac, pulmonary, myenteric, and mucosal. The afferent fibers of the parasympathetic system travel from the area they are monitoring to their cell bodies. The cell bodies of the cranial portion are in the sensory ganglia of the cranial nerves; the cell bodies of the sacral portion are in the posterior root ganglia of the spinal nerves. The major difference between the sympathetic and parasympathetic systems (aside from their antagonistic effects on various organs) is that the sympathetic system has a wide, diffuse effect due to its remote ganglia and multiple, branching postganglionic fibers, whereas the parasympathetic system, due to its few ganglia located near the organ affected and its short postganglionic fibers, has a more local, discrete effect. See Autonomic nervous system, Cranial nerves.

PARASYMPATHETIC NERVOUS SYSTEM: See Autonomic nervous system.

PARASYMPATHETIC TONE: See Sympathetic tone.

PARAVERTEBRAL BLOCK: The introduction of a local anesthetic alongside the vertebrae with the purpose of blocking the injected level of the sympathetic chain. See Paravertebral lumbar sympathetic block.

PARAVERTEBRAL LUMBAR SYMPATHETIC BLOCK: The injection of a local anesthetic into the area of the first or second lumbar vertebra (unilateral or bilateral) to block the sympathetic chain. This technique provides excellent analgesia for the first stage of labor but is inadequate for delivery. (Local anesthetics cross the placental barrier and high levels may cause circulatory and central nervous system depression in the fetus.) The paravertebral lumbar block is also useful in treating vascular disorders in the lower limbs. It relieves vascular spasms and dilates blood vessels.

PARENTERAL FLUIDS: Those solutions composed of various proteins, calories, and essential minerals and designed to be administered by direct intravenous injection usually on a continuous basis, with the prime purpose of restoring and maintaining circulating volume. See Transfusion therapy.

PARESTHESIA: An inappropriate sensation in a body part or over a portion of the body surface, usually described as burning, stinging, or tingling. It can be a symptom of neurologic disease. In regional anesthesia, "eliciting paresthesia" by probing for a nerve trunk with a needle prior to injection is a technique for determining proper deposition of a local anesthesia solution.

PARGYLINE (EUTONYL): A monoamine oxidase inhibitor that is useful as an anti-hypertensive agent. Administration of pargyline is contraindicated in patients taking antidepressants or indirect sympathomimetics, or following ingestion of tyramine-containing foods.

PARTIAL PRESSURE: The contribution to the total pressure made by each gas in a mixture of gases. In a fixed volume, each gas exerts the pressure which it would exert if it were alone. See Vapor pressure.

PARTIAL PRESSURE CROSSOVER POINT: See Respiratory failure.

PARTIAL THROMBOPLASTIN TIME (PTT): A test of the clotting mechanism which determines the relative intactness of the intrinsic clotting system. The measurement is of the time necessary for recalcified citrated plasma to clot in the presence of a standardized platelet substitute (cephalin) and standardized activating surface (provided by kaolin).

PARTITION COEFFICIENT: The ratio of the concentrations in each phase of a substance in equilibrium between two phases. For example, the drug methoxyflurane has a fat/blood partition coefficient of 49, i.e., at equilibrium there will be 49 times the number of molecules of methoxyflurane in fat versus the number of molecules of methoxyflurane in the blood flowing through the fat. Because a partition coefficient can be determined for any two phases in contact with one another, one can determine the blood/gas partition coefficient, the tissue/blood partition coefficient, or the oil/gas partition coefficient. Any determination of the partition coefficient assumes that equilibration of partial pressures of the gas in question has occurred in the two phases. See Ostwald solubility coefficient.

PASCAL: The standard international unit of pressure. It is the pressure that results from the force of 1 newton **acting** uniformly over an area of 1 m^2. See Pressure.

PASSWORD: The unique set of characters or digits used to identify a particular individual or user of a computer facility. It can be used to restrict an individual to only certain parts of a computer facility or parts of a computer memory and is usually used to upgrade the security of a computer facility.

PATCHY ATELECTASIS: See Atelectasis.

PATENT: A synonym for open or unblocked. It is also a government guarantee to an inventor that his or her invention, because of its uniqueness, is solely exploitable by him or her for a given period. (A United States patent confers this right for 17 years.)

PATENT DUCTUS ARTERIOSUS (PDA): The abnormal persistence in the newborn of an opening in the ductus arteriosus connecting the pulmonary artery with the thoracic aorta. This condition, common in premature infants, can be life threatening as it can act as a left-to-right shunt (to a variable degree) causing severe cardiac decompensation and increased pulmonary blood flow. In normal infants, the ductus closes shortly after birth, probably due to local prostaglandin activity. See Fig. See Fetal circulation.

PATHWAY: The route that a nerve impulse takes from the periphery to the spinal cord and upward into the brain. Depending on the type of signal and the require-

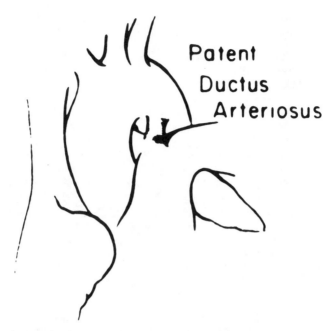

Patent Ductus Arteriosus: Patent ductus arteriosus connecting the thoracic aorta with the pulmonary artery.

ments for the body to respond to it, the pathway can be made up of a single long nerve fiber or tract or numerous short fibers which communicate between multiple junctions (synapses).

PATIENT POSITIONING (POSTURE): The position in which the patient is placed during anesthesia. In order to meet the requirements for access of a particular surgical procedure, modern operating room tables can fold the human body into a number of positions. In most regions of the United States, it has been determined that the anesthesia personnel are legally responsible for proper positioning of the patients. Reported complications of patient positioning include nerve palsies, pressure atrophy of the skin, bone breaking, i.e., limbs caught between folding table parts, and special conditions, e.g., electrosurgical burns and direct damage caused by the weight and position of such items as endotracheal tube connectors, hoses, and head straps. Position is usually noted by a stick figure drawn on the anesthesia record. See Figs.

PATTERN RECOGNITION: The ability to identify one symbol or object among many symbols or objects. Pattern recognition appears to be one of the basic functions of intelligence.

PAULING ANALYZER: See Oxygen analyzer.

PAVULON: See Pancuronium bromide.

PEAK FLOWMETER: A device for measuring (in L/min) the amount a patient can exhale at forced expiration.

PEAK POWER FREQUENCY (PPF): See Median power frequency.

310

Supine
Arms at side, face up

Supine
Arms out, face up

Sitting
Arms on chest

Trendelenburg

In Operating Room Parlance,
head down, body straight.
True Trendelenburg, patient supine
on a surface at a 45° angle, head at
lower end, knees flexed over upper end.

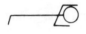

Reverse Trendelenburg

In Operating Room Parlance, head
up, body straight. True Reverse
Trendelenburg, patient supine on
surface at 45° angle, head at highest end.

Lithotomy
Patient supine with hips
and knees flexed, thighs
abducted and externally
rotated.

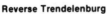

Prone
Face down

I

Nerve	Site of lesion	Cause
Supraorbital	Orbital ridge	Pressure of a face mask; pressing on nerve to provide a painful stimulus for assessment of coma.
Brachial plexus	Stretching over head of humerus	Shoulder rests placed in root of neck. Over 90° abduction of the supinated arm. Hyperextension of head.
Radial	Radial groove in humerus	Arm falling down during surgery. Badly applied tourniquet.
Radial	At wrist	Placing patient's hands under buttocks.
Ulnar	Epicondylar groove	Resting arm on unpadded arm board.
Sciatic	Posterior roots	Failing to flex both legs together when adopting lithotomy position.
Lateral popliteal	Head of fibula	The unpadded knee in the lateral position: pressure from lithotomy poles on unprotected knee.
Lingual	Tip of tongue	Biting of tongue following laryngeal spasm.
Cervical cord	C3-4	Extension of head in the presence of subluxation of cervical vertebrae (e. g., injury or rheumatoid arthritis)

II

Patient Positioning: (I) Stick drawings of the various positions of the
patient on the operating table. (II) Some of the affected nerves and the
sites of lesions caused by poor patient positioning.

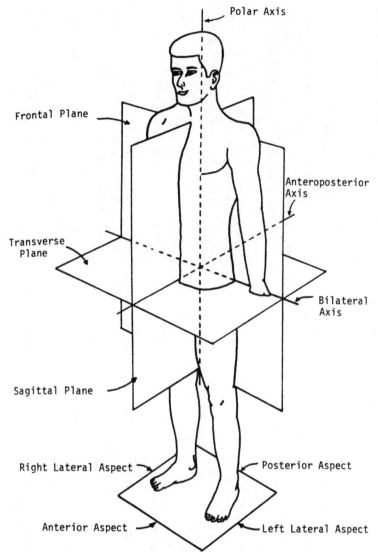

Polar Axis

Frontal Plane

Anteroposterior
Axis

Transverse
Plane

Bilateral
Axis

Sagittal Plane

Right Lateral Aspect

Posterior Aspect

Anterior Aspect

Left Lateral Aspect

III

Patient Positioning: (III) Cardinal planes and axes of the human body.

PEEP: See Positive end expiratory pressure.

PELTIER EFFECT: See Thermocouple.

PENDELLUFT: A pendulum-like movement of the lungs seen when the patient is breathing spontaneously in the presence of an open pneumothorax. On inspiration, the normal side fills partially from the trachea and partially from the lung on the injured side. On expiration, air returns up the trachea and into the partially deflated lung on the injured side.

PENICILLIN: The first available effective biologic antibiotic, discovered by Alexander Fleming in 1928. Its use has been limited in recent years because of the proliferation of resistant strains of microorganisms. Multiple derivatives of the drug

Penicillin and Penicillin Derivatives.

Generic Name (Representative Trade Name*)	Spectrum	Penicillinase-Resistant	Acid-Stable	Route	Comments
Penicillin G (Pentids) Potassium Sodium	G⁺, some G⁻ (Escher-ichia coli, Proteus mirabilis, Hemophilus influenzae, Salmonella, Shigella, and strains of Enterobacter aerogenes), Leptospira, and Treponema.	No	No	PO	Penicillin and its derivatives are bactericidal in action. The penicillins can cause various side effects, including anaphylaxis, skin rash, Coombs-positive hemolytic anemia, fever, interstitial nephritis, angioedema, and serum sickness.
Benzathene (Bicillin)				IM	
Procaine (Wycillin)				IM	
Penicillin V (Pen-Vee K)	Same as penicillin G	No	Yes	PO	Penicillin V is well-absorbed orally.
Ampicillin (Omnipen)	Broad spectrum, especially against G⁻ rods.	No	Yes	PO IM IV	Ampicillin is well-absorbed orally. Side effects include GI upset, anaphylaxis, increased SGOT, and skin rash.
Hetacillin (Versapen)	Same as ampicillin	No	Yes	PO	Hetacillin is metabolized to ampicillin in the body.
Cyclacillin (Cyclapen)	Similar to ampicillin though less broad.	No	Yes	PO	Cyclacillin may show less incidence of GI upset and skin rash than ampicillin.
Amoxicillin (Amoxil)	Broad spectrum	No	Yes	PO	Amoxicillin is absorbed better orally than ampicillin. It is reported to show higher blood levels, and less incidence of diarrhea than ampicillin.

Drug (trade name)	Spectrum			Route	Comments
Carbenicillin (Pyopen)	Broad spectrum with a high activity against Proteus and Pseudomonas and occasional strains of G⁻ rods such as <u>Bacillus fragilis</u>	No	Yes	IM IV	Carbenicillin's side effects are similar to other penicillins but also include possible abnormalities in coagulation tests. It is very useful for severe urinary tract infections. Nephrotoxicity may be seen in large doses.
Ticarcillin (Ticar)	Similar to carbenicillin including G⁻, especially Pseudomonas	No	No	IM IV	
Methicillin (Celbenin)	G⁺, including penicillinase-resistant Staphylococci	Yes	No	IM IV	One of the first penicillinase-resistant penicillins.
Bacillin (Bactocill)	Same as methicillin	Yes	Yes	PO IM IV	Side effects include GI upset, fever, skin rash, decreased hemoglobin, neutropenia, increased SGOT, and transient hematuria in infants.
Cloxacillin (Tegopen)	Same as methicillin	Yes	Yes	PO	Cloxacillin and dicloxacillin do not show complete cross-sensitivity with penicillin G.
Dicloxacillin (Dynapen)	Same as methicillin	Yes	Yes	PO IM	Dicloxacillin is the best orally absorbed penicillinase-resistant penicillin.
Nafcillin (Nafcil)	Same as methicillin	Yes	Variable	PO IM	Nafcillin is not particularly well-absorbed orally. Its side effects are similar to those of oxacillin.

* Particularly for the older preparations many trade names exist for the same product. At times the trade name covers all forms of administration, other times it does not.

all have the potential for causing allergic reactions in susceptible individuals. The various preparations can carry a significant ionic load (sodium, potassium) upon massive injection. See Fig. See Antibiotic.

PENTAZOCINE (TALWIN): A synthetic analgesic with moderate potency and short duration. Originally believed to be completely nonaddictive, it has been shown to have a low addiction capability. It is available for use in subcutaneous, intravenous, and intramuscular injection form. In oral tablet form the drug is only one-third as effective as in the parenteral route. Pentazocine has been used as a premedicant and for pain relief in the recovery room. It may cause discomforting hallucinogenic activity. See Narcotic.

PENTHRANE: See Methoxyflurane.

PENTOBARBITAL (NEMBUTAL): A popular barbiturate for preanesthetic medication. See Barbiturate.

PENTOLINIUM (DRUG C-5): A ganglionic blocking agent no longer available clinically.

PENTOTHAL: See Thiopental sodium.

PENTYLENETETRAZOL (METRAZOL): A central nervous system stimulant which is useful as a diagnostic aid in epilepsy. A patient's response to the drug is monitored with an electroencephalogram to evaluate the cerebral disorder.

PERFUSION: The passage of a fluid through a vessel, tissue, or specific organ of the body. The fluid usually perfusing the body tissue is blood, but techniques have been recently developed in which an organ or limb is isolated as to its arterial inflow and venous return and perfused with various solutions or drugs, such as chemotherapeutic agents. The definition of perfusion has been extended to include cardiopulmonary bypass. (The technician operating the cardiopulmonary bypass pump and oxygenator apparatus is known as a perfusionist.)

PERFUSION ABNORMALITY: See Ventilation/perfusion abnormality.

PERFUSION LIMITATION: See Diffusion limitation.

PERFUSION, PULMONARY: See Pulmonary perfusion, zones of.

PERIDURAL ANESTHESIA: See Epidural anesthesia.

PERIOD (T): The duration of a single repetition of a cyclic phenomenon or the time occupied in one complete to-and-fro movement of a given oscillation or vibration.

PERIODIC BREATHING: A period of apnea followed by a gradual crescendo and then decrescendo of respiratory volume, terminating again in apnea. In healthy individuals, periodic breathing can be demonstrated after a period of deliberate hyperventilation. The hyperventilation causes hypocapnia. This lack of CO_2 causes apnea. During this apneic period, arterial O_2 tension falls off. There then arises a situation of relative hypoxia which drives respiration to begin again. The hypoxic drive is satisfied by a few good respirations; however, the CO_2 has not yet built up due to tissue metabolism and respiration therefore ceases. This cycle continues until CO_2 is built up to a normal range again, whereupon it resumes control of respiration.

PERIODIC FHR: See Fetal heart rate terminology.

PERIODIC TABLE: A table of the elements displayed in sequence according to atomic number and atomic weight and arranged in horizontal rows (periods) and vertical columns (groups). See Fig.

Periodic Table: Periodic table of the elements.

PERIPHERAL CHEMORECEPTORS: A small mass of cells (carotid and aortic bodies) which respond to changes in PCO_2, PO_2, and the pH of blood. They appear to be most sensitive to the PO_2. A fall in O_2 tension causes a rise in ventilation.

PERIPHERAL NERVE STIMULATOR: A device which can deliver precise amounts of electric current to excite a peripheral nerve. The stimulators may be used to evaluate neuromuscular blockade and to prevent overdose with blocking agents. A supramaximal stimulus is applied to the skin electrodes (previously needle electrodes) and the movements of the tested areas, e.g., fingers, are observed. The output voltage under no-load conditions of a typical device can be in excess of 250 V. The output current is usually adjustable between 0 and 50 mA. See Fig. See Blockade monitor; Neuromuscular blockade, assessment of.

PERIPHERAL NERVOUS SYSTEM (PNS): The part of the nervous system exclusive of the brain and spinal cord. See Autonomic nervous system.

PERIPHERAL VASCULAR RESISTANCE: See Total peripheral resistance.

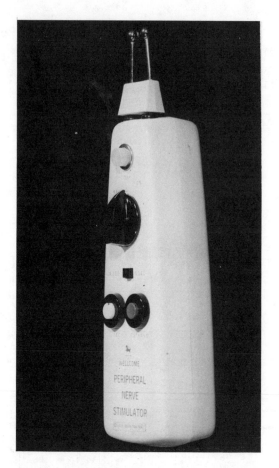

Peripheral Nerve Stimulator: Typical bipolar peripheral nerve stimulator used for assessing neuromuscular blockade.

PERITONEAL DIALYSIS: A procedure, useful in patients with acute or chronic renal failure, which aids in the removal of toxic waste material from the blood and maintenance of fluid, electrolyte, and acid-base balance. It is accomplished by means of selective exchange or diffusion across the peritoneal surface (a semipermeable membrane). Peritoneal dialysis involves passing a large volume of dialyzing fluid (dialysate) through the abdominal wall, waiting while exchange takes place, then removing the introduced fluid. Although peritoneal dialysis is easier than hemodialysis, it is a more time-consuming procedure. See Hemodialysis.

PERITONEAL INSUFFLATION: See Insufflation, intraperitoneal.

PERITONEOSCOPY: See Laparoscopy.

PERMANENT GAS: A gas that can only be liquefied by the combination of extreme pressure and cooling below normal temperatures.

PERMEABILITY THEORY OF ANESTHESIA: The theory that proposes that anesthetics reduce permeability to ions affecting synaptic transmission of the central nervous system. In experimental systems, some anesthetics can change membrane permeability. Other drugs, however, which are not anesthetics are able to affect this alteration as well. Therefore, this theory does not fully explain the anesthetic state. See Lipid solubility theory of anesthesia.

PERSISTENCE (AFTERGLOW): The faint glow seen in certain gases for a considerable time after the passage of an electric current. The term also refers to the faint light emitted from the screen of a cathode-ray tube after electron bombardment has ceased.

PETHIDINE: The British term for meperidine (Demerol).

PETROLATUM (PETROLEUM JELLY): A hydrocarbon obtained in the fractional distillation of petroleum. It is used as an emollient, lubricant, and ointment base.

$$pH = - \log H^+$$

Normal $H^+ = 40 \times 10^{-9}$ Eq/L (40 nEq/L)

$$pH = - \log 40 \times 10^{-9}$$

$$= - (\log 40 + \log 10^{-9})$$

$$= - (\log 4.0 + \log 10^{-8})$$

$$= - (0.59 - 8)$$

$$= - (-7.4) = 7.4$$

I

$[H^+]$ (nEq/L)	pH
125	6.8
100	7.0
40	7.4
25	7.8
15	8.0

II

pH: (I) Normal blood pH derivative. (II) Hydrogen ion nEq/L related to pH.

pH: A symbol indicating hydrogen ion concentration. It is the negative logarithm to the base 10 of the hydrogen ion concentration and is used in measuring acidity and alkalinity on a scale of 0-14 with 7 indicating neutrality. The system serves the useful purpose of restating very small values within a narrow range of larger numbers. For example, the hydrogen ion concentration of the extracellular fluid is normally 4×10^{-8} Eq/L. The pH is inversely proportional to the hydrogen ion concentration, i.e., as the pH increases, the hydrogen ion concentration decreases. A suggestion has been made that hydrogen ion concentration be reported directly in the linear system of nanoequivalents. See Fig.

PHANTOM LIMB: A phenomenon occurring in recent amputees in which the patient claims that he or she can still feel, locate in space, and experience pain in the missing limb. It is sometimes reported by patients who have had adequate regional anesthetics. The "phantom" position most often reported is the limb position at the onset of motor blockade. Phantom limb pain is a particularly perplexing problem because regional block done in amputees often does not alleviate the pain and actually makes it worse.

PHARMACODYNAMICS: The measurement of what a drug does in the body, specifically, its therapeutic, toxic, and pharmacologic effects. This includes analysis of the mechanism of drug action and measurement of response versus dose or plasma concentration.

PHARMACOKINETICS: The study of the relationship between the time and serum concentration of a drug and its metabolites. It is usually broken down into subcategories of absorption, distribution, and elimination. The latter is a combination of metabolism and excretion.

PHARYNX: The mucous membrane-covered muscular sac which is the communication between the nares and mouth superiorly and the esophagus and larynx inferiorly. Specifically, the nasopharynx is the part of the pharynx above the level of the soft palate which is continuous with the nasal passages and contains the opening for the eustachian tubes to the inner ear. The lower part of the pharynx from the soft palate to the upper edge of the epiglottis forming the rear of the mouth is called the oropharynx. The laryngopharynx (hypopharynx) is that part of the pharynx contained between the upper edge of the epiglottis continuous with the larynx and the esophagus.

PHASE I BLOCK: The normal neuromuscular blocking effect of depolarizing muscle relaxants on the motor endplate area. Agents such as succinylcholine react with the receptors of the motor endplate and depolarize the endplate membrane. The depolarization of the endplate region persists until succinylcholine is metabolized. This continuous action eventually leads to inexcitability in the muscle membrane adjacent to the endplate and to neuromuscular blockade. In phase I block, there is prolonged response to a single twitch, sustained tetanus, no posttetanic facilitation, and train-of-four, each of which is equally depressed. Initial onset of a phase I block causes muscle twitching (fasciculation). See Neuromuscular blockade, assessment of.

PHASE II BLOCK (DESENSITIZATION BLOCK, DUAL BLOCK): A poorly understood phenonemon which occurs after prolonged depolarizing neuromuscular blockade. In this block the muscle membrane becomes at least partially repolarized but will not normally respond to acetylcholine by depolarizing. A phase II block resembles a nondepolarizing block in that tetanus is poorly sustained, post-tetanic facilitation is present, and a train-of-four ratio of less than 50% has been observed. Response to anticholinesterase reversal is variable, however. See Neuromuscular blockade, assessment of.

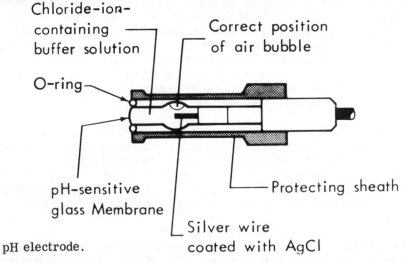

pH electrode.

pH ELECTRODE: A device which determines the hydrogen ion concentration in a solution as the ions cross a glass membrane to reach an electrode, thereby causing or forming an ion current. This current is proportional to the pH of the solution. The current is read out in units of pH or hydrogen ion concentration. See Fig. See Carbon dioxide electrode.

PHENACETIN: An analgesic and antipyretic agent often used in conjunction with salicylates. It is an aniline (coal-tar) derivative in which the active metabolite is acetaminophen. These agents offer only weak anti-inflammatory activity. Overdosage

KETAMINE   **PHENCYCLIDINE**

Phencyclidine: Molecular diagrams of ketamine and phencyclidine showing the similarity.

with phenacetin may lead to methemoglobinemia, cyanosis, respiratory depression, and cardiac arrest. See Acetaminophen.

PHENCYCLIDINE (SERNYLAN; "ANGEL DUST"; PCP): A nonbarbiturate compound originally proposed as a human anesthetic but not used clinically because of the high incidence of hallucinations. (It is, however, used as a veterinary anesthetic.) It is chemically related to ketamine. A widely abused drug which can be easily manufactured, it can cause severe toxic psychosis, convulsions, and death. Some anecdotal evidence exists that it can cause permanent personality changes after single- or short-term use, an attribute which would make it a unique pharmacologic entity. See Fig.

PHENERGAN: See Phenothiazine, Promethazine hydrochloride.

PHENOBARBITAL (LUMINAL, PHENOBARB): A barbiturate used as a sedative, hypnotic, and anticonvulsant. It is more potent as an anticonvulsant than as a sedative. After even short-term use, phenobarbital stimulates liver enzyme systems which metabolize many similar drugs. It can therefore, theoretically at least, shorten the action of those agents which depend on metabolism to terminate their actions. See Barbiturate.

PHENOL (CARBOLIC ACID): The first widely used antiseptic. Many dilute phenol derivatives are employed in disinfecting equipment and furniture surfaces that do not come in contact with patients. Phenol is extremely toxic and may cause convulsions and renal damage. It may be used clinically for neurolytic injection in the treatment of intractable pain. See Neurolysis.

PHENOPERIDINE: A narcotic related to meperidine. Approximately 10 times more potent than morphine, it is available in England under the trade name of Operidine. The drug is a very long-acting respiratory depressant. See Narcotic.

PHENOTHIAZINE: A widely used group of drugs which are employed primarily in the treatment of psychiatric disorders and are also important as antiemetic and antihistaminic agents. Although not addictive, they can produce some degree of physical dependence. The phenothiazines are weak alpha-adrenergic blocking agents and can therefore enhance hypotension seen during anesthesia. They can produce acute parkinson-like rigidity which can lead to respiratory embarrassment. See Antipsychotic agent.

PHENOXYBENZAMINE (DIBENZYLINE): An alpha-adrenergic blocking agent, close-ly related to the nitrogen mustards, which effectively prevents responses that are mediated by alpha receptors, producing a "chemical sympathectomy." Phenoxyben-zamine lowers blood pressure and may produce orthostatic hypotension. It is used in the presurgical treatment of pheochromocytoma. In this role it controls the epi-sodic hypertension and sweating which characterize this disease. It has also been used to alleviate vasospastic peripheral vascular disease. Adverse side ef-fects of phenoxybenzamine include tachycardia, miosis, and orthostatic hypotension.

PHENTOLAMINE (REGITINE): An imidazoline with a wide range of pharmacologic actions, the most important of which is its alpha receptor blockade. It is used to prevent or control the hypertensive episodes of a patient with pheochromocytoma. It is also used in the Regitine test to assist in the diagnosis of pheochromocytoma. An intravenous injection of phentolamine produces a rapid fall in blood pressure in a patient with the adrenal tumor. An alternate use of the drug is in the treatment of dermal necrosis caused by extravasation of norepinephrine from an intravenous site. Adverse side effects include tachycardia, cardiac arrhythmia, angina, abdom-inal pain, nausea, vomiting, diarrhea, and exacerbation of peptic ulcer. See Phen-oxybenzamine.

PHENYLEPHRINE (NEO-SYNEPHRINE): A potent pressor agent (raises blood pres-sure) and a powerful alpha receptor stimulant with little effect on beta receptors. It produces a marked reflex bradycardia, increases peripheral resistance, and slight-ly decreases cardiac output. Because of its potency, it is administered in highly di-lute form in an intravenous bolus or drip; because of its rapid onset, it requires extremely careful management. It is also used topically as a nasal decongestant and as a mydriatic agent.

PHEOCHROMOCYTOMA: A tumor arising from the chromaffin cells in sympathetic ganglia. It is capable of secreting vasoactive substances, particularly epinephrine and norepinephrine, and may be found anywhere in the body where sympathetic ner-vous tissue is found, most typically in the adrenal medulla. This type of tumor is particularly significant to anesthesia; premedication with alpha-blocking agents, e.g., phenoxybenzamine, to block the action of the agents secreted by the tumor is absolutely essential. At times, even in the face of adequate long-term blockade, the anesthetic course is extremely uneven with wild shifts in the blood pressure and cardiac output as the tumor is manipulated. Pheochromocytoma tends to be familial and is often associated with medullary carcinoma of the thyroid gland. See Fig. See Phenoxybenzamine, Phentolamine.

Pheochromocytoma: Symptoms and signs.

Hypertension	Psychosis
Palpitations	Syncope
Sweating	Convulsions
Pallor	Tinnitus
Flushing	Blurred vision
Angina	Weight loss
Dyspnea	Anorexia
Headache	Nausea
Nervousness	Epigastric pain
Weakness	Back pain
Dizziness	Neck pain
Tremors	Flank pain

PHISOHEX: See Hexachlorophene.

PHOSGENE (CARBONYL CHLORIDE): A highly toxic, colorless gas ($CoCl_2$) that condenses at 0 degrees Celsius to a fuming liquid. It is a breakdown product of tri-chloroethylene (an obsolete anesthetic). Phosgene was used as a poisonous gas during World War I and is now used in the manufacture of organic compounds. See Tri-chloroethylene.

PHOSPHOLINE: See Echothiophate iodide.

PHOSPHOR: A substance capable of emitting light when excited by radiant energy.

PHOSPHORESCENCE: The luminescence seen after bombardment with electromag-netic energy and visible for a time after the excitement has ceased. See Lumines-cense.

PHOTOCELL (PHOTOELECTRIC CELL): A solid-state photosensitive electronic device. Its resistance to electric current flow is a function of incident radiation. It is also known as an electric eye, because of its use as a sensor in burglar alarm systems. See Photoconductivity.

PHOTOCONDUCTIVITY: A subclass of the photoelectric effect which describes the ability of specific elements or compounds to change (usually by lowering) their elec-tric resistance when illuminated by a light frequency specific to the compound. It is the basic process which makes photocells possible.

PHOTOELECTRIC DETERMINATION OF BLOOD PRESSURE: A technique for de-termining blood pressure using a light source, a photocell, and a blood pressure cuff. A light source is aimed at a particular area of tissue. The amount of light reflected or transmitted through the tissue changes with each pulse. The amount of light received by a photoconductive cell fluctuates. Since the resistance of the cell changes with light striking it, current flowing through it will pulsate with tissue blood flow. Quantitating pressure changes requires the slow deflation of a proximal blood pressure cuff while watching for a pulse indication from the photocell. See Arterial blood pressure.

PHOTOELECTRIC EFFECT: The physical property which allows certain substances to use energy contained in incident electromagnetic radiation (particularly light) to raise the energy level of electrons in the substance. This is the phenomenon under-lying photoconductivity and photoelectric emission.

PHOTOELECTRIC EMISSION (PHOTOEMISSION): The physical property of certain substances that causes electrons to be randomly emitted when the substance is struck in a vacuum by electromagnetic energy such as light. Elements which exhib-it this property include barium, cesium, and lithium. See Photovoltaic effect.

PHOTOMULTIPLIER: A device which detects light by converting light energy to an electric current and then amplifying the current. For example, in liquid scintilla-tion counters light flashes strike a photocathode which exhibits the photoelectric ef-fect (photons of light energy are converted to free-moving electrons). These elec-trons are then accelerated by a magnetic field and are used to strike subsequent cathodes liberating more electrons. The strength of the ultimate electron cascade is the function of the strength of the magnetic field used to guide it and the number of cathodes.

PHOTON: A discrete unit of electromagnetic radiation which has no rest mass and travels at the speed of light. Its energy is the product of its frequency, in cycles per second, times Planck constant, i.e., $E = h\nu$.

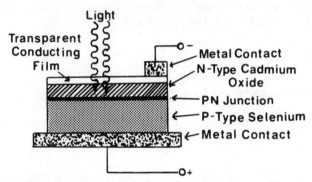

Photovoltaic Effect: Simple photovoltaic cell showing the various components.

PHOTOVOLTAIC EFFECT: The production of an electric field or voltage in a substance by the absorption of the energy contained in the light striking the substance. As a subclass of the photoelectric effect, it is the phenomenon underlying solar cells. The efficiency of the process of converting one form of energy to another is at best 20-25%. See Fig. See Photocell.

PHRENIC NERVE: The paired main motor nerves which arise from the cervical plexus at levels C3-C5 and innervate the diaphragm. Paralysis of the phrenic nerve(s) may result from neck fracture or inadvertently from brachial plexus block, high epidural, or high spinal anesthesia. Deliberate phrenic nerve block was an old method of treating intractable hiccup. See Electrophrenic respiration.

PHYSICAL STATUS CLASSIFICATIONS, ASA: The evaluation of the patient's overall health as it would influence the conduct and outcome of anesthesia and/or surgery. Physical status can be defined within one of five assigned classes. (1) Class 1 patients have no organic, physiologic, biochemical, metabolic, or psychiatric disturbance. The operation to be performed is for a local pathologic process and has no systemic effect. An example of a class 1 patient is an athlete who requires repair of an inguinal hernia. (2) A class 2 patient has a systemic disturbance which may be of a mild to moderate degree but which is either controlled or has not changed in its severity for some time. Examples are patients with controlled diabetes, controlled hypertension, or mild nonlimiting organic heart disease. Often, anesthetists consider healthy individuals at the extremes of age (neonate or octogenarian) to be class 2 patients. (3) Class 3 patients suffer from significant systemic disturbance, although the degree to which it limits the patient's functioning or causes disability may not be quantifiable. Examples include severe organic heart disease, severe diabetes with vascular or kidney involvement, pulmonary insufficiency, angina pectoris, or an old myocardial infarction. (4) Class 4 patients have severe systemic diseases that are already life-threatening and may or may not be correctable by surgery. An example is a patient with initial signs of cardiac failure, advanced liver or renal disease, or intractable angina. (5) The class 5 patient is considered to have little or no chance of survival in the short term (less than 24 hr) and is submitted to operation in desperation. An example of a class 5 patient is an individual with a massive pulmonary embolus, major cerebral trauma, or severe and progressive compromised respiratory gas exchange. As a further subclassification of physical states, any patient falling naturally into one of the five classes who comes to an operation as an emergency has the letter E placed after the classification number. For example, the patient scheduled for emergency nephrectomy due to rejection of a transplanted kidney would be classified as 4E.

PHYSICIAN-PATIENT RELATIONSHIP: When a patient has entered into a contract with a physician for services, the relationship contains the following legal considerations. (1) The physician must personally render the care agreed upon; the patient suffers legal injury if another physician is substituted without permission of the patient. (2) The physician has the responsibility of working to the standard set by similarly trained physicians with similar experience in similar communities. (3) The physician has a duty or obligation not to cease rendering care without the permission of the patient. (4) The physician must maintain the trust of the patient and not reveal publicly details of the patient's care which are of a confidential nature. When a contract for care has been established with a physician, the patient has the following obligations and duties. (1) The patient is required to follow the instructions, prescriptions, and advice of the physician. (2) The patient is obligated to pay for the services he or she receives. If any of the above duties are not carried out, one or the other of the parties to the agreement may have legal recourse.

PHYSIOLOGIC DEAD SPACE: The portion of a tidal volume which is not available for gas exchange. It includes the anatomic dead space and those alveoli which, although ventilated, are not perfused. See Alveolar dead space, Anatomic dead space.

PHYSOSTIGMINE; ESERINE (ANTILIRIUM): An anticholinesterase agent useful in the treatment of glaucoma. It is capable of penetrating the blood-brain barrier. It has been used to reverse the cardiovascular and central nervous system (CNS) effects of acute atropine and scopolamine overdose. It has also been reported to be an effective antidote to a variety of CNS depressants; however, it can cause profound bradycardia.

PICKUP: A device that converts a sound or other form of mechanical vibration into an electric signal. Such devices include microphones and phonograph cartridges.

PICKWICKIAN SYNDROME: A condition involving morbid obesity with various associated problems such as somnolence, cyanosis, intermittent respiration, secondary polycythemia, and right-sided cardiac failure. Total lung capacity, vital capacity, and respiratory reserve volume are all decreased. The work of breathing is increased as the amount of energy required to move the chest mass is elevated.

PICO-: The prefix meaning 10^{12}. (This term replaces micromicro-.) See SI unit.

PIERRE ROBIN SYNDROME: A congenital syndrome which combines micrognathia with cleft palate and glossoptosis. Glossoptosis, the displacement or retraction of the tongue into the hypopharynx, may produce intermittent airway obstruction.

PIEZOELECTRIC EFFECT: The property of certain crystals to produce an electric charge when subjected to mechanical stress (pressure, expansion, twisting). The electric charges are proportional to the tension applied. Depending on size, shape, and composition (quartz, barium tartrate), the frequency at which a crystal oscillates is extremely controllable and exact. Crystals are therefore used for precision clocks or timing circuits.

PILOCARPINE: A naturally occurring alkaloid which mimics the effects of acetyl-choline in the heart, salivary glands, and sweat glands. It is most commonly used as a miotic agent.

PIN-INDEX SAFETY SYSTEM: A safety system which prevents the wrong gas cylinder from being placed in a yoke. The pin-index safety system is used with small cylinders (size E or less) and consists of two pins on the yoke which fit into two corresponding holes in the cylinder valve. If the pins and holes cannot be aligned, the cylinder port will not fit against the washer of the yoke. The system uses various combinations of six locations of holes and pins. Anesthetic disasters have occurred when the pin-index system was deliberately defeated by extracting the pins or using double washers as a temporary convenience.

PINK PUFFER AND BLUE BLOATER: The classic description of the two ends of the spectrum of chronic obstructive pulmonary disease. In clinical practice, however, a pure case of either is rare. The "pink puffer" is the pure emphysemic whose major pathologic findings are critical loss of alveolar walls, little airway inflammation, and little right ventricular hypertrophy. The patient has signs and symptoms of mild hypoxia, hypocapnia, increased total lung capacity and residual volume, markedly decreased diffusion, and some rise in airway resistance not amenable to treatment. The "blue bloater" is the archetypical chronic bronchitis patient. The pathologic findings are minimal loss of alveolar walls but marked bronchitis with mucous gland hyperplasia, bronchiolitis, and right ventricular hypertrophy. Signs and symptoms are severe hypoxia, hypercapnia, polycythemia (coupled, however, with a relatively normal total lung capacity), a preserved diffusion capacity of the lung, and elevated airway resistance which does respond to some degree of treatment. The "blue bloat" refers to venous distention, hepatomegaly, edema, and some degree of cyanosis. See Chronic obstructive pulmonary disease.

PIN VALVE: See Flow control valve.

PIPEROCAINE (METYCAINE): A local anesthetic agent with properties similar to procaine. See Local anesthetic.

PLANCK CONSTANT (h): A universal constant that relates the frequency of radiation to its quanta of energy and has a value of 6.25×10^{-27} erg sec.

PLANCK LAW: The basis of quantum theory used to describe the behavior of electromagnetic radiation. It states that the energy of electromagnetic radiation is in the form of small individual packets called photons. See Photon.

PLASMA: The clear straw-colored liquid portion of the blood which contains erythrocytes, leukocytes, platelets, and various proteins.

PLASMA EXPANDER: A solution used to replace critical loss of blood plasma. Plasma expanders may be non-blood-derived starch solutions such as dextran or hetastarch and are administered intravenously. See Albumin, Dextran, Hetastarch.

PLASMA KININ: See Bradykinin.

PLATELET (THROMBOCYTE): An anucleate, disc-shaped cell from 2 to 4 μm in diameter which is a constituent of mammalian blood and important in coagulation. Normal levels range from 200,000-400,000 platelets/mm^3 blood. Platelets can change shape and accumulate at the site of vascular injury (platelet aggregation). Platelet aggregation and adhesion occur in response to the contact of platelets with a nonvascular surface. These two processes cause many products to be released from cytoplasmic granules in the platelets, the most important being adenosine diphosphate (ADP). (Other substances released include serotonin, epinephrine, calcium, and clotting factors.) ADP is a potent agent for causing further platelet aggregation. Aggregation, adhesion, and release are collectively called platelet activation and, once having reached a threshold, it is a self-sustaining process. See Blood coagulation.

PLATELET CONCENTRATE: A pooling of platelet-rich plasma produced by the differential centrifugation of several units of whole blood. Stored at room temperature, the concentrate contains a significant number of viable platelets for 72 hr. Platelets stored at 4 degrees Celsius retain viability for only 24 hr. The concentrate, used in platelet transfusion, temporarily prevents or reduces bleeding associated with platelet-deficient diseases, such as acute leukemia, thrombocytopenia, and aplastic anemia.

PLATINUM: A grayish white metallic element which, due to its malleability and high electric and corrosive resistance, is used in alloys, jewelry, and electric and electronic equipment. It acts as a catalyst for many chemical reactions. See Oxygen analyzer.

PLETHYSMOGRAPH: See Blood flow, methods for measuring; Body plethysmograph.

PLEURA: The collective name for the two layers of serous membrane which enclose and protect the lungs. The parietal pleura, the outer layer, is attached to the walls of the pleural cavity; the visceral pleura, the inner layer, lines the lungs. The potential space between the two layers of the pleura is called the pleural cavity and contains a lubricating fluid secreted by the membranes.

PLEXUS: See Ganglion.

PNEUMATICS: The branch of physics that deals with the mechanical properties of gas.

PNEUMOCARDIOGRAPHY (PNCG); THORACIC AIR PLETHYSMOGRAPHY: The recording of variations in heart functions via monitoring of respiration. The pneumocardiograph senses changes in thoracic cavity dimensions and changes in bronchial pressure with each heartbeat. This procedure is most conveniently done in the apneic patient.

PNEUMOCYTE: See Alveolar cell types.

PNEUMOTACHYGRAPH (FLEISCH PNEUMOTACHYGRAPH): A device for measuring gas flow during general anesthesia. It operates by placing a mesh screen in the path of a moving gas. The resistance of the mesh screen causes a pressure drop across its surface and the magnitude of this decrease in pressure is related to the volume of gas passing the screen. By measuring the pressure difference, an approximation can be made of the volume of gas which has passed the screen per unit of time. The device tends to become inaccurate at low flows or if the screen becomes obstructed.

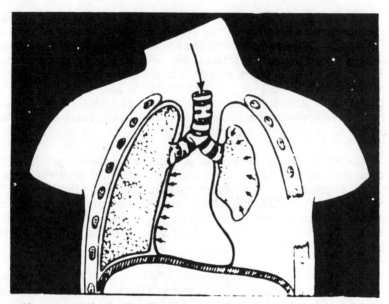

Pneumothorax: Effect of pneumothorax on mediastinum upon inspiration. The mediastinum moves toward the normal lung. On expiration it moves back toward the normal position (mediastinal flap).

PNEUMOTHORAX: The presence of free air in the pleural cavity. It may occur traumatically after a puncture or penetration of the chest wall or pleura or spontaneously following the blowout of a bleb on the surface of the lung. An open pneumothorax occurs when the wound of external entry remains exposed. The air space will then enlarge with each inspiration as the negative pressure in the chest sucks air simultaneously down the trachea and through the hole in the chest wall. A closed pneumothorax is the aforementioned air space with no communication with either the external chest wall or the air passageways of the lung. The closed pneumothorax may become a tension pneumothorax if the pressure of the air in the pleural cavity rises above that in the lung. The best explanation of the mechanism of tension pneumothorax is to consider the communication with the pleura as a ball valve which enlarges the pneumothorax space at peak inspiratory pressure but closes when expiratory pressure pushes air out of the cavity. The trapped air compresses the affected lung. Tension pneumothorax can be exacerbated by the use of N_2O during anesthesia. Nitrous oxide, because it diffuses across membranes so rapidly (faster than the N_2 it replaces), diffuses into the closed air space continually pressurizing and expanding it. This will progressively encroach on the lung volume and may lead to severe respiratory embarrassment. Signs and symptoms of pneumothorax include pain, dyspnea, effusion (hydropneumothorax), and absence of breath sounds. See Fig.

POISEUILLE LAW: A physical principle determining flow of fluid in a tube or vessel. Flow rate is directly proportional to (1) the pressure drop along the length and (2) the fourth power of the tube radius. Flow is inversely proportional to tube length and fluid viscosity. In practical terms, doubling the height of an intravenous bottle roughly doubles flow; doubling the radius of an intravenous cannula increases flow 16 times.

POLARIZATION: A state of matter in which two surfaces have opposite, and often equal, electric charges. For example, in a polarized membrane of a nerve cell the outside surface is positive and the inside surface is negative. Differences in electric potential are normally measured in volts. Generally, when a skin electrode is polarized, difference measurable in volts (millivolts) exists between the electrodes and the skin.

POLAROGRAPHY: An electrochemical technique of analysis in which changes in the chemical or physical composition of a solution create changes in its electric conductivity, thereby effecting a change in any electric current passing through the solution. Thus, in accordance with Ohm law, changes in the voltage difference across the solution can be measured and reflect the changing conditions in the solution. Polarography is most immediately applicable to O_2 analysis where the presence or absence of O_2 changes the electric conductivity of an ionic solution and this in turn is used to measure the O_2 concentration. See Oxygen analyzer.

POLIO BLADE: An adaptation of the Macintosh laryngoscope blade which sits at an obtuse angle on the handle to allow intubation of a patient in an iron lung.

POLYMERIZATION: The process of forming a polymer by bonding monomers of repeating structural units. Polymers may be naturally occurring (e.g., rubber, proteins, starches) or man-made (e.g., nylon, Teflon, polyvinyl chloride).

POLYMYXIN B (AEROSPORIN): A potent peptide antibiotic agent of the polymyxin group produced from a strain of soil bacillus (Bacillus polymyxa). It is active against gram-negative bacteria. Polymyxin B is administered parenterally [intravenous (IV), intramuscular (IM), intrathecal], topically (usually in combination with bacitracin as an ointment), or orally. Untoward side effects include pain (after IM injection), renal toxicity, nausea, vomiting, diarrhea, headache, meningeal irritation (after intrathecal injection), diplopia, ptosis, and generalized areflexia. Polymyxin E, commonly known as colistin (Coly-Mycin), is another member of the antibiotic group. See Fig.

POLYPEPTIDE: A peptide composed of three or more amino acids joined by peptide bonds, i.e., a carbon atom linked to a nitrogen atom in an alternating chain. The size of the polypeptide depends on the number of amino acids in the chain.

PONTOCAINE: See Tetracaine hydrochloride.

POP-OFF VALVE (EXPIRATORY VALVE; HIGH-PRESSURE RELIEF VALVE): A valve, downstream from the patient in a gas delivery system, which relieves the excess volume that continuously builds up when the fresh gas flow into the system exceeds the O_2 uptake of the patient. See Fig.

PORPHYRIA: A hereditary disease which involves errors in the formation or excretion of the porphyrins. Porphyrins are molecular components of hemoglobin, myoglobin, various enzymes concerned with oxidation reactions such as the cytochromes, and other proteins concerned with oxidation and electron transport. They are chemically related to plant chlorophyll. There are two basic types of porphyrias: (1) erythropoietic, in which the metabolic disturbance is in the bone marrow, and (2) hepatic, in which the metabolic disturbance is in the liver. Hepatic porphyrias, of clinical interest to the practice of anesthesia, are divided into three types: acute intermittent porphyria, variegate porphyria, and hereditary coproporphyria. The latter is an extremely rare type which clinically mimics either of the first two. Acute intermittent porphyria is characterized by attacks which are irregular and unpredictable. The acute type can consist of abdominal pain, various moderate to severe neurologic abnormalities involving both central and peripheral nervous sys-

Polymyxin B: Polymyxins.

Generic Name (Trade Name)	Spectrum of Activity	Comments
Polymyxin B (Aerosporin) Topical IM PO Otic Solution	G⁻ bacilli, including Pseudomonas, Escherichia, Enterobacter, Klebsiella, Hemophilus, Salmonella, and Shigella. Proteus is resistant.	Polymyxin B, like the other polymyxins, is bactericidal and is associated with certain side effects, including nephrotoxicity and neurologic disturbances such as vertigo, paresthesias, and neuromuscular blockade. It is not absorbed orally but is used orally for the treatment of GI infections.
Colistin (Coly-Mycin S) PO Otic Solution	Similar to polymyxin B.	Colistin is used in treating diarrhea caused by E. coli and Shigella in children with enteritis. Side effects include superinfection within the GI tract, especially by Proteus.
Colistimethate (Coly-Mycin M) IM IV	Similar to polymyxin B.	Colistimethate can cause nephrotoxicity, neuromuscular blockade, and transient neurologic disturbances. Its therapeutic uses are essentially the same as polymyxin B.

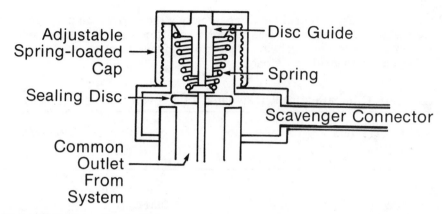

Pop-Off Valve: Typical spring-loaded pop-off valve showing the various internal parts.

tems, motor disturbances, **seizure** activities, psychiatric aberrations, and cardiovascular involvement. The patients ultimately die from the additive effect of multiple central nervous system lesions. Anesthetic interest lies in the fact that intravenous barbiturates in the dose used for anesthesia induction allegedly can trigger an attack of acute intermittent porphyria which can lead to cardiovascular collapse.

POSITIVE END EXPIRATORY PRESSURE (PEEP): A modality for the treatment of patients who require ventilatory support. When PEEP is employed, the airway pressure is never allowed to return to "zero" (atmospheric). At the end of expiration, when airway pressure would normally be at its lowest point, it is artificially held at positive pressure by the PEEP apparatus. This can be done simply by a water trap into which the exhalation hose is dipped. The amount of pressure placed on the gas in the hose is directly readable as the number of centimeters the hose dips below the surface of the water. The prime purpose of PEEP is to keep the small airways open and stabilize the structural integrity of the lung. The positive pressure "splints" open airways that would otherwise close (due to loss of support) and thereby trap air.

POSITIVE WATER BALANCE: See Negative water balance.

POSITRON: An elementary particle with an identical mass and positive charge equal in strength to the negative charge of an electron.

POSTANESTHETIC RECOVERY ROOM (PAR): See Recovery/recovery room.

POSTOPERATIVE VISIT: The bedside visit by the anesthetist to the postoperative patient with the purpose of evaluating the outcome of anesthesia and recording appropriate remarks on the patient's chart. A postoperative visit is a requirement for hospital accreditation, particularly for those patients who are in the hospital for at least 24 hr postoperatively.

POSTSYNAPTIC MEMBRANE: See Neuromuscular blockade, assessment of.

POSTSYNAPTIC POTENTIAL: See Neuromuscular blockade, assessment of.

POST-TETANIC FACILITATION: See Neuromuscular blockade, assessment of.

POSTURAL DRAINAGE: A technique of respiratory therapy which uses gravity to mobilize excess lung secretions. The patient is positioned so that the affected area of the lung is superior to the trachea. Postural drainage is often used with chest percussion to "shake" secretions loose.

Potassium: Clinical entities associated with serum potassium changes.

Causes of Potassium Elevation	Causes of Potassium Depletion
Excess intake	Dietary lack
Use of K-sparing diuretics, i.e., aldactone, dyrenium	Diarrhea
	Alkalosis
Acidosis	K-losing renal disease
Renal insufficiency	Diuretic therapy
Acute hemolysis	Aldosteronism
Muscle necrosis	Nasogastric suction
Addison disease	Secondary to glucose and insulin administration
Hypoaldosteronism associated with diabetes	Villous adenoma (bowel)

POTASSIUM (K): An element which occurs abundantly in nature and the principal cation of intracellular fluids. It has an atomic number of 19 and an atomic weight of 39. The potassium balance of the body is exquisitely important to both the integrity of cellular function and, more specifically, the maintenance of normal cardiac rhythmicity. The normal 70-kg man has a total body content of exchangeable potassium of approximately 3200 mEq; of this amount about two-thirds is intracellular. The concentration of intracellular water is approximately 160 mEq/L. Extracellularly, the serum potassium normally ranges from 3.5 to 5.5 mEq/L. Under normal circumstances with normally functioning kidneys, the minimum daily requirement approaches 30 mEq/L. Problems arise with potassium control that do not exist with the control of sodium concentration because the kidney is not as well equipped to conserve potassium as it is sodium. There appears to be a minimum obligatory loss of potassium when potassium is depleted in the body. This loss is in the range of 20 mEq/24 hr. Particularly in those instances where a normal adult continues to receive sodium but is restricted in potassium intake for as little as 7 days, significant potassium depletion can occur. Potassium and hydrogen ions compete for exchange with sodium ions in renal tubules and, when sodium is provided, adrenal steroids increase renal potassium loss. When the patient is stressed and has normal kidneys, excretion may reach levels in excess of 100 mEq/24 hr. Of particular interest to individuals managing patients with acid-base imbalances is the fact that plasma potassium increases approximately 0.6 mEq/L for each 0.1-unit fall in blood pH. Conversely, plasma potassium decreases about 0.6 mEq/L for each 0.1-unit rise in blood pH. It is extremely difficult to raise serum potassium levels in alkalotic patients. This is due to the interchangeability, as far as the body is concerned, of potassium and hydrogen. See Fig. See Cardiac glycosides, Electrocardiogram.

POTASSIUM CHANNEL (POTASSIUM TUNNEL): The name given to the opening in the membrane of a nerve which allows for the passage of the potassium ion outward into the extracellular fluid during depolarization. The potassium channel is a theoretic entity. Unlike the sodium pore, which appears to occur in areas of the membrane that are thin, the potassium pore or channel occurs in areas of the membrane which are of normal thickness. The nature of the gate in the potassium tunnel is not well-defined. See Sodium channel.

POTENCY: The relative strength of a drug determined by the dose (measured by weight) which produces pharmacologic effects (especially intensity and duration of action) equal to those of a reference compound. For example, milligram for milligram, tetracaine has been determined to be approximately 10 times more potent than procaine.

POTENTIAL ENERGY: The energy which a body or system has by virtue of its position. It is equal to the work that was done in bringing that system to its current position.

POTENTIATION: An increase in the power of an activity, e.g., the greater force of contraction of the heart on administration of a positive inotropic drug. It is used frequently but less correctly as a synonym for synergism in reference to drug interaction. See Synergism.

POTENTIOMETER: A variable resistor in electronic circuits with resistance changes from zero up to its rated resistance in ohms, depending on the position of a moving contact. It is also an instrument for measuring voltage.

POTTS SHUNT: A side-to-side anastomosis of the descending thoracic aorta and the left pulmonary artery. It is performed as a palliative surgical procedure to help patients with reduced pulmonary blood flow, e.g., congenital pulmonary artery stenosis. It has been largely replaced by the Blalock-Taussig shunt because of the difficulty in controlling the blood flow through the anastamosis.

POYNTING EFFECT: The ability of N_2O and O_2 in a premixed cylinder to exist as a single-phase gas at a pressure below 2000 psi at room temperature. This effect is due to the solvent action of O_2.

PRACTOLOL (ERALDIN): A beta-adrenergic blocking agent said to have a predilection for beta sites in the myocardium. It has been used to treat hypertension but produces toxic side effects after long-term use. It is not presently available for use in the United States.

PRALIDOXIME (PROTOPAM; 2-PAM): The specific drug used to treat organophosphate poisoning. It reactivates cholinesterase by causing its release from the organophosphate to which it has been bound. Without 2-PAM, nonspecific cholinesterase is regenerated by the liver in about 2 weeks whereas acetylcholinesterase may take up to 3 months to be regenerated. See Organophosphorus compounds.

PREAMPLIFIER: An amplifier used to provide moderate amplification of an incoming signal before it reaches the main amplifier. Using one amplifier to power another allows for a better signal-to-noise ratio; by placing the preamplifier close to the signal source, the initial signal is amplified before noise from transmission lines can occur.

PREANESTHETIC VISIT (PREOPERATIVE EVALUATION): The introduction of the anesthetist to the patient prior to surgery. Aside from any social purpose which the preoperative visit may accomplish, it allows the patient to see and identify the individual who will have a profound effect upon his or her immediate future. This alone often allays patient anxiety. The preoperative visit also allows the anesthetist to evaluate the patient's medical history and review pertinent operative and hospital records. A physical examination can be done as required and subtle clues, such as respiratory rate, skin color, motor coordination, and emotional level, can be ascertained. The preoperative visit is always a good idea and is the only way that the anesthetist can obtain informed, intelligent consent to anesthetic procedures.

PRECISION VAPORIZER: See Vaporizer.

PREDNISOLONE (DELTA-CORTEF; METICORTELONE): A glucocorticoid with a higher anti-inflammatory potency than cortisol. Prednisolone has a slightly lower tendency than cortisol to cause sodium retention. See Corticosteroid.

PREDNISONE (METICORTEN; DELTASONE): A glucocorticoid with a higher anti-inflammatory potency than cortisol. It also has less tendency than cortisol to cause sodium retention. See Corticosteroid.

PREECLAMPSIA: A toxemia of unknown etiology occurring in late pregnancy and characterized by generalized hypertension, edema, and the appearance of albumin in the urine. When these phenomena are accompanied by seizure activity, the patient is considered to be eclamptic. Preeclampsia and eclampsia are obstetric emergencies; patients manifesting these symptoms are considered increased anesthetic risks.

PREEJECTION PERIOD (PEP): The time interval between the onset of ventricular depolarization (QS_2) and the onset of left ventricular ejection time (LVET) on the electrocardiogram. The PEP is used as a qualitative estimate of left ventricular performance. See Systolic time intervals.

PREMEDICATION: The concept that appropriate administration of drugs will facilitate anesthetic induction. In many ways it is an idea which grew up with and was made mandatory by the use of diethyl ether as an anesthetic, since one of diethyl ether's outstanding characteristics is irritation to the respiratory tree on inhalation. The initial purpose of premedication was to prevent the outpouring of secretions in the respiratory tree which could precipitate respiratory obstruction. Therefore, atropine and scopolamine, which decrease salivation and other secretions, were important in early premedicant regimens. In addition, because of the irritation, diethyl ether anesthetic inductions were often stormy. This led to the use of sedative drugs to allay anxiety and make the perioperative experience smoother. With the use of intravenous induction agents and the more modern, less irritating halogenated hydrocarbon general anesthetics, the absolute requirement for premedication and, in particular, the antisecretory drugs has diminished, but ritualistic dousing of patients with premedication has continued to be a part of anesthetic practice and appears to have a firm hold into the future. See Atropine, Basal anesthesia, Preanesthetic visit.

PREOPERATIVE EVALUATION: See Preanesthetic visit.

PREOXYGENATION: See Denitrogenation.

PRESERVATIVE: A chemical additive which prevents decomposition and growth and multiplication of microorganisms. Benzoic acid (0.1%) is a common pharmacologic preservative as are its parahydroxy variations, such as methylparaben, ethylparaben, propylparaben, and butylparaben (all used in concentrations from 0.1 to 0.3%).

All preservatives are justifiably considered to have a low systemic toxicity but allergies to preservatives are encountered in medical practice. Preparations without preservatives are available, although these have a very short shelf-life once exposed to room air. They are used in those circumstances in which any irritation or toxicity must be avoided, such as spinal anesthesia or intravenous therapy for cardiac arrhythmias.

PRESSORECEPTOR: See Baroreceptor.

PRESSURE (P): The force exerted per unit area in any direction from any point. In a liquid the pressure varies with the depth. While the standard international (SI) unit of pressure is the pascal, pressure can also be measured in millibars, millimeters of mercury (mmHg), atmospheres, centimeters of water (cm H_2O), or pounds per square inch (psi).

PRESSURE EFFECT: See Pumping effect; pressure effect.

PRESSURE-EQUALIZING VALVE: A combination valve which can be set to act either as a low-pressure relief valve or as a safety feature to prevent a pressure buildup in the system. This function is dependent on the position of the toggle handle which controls an internal valve disc in the valve body.

PRESSURE HEAD: The height of a column of liquid necessary to exert a specific pressure.

PRESSURE-LIMITED VENTILATOR: See Ventilator.

PRESSURE-REDUCING VALVE; PRESSURE REGULATOR: A device which converts the high, variable pressure within a gas cylinder to a lower, more constant gas pressure. For example, a standard O_2 regulator reduces the input pressure of a full tank of O_2 at 2200 psi to an output pressure of approximately 50 psi.

PRESSURE REVERSAL OF ANESTHESIA: See Anesthesia, pressure reversal of.

PRILOCAINE (CITANEST): An amide-type local anesthetic which undergoes rapid biotransformation in the liver and kidney. See Local anesthetic.

PRIMARY ATELECTASIS: See Atelectasis.

PRIMARY FIBRINOLYSIS: A rare disorder in which the fibrinolytic system is inappropriately activated without the prior existence of large-scale clotting. The clinical picture resembles disseminated intravascular coagulation (DIC). The differential diagnosis is often made by a platelet count, a normal count ruling out DIC. The clinical course is complicated by the fact that severe primary fibrinolysis can drop the platelet count as fibrin degradation products tend to clump platelets. Secondary fibrinolysis is an appropriate response to DIC as it is an attempt by the body to compensate for inappropriate clotting. E-Aminocaproic acid (EACA) blocks the fibrinolytic system and is a specific treatment for primary fibrinolysis but can cause a disaster in secondary fibrinolysis because the clotting mechanism of the underlying DIC is unchecked. Since primary fibrinolysis usually does not cause massive bleeding and is quite rare, EACA should not be empirically administered for emergency treatment of hemorrhage. See Blood coagulation, Disseminated intravascular coagulation.

PRIMARY WINDING: See Transformer.

PRINTER: A device using characters which reproduces copy interpretable by a human user. Subcategories are determined by the manner in which the printer converts encoded signals into characters, e.g., electrostatic, type face, heat, etc.

PRISCOLINE: See Tolazoline hydrochloride.

PRIVILEGED COMMUNICATION: The right of the patient, in a medicolegal context, to expect that the physician will not divulge any personal information concerning the patient to the public. It forms part of the physician-patient relationship. The extent to which the doctrine of privileged communication applies depends on state law.

PROBABILITY: The likelihood that a stated result will occur. Probability is expressed as a number between 0 and 1. If the result cannot occur, its probability is 0. If it must occur, then it is a certainty and its probability is 1.

PROCAINAMIDE (PRONESTYL): An effective, quinidine-like antiarrhythmic agent that is pharmacologically similar to procaine. The drug decreases cardiac automaticity. It retards electric conduction in the atrium and ventricle and enhances atrioventricular (AV) block. Effective against a wide range of arrhythmias, procainamide can cause, on rapid intravenous injection, a precipitous drop in blood pressure. The drug can be administered intravenously, intramuscularly, or orally.

PROCAINE HYDROCHLORIDE (NOVOCAIN): The first successful local anesthetic to be synthesized (by Einhorn in 1905). It is an ester-type drug. It is the standard measure of relative potency for other local anesthetic agents. See Local anesthetic.

PROGRAM, COMPUTER: The sequence of instructions by which a computer manipulates the data which it receives. Programs can range from simple and direct, e.g., hand-held calculators, to thoroughly complex so that it is necessary to use a small computer to program a larger computer.

PROLAPSE: The falling down or sinking of a part or an organ. For example, in the multiparous patient weakening of the pelvic floor can lead to uterine prolapse, a condition in which the uterus appears outside the lower abdominal cavity.

PROMETHAZINE HYDROCHLORIDE (PHENERGAN): A phenothiazine derivative that, in addition to being a potent antihistamine and sedative, can be used as a mild tranquilizer and hypnotic. While its mechanism of action is unknown, promethazine clearly enhances the actions of drugs which depress the central nervous system. See Antipsychotic agent.

PRONESTYL: See Procainamide.

PROPANIDID (EPONTOL): A eugenol (oil of cloves) derivative used in Europe as an intravenous anesthetic, but not available in the United States. As fast-acting as thiopental, electroencephalogram changes seen with its use are similar to those of barbiturates. Excitatory muscle movements in patients receiving propanidid appear to be dose-related. Hypersensitivity reactions to the drug have been reported. Propanidid increases apnea caused by succinylcholine transiently decreasing serum pseudocholinesterase levels. (Pseudocholinesterase breaks down nearly all the injected propanidid.)

PROPOXYPHENE (DARVON): A close chemical derivative of the narcotic methadone. Although no longer considered as potent as codeine, it is known to be an abused drug. Overdose resembles narcotic poisoning and is treated with narcotic antagonists. Abrupt termination of drug administration (following chronic ingestion of high doses) may produce withdrawal symptoms.

PROPRANOLOL (INDERAL): A competitive antagonist of catecholamines at beta receptors throughout the body. It precipitates bronchoconstriction, can have a negative chronotropic effect, and can decrease the strength of cardiac contractions. Currently, it is used to treat arrhythmias, hypertension, angina, thyrotoxicosis, pheochromocytoma, and some intrinsic cardiac diseases. In high concentrations, it attenuates the fight-or-flight reaction. It was originally believed to be quite dangerous to anesthetize patients taking propranolol. Recently, however, it has been shown that, at least in cases in which it is given for legitimate hypertensive disease and/ or angina, withdrawal of the drug can cause a precipitous crisis of the original condition.

PROPRIETARY PHARMACEUTICAL: A drug or chemical which is exclusively or privately owned, usually by patent.

PROPYLPARABEN: See Preservative.

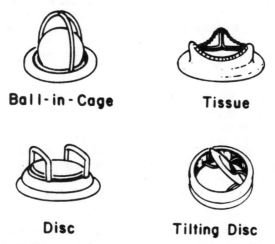

Prosthetic Heart Valves: Common types of valve prostheses.

PROSTHETIC HEART VALVE: A device which can be surgically implanted to replace a diseased heart valve, particularly aortic or mitral valves. They are available in various designs and with continued refinement have become functionally more efficient as replacements for stenosed (narrowed) or regurgitant (permitting backflow) valves. See Fig.

PROSTIGMIN: See Neostigmine.

PROTAMINE SULFATE: A naturally occurring (found in certain fish sperm) low molecular weight protein used to block and reverse the anticoagulant action of heparin. Protamine is used clinically to antagonize heparin after extracorporeal circulation. Rapid intravenous injection may cause direct peripheral dilatation, cardiac depression, and severe hypotension. See Anticoagulant, Heparin.

PROTEIN HYDROLYSATE: See Amigen.

PROTHROMBIN TIME, ONE-STAGE PROTHROMBIN TIME (PT): A test of the clotting mechanism which determines the relative intactness of the extrinsic clotting system. The measurement is of the time necessary for recalcified citrated plasma to clot in the presence of tissue thromboplastin. See Blood coagulation, Extrinsic pathway, Intrinsic pathway.

PROTON: A positively charged elementary particle which is a constituent of all nuclei and forms the nucleus of the hydrogen atom. It is approximately 1836 times heavier than the electron.

PROTOPAM: See Pralidoxime.

PROXIMATE CAUSE: An action which immediately precedes and gives rise to an effect. For example, in the case of a patient death due to drug allergy, the actual injection, rather than the preparation of the injection itself, would be the proximate cause of death.

PRUNE-BELLY SYNDROME: A congenital syndrome characterized by a protruding abdomen with wrinkled, thin skin. This appearance is due to the absence of the lower portion of the rectus abdominis and the medial parts of the oblique muscles. Usually, along with this defect, the bladder and ureters are dilated and the kidneys are small, dysplastic, and hydronephrotic. In males, the testes are undescended.

PSEUDOCHOLINESTERASE: See Acetylcholinesterase, Dibucaine number, Succinylcholine.

PSYCHOGENIC: Having an origin in the mind. Psychogenic pain, for example, refers to pain which, due to the absence of a satisfactory organic cause, is considered of psychologic or emotional origin.

PSYCHOTROPIC (PSYCHOACTIVE) DRUG: A pharmacologic agent used in the treatment of psychiatric disorders. Examples of psychotropic drugs are antipsychotics (phenothiazines, thioxanthenes, butyrophenones), antidepressants, antianxiety-sedatives (benzodiazepines), and mood stabilizers. See Antipsychotic agents, Benzodiazepine.

PULMONARY ALVEOLAR PROTEINOSIS: A chronic lung disease of unknown etiology. Clinical manifestations of the disease range from asymptomatic involvement to total disability or death from respiratory insufficiency, secondary infection (e.g., Nocardia), or cor pulmonale. Pulmonary alveolar proteinosis is characterized pathologically by alveoli which are filled with periodic acid-Schiff-positive dense granular material (a lipoprotein). Bronchopulmonary lavage is an effective treatment for patients with significant symptoms. See Pulmonary lavage.

PULMONARY ARTERY BANDING: An operation performed to correct excessive pulmonary blood flow, as in the congenital disorder of common ventricle. A band is tightened around the external circumference of the pulmonary artery, thereby increasing pulmonary outflow resistance.

PULMONARY ARTERY CATHETER: See Swan-Ganz catheter.

PULMONARY BLOOD VESSELS: The vessels, i.e., arteries, arterioles, capillaries, veins, and venules, which transport blood through the pulmonary circulation, starting at the pulmonary artery outflow and returning via the pulmonary veins to the left atria.

PULMONARY CAPILLARIES: The minute blood vessels connecting the pulmonary metarterioles and venules. The pulmonary capillaries actually form a continuous network of blood (flowing sheet) in the alveolar wall. This network constitutes an effective arrangement for pulmonary gas exchange.

PULMONARY CAPILLARY TRANSIT TIME: The length of time it takes (usually less than 1 sec with normal cardiac output) for blood to traverse the pulmonary capillaries. A single red blood cell traverses two or three alveoli in this time period. Oxygen equilibration is essentially complete in approximately 0.3 sec. Carbon dioxide equilibrium is even faster.

PULMONARY CAPILLARY WEDGE PRESSURE (PCWP): The pressure distal to the inflated balloon tip of a Swan-Ganz catheter. This reading approximates left atrial pressure. See Swan-Ganz catheter.

PULMONARY EDEMA: The presence of excessive amounts of fluid in the interstitial spaces of the lung or in the alveoli. Pulmonary edema is usually the result of left-sided heart failure, which tends to increase pulmonary capillary pressure to such a degree that the interstitial spaces are overloaded. Pulmonary edema may also be due to destruction of the capillary membranes by noxious vapors or can be caused by aspiration pneumonitis. Severe pulmonary edema of the alveoli often leads to death by suffocation. See Congestive heart failure.

PULMONARY FUNCTION TESTS (PFT): A combination of clinical and laboratory tests designed to assess the patient's ability to perform the functions of ventilation, i.e., arterialize venous blood. PFTs also establish the norms of the various lung volumes for a particular patient and his or her ability to move air at maximal rates. In their simplest form, PFTs consist of the measurement of vital capacity and arterial blood gases. At a more sophisticated level, the next test usually performed is the measurement of forced expiratory volume (FEV) in 0.5 sec ($FEV_{0.5}$) or 1 sec (FEV_1). The results from a particular patient can be compared with standards for age, sex, and body size. It must be kept in mind, however, that normal problems with the apparatus, such as maintenance of an air-tight seal at the machine-patient interface, as well as patient motivation, are critical factors in obtaining an accurate, repeatable result. See Forced expiratory volume, Maximum voluntary ventilation, Vital capacity.

PULMONARY HYPERTENSION: A morbid condition said to be present when the systolic pressure in the pulmonary artery rises above 30 mmHg. This rise can be due to an increase in pulmonary-vascular resistance or to blood backup behind a failing left side of the heart.

PULMONARY LAVAGE: The therapeutic "washing out" or irrigating of the air passages of a lung performed with general anesthesia via a double-lumen tube. A hazardous procedure usually employed as a specific treatment for pulmonary alveolar proteinosis, it is performed on one lung at a time with a recovery period between procedures. Recovery is complicated by the fact that surfactant is also "washed out," making reinflation of the washed lung difficult. See Double-lumen tube, Pulmonary alveolar proteinosis.

PULMONARY PERFUSION, ZONES OF: A model for the way in which blood flow from the right side of the heart perfuses the lung. In this model, the lung is divided into three zones. The superior zone is that area in which alveolar gas pressure is higher than pulmonary artery pressure (due to gravitational forces). In this abnor-

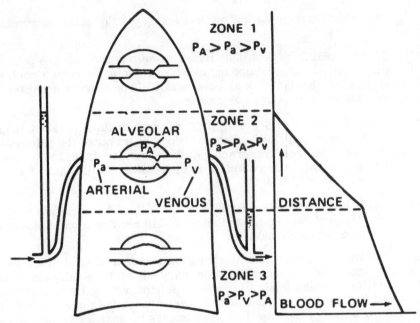

Pulmonary Perfusion, Zones of: Supposed behavior of the small vessels in various parts of the lung which cause regional differences in the blood flow. The lung is shown in a vertical position.

mal state the alveolar capillaries are so constricted that blood flow is prevented. This gives rise, therefore, to a portion of the lung which is ventilated but not perfused (alveolar dead space). In zone 2, further down in the lung, pulmonary arterial pressure rises and exceeds alveolar pressure. In this zone, flow is determined by the difference between arterial and alveolar pressures rather than arterial and venous pressures. Flow occurs when arterial pressure becomes higher than alveolar pressure for part of the cardiac cycle and ceases as systolic pressure wanes toward diastolic pressure. The effect seen in zone 2 is called a Starling resistor, sluice, or waterfall effect. In zone 3, still further down the lung, not only is pulmonary arterial pressure higher than alveolar pressure, but venous pressure is now high enough for flow to be determined in the normal manner, i.e., the difference between arterial and venous pressures. There are no sharp distinctions between zones; they are dependent on the patient's body position. See Fig. See Ventilation/perfusion abnormality.

PULMONARY PHYSIOLOGY SYMBOLS: See Fig.

PULMONARY STENOSIS: A narrowing in the pulmonary vasculature which causes raised right ventricular pressure.

PULMONARY VASCULAR RESISTANCE: The resistance to blood flow from the right ventricle. This can be calculated given the fact that the pulmonary vasculature carries the same volume of blood as the systemic vasculature over time (conveniently calculated at 1 min). Under normal circumstances the pulmonary pressure drop from the pulmonary artery to the left atrium is only 1/8 to 1/10 that of the pressure drop in the systemic circulation. Pulmonary vascular resistance is therefore 1/8 to 1/10 the systemic vascular resistance.

PULSE: The physical manifestation of the blood pressure as it waxes and wanes in a palpable artery. The pulse can be counted to determine the number of heartbeats

SPECIAL SYMBOLS

— Dash above any symbol indicates a *mean value*.

. Dot above any symbol indicates *a time derivative*.

FOR GASES

PRIMARY SYMBOLS (Large Capital Letters)	EXAMPLES
V = gas volume	V_A = volume of alveolar gas
V̇ = gas volume/unit time	$\dot{V}_{O_2}$ = O_2 consumption/min
P = gas pressure	P_{AO_2} = alveolar O_2 pressure
P̄ = mean gas pressure	$\bar{P}_{CO_2}$ = mean capillary O_2 pressure
F = fractional concentration in dry gas phase	F_{IO_2} = fractional concentration of O_2 in inspired gas
f = respiratory frequency (breaths/unit time)	
D = diffusing capacity	D_{O_2} = diffusing capacity for O_2 (ml O_2/min/mm Hg)
R = respiratory exchange ratio	R = $\dot{V}_{CO_2}/\dot{V}_{O_2}$

SECONDARY SYMBOLS (small capital letters)	EXAMPLES
I = inspired gas	F_{ICO_2} = fractional concentration of CO_2 in inspired gas
E = expired gas	V_E = volume of expired gas
A = alveolar gas	$\dot{V}_A$ = alveolar ventilation/min
T = tidal gas	V_T = tidal volume
D = dead space gas	V_D = volume of dead space gas
B = barometric	P_B = barometric pressure
STPD = 0°C, 760 mm Hg, dry	
BTPS = body temperature and pressure saturated with water vapor	
ATPS = ambient temperature and pressure saturated with water vapor	

FOR BLOOD

PRIMARY SYMBOLS (Large Capital Letters)	EXAMPLES
Q = volume of blood	Q_c = volume of blood in pulmonary capillaries
Q̇ = volume flow of blood/unit time	$\dot{Q}_c$ = blood flow through pulmonary capillaries/min
C = concentration of gas in blood phase	C_{aO_2} = ml O_2 in 100 ml arterial blood
S = % saturation of Hb with O_2 or CO	$S_{\bar{v}O_2}$ = saturation of Hb with O_2 in mixed venous blood

SECONDARY SYMBOLS (small letters)	EXAMPLES
a = arterial blood	P_{aCO_2} = partial pressure of CO_2 in arterial blood
v = venous blood	$P_{\bar{v}O_2}$ = partial pressure of O_2 in mixed venous blood
c = capillary blood	P_{cCO} = partial pressure of CO in pulmonary capillary blood

FOR LUNG VOLUMES

VC = Vital Capacity	= maximal volume that can be expired after maximal inspiration
IC = Inspiratory Capacity	= maximal volume that can be inspired from resting expiratory level
IRV = Inspiratory Reserve Volume	= maximal volume that can be inspired from end-tidal inspiration
ERV = Expiratory Reserve Volume	= maximal volume that can be expired from resting expiratory level
FRC = Functional Residual Capacity	= volume of gas in lungs at resting expiratory level
RV = Residual Volume	= volume of gas in lungs at end of maximal expiration
TLC = Total Lung Capacity	= volume of gas in lungs at end of maximal inspiration

Pulmonary Physiology Symbols: Symbols and abbreviations used by pulmonary physiologists.

per minute. In electronics a pulse is considered to be a discrete, transient phenomenon of short duration.

PULSE PRESSURE: The difference between diastolic and systolic pressure extremes in the arterial circulation. If the blood pressure is recorded as 120/80, the pulse pressure would be 40 torr.

PULSE PRESSURE TRACING: The oscillographic or paper representation of the pulse pressure contours as recorded with the Y axis representing pressure and the X axis representing time. The shape of the generated tracing changes with the location at which it is transduced (aortic arch, peripheral artery), the force of cardiac contraction, and the peripheral vascular resistance. A qualitative interference of myocardial function can be derived from the changing shape of this tracing.

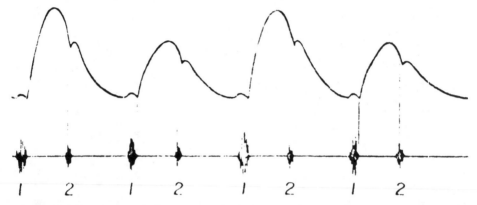

Pulsus Alternans: A diagrammatic representation of the carotid artery pressure and heart sound tracings in pulsus alternans. The cardiac rhythm is regular but the strength of the ventricular beat alternates between strong and weak.

PULSUS ALTERNANS (ALTERNATING PULSE): A pulse in which a weak beat alternates with a strong beat. It is most often found in conjunction with left ventricular failure. A failing ventricle changes its strength of contraction with minor changes in left ventricular muscle fiber length. See Fig.

PUMPING EFFECT; PRESSURE EFFECT: Two effects reported with the variable bypass vaporizer (precision vaporizers, agent-specific vaporizers) in which back pressure to the vaporizer changes the anesthetic output delivered. The pumping effect is seen when the vaporizer output is increased, whereas the pressure effect is seen when the vaporizer output is decreased. Three factors influence which effect predominates: the magnitude of the back pressure fluctuations, the amount of flow of the vaporizer, and the vaporizer dial setting. Design changes in vaporizers produced over the last 5 or 6 years have eliminated, or significantly attenuated, these variations in vaporizer output. The simplest modification for preventing the pressure and pumping effects is to place a backflow check device between the vaporizer and the patient circuit. See Figs.

PUMP LUNG: A ventilatory dysfunction seen in patients following cardiopulmonary bypass machine usage. It appears to be caused by a group of unrelated factors including massive blood transfusion, concomitant infection, and altered hemodynamics following bypass. Pump lung is characterized by diffuse pneumonitis and/or pulmonary edema. Its severity is related to the following factors: total time the patient remains on extracorporeal circulation, total blood loss, and total blood replacement See Cardiopulmonary bypass.

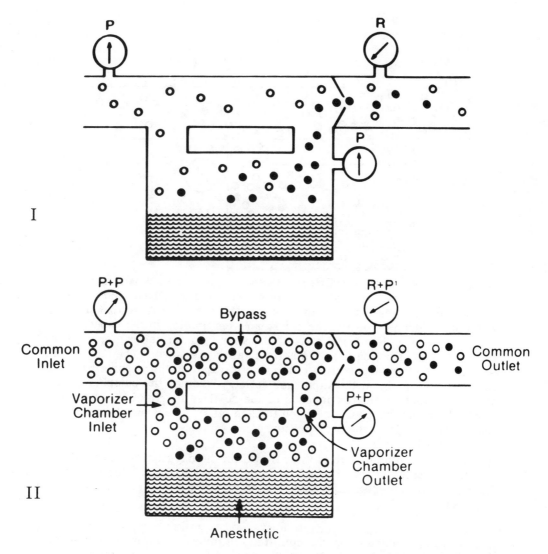

Pumping Effect; Pressure Effect: (I) Vaporizer is shown with gas freely exiting to the atmosphere. P, pressure in the vaporizing chamber and
in the bypass; R, gas pressure at the outlet. The number of molecules
of anesthetic agent which joins the outflow is solely dependent on the
vapor pressure of the liquid which in turn is dependent on the temperature. This is not affected by the alterations in atmospheric pressure.
Pumping effect: (II) The backflow of anesthetic-laden gas fills the bypass as well as the vaporizing chamber. Since the final output of the
vaporizer depends on dilution from the bypass, the total output of the
vaporizer will have increased as this dilution no longer takes place.

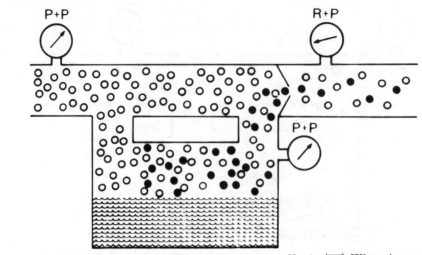

III

Pumping Effect; Pressure Effect: Pressure effect: (III) When increased pressure (P^1) flows into the vaporizer from the downstream side (due to back pressure), the increase compresses the carrier gas so that there are more molecules of carrier per square centimeter in the vaporizer. The number of molecules of anesthetic vapor remains the same, however, as there is no effect on the anesthetic's vapor pressure. The net outcome is a decrease in concentration of anesthetic vapor in the vaporizing chamber and, therefore, at the vaporizer outlet. Whether the pumping or pressure effect dominates depends on the relative length of the passageways, their resistances in relation to each other, backflow check valves, and the magnitude of the back pressure.

PUMP PRIME: The volume of fluid initially within the oxygenator and fluid circuits of a heart-lung machine at the start of cardiopulmonary bypass. Pump primes are often whole blood but other solutions are becoming more popular. See Cardiopulmonary bypass.

PUNITIVE DAMAGES: The compensation awarded to an injured party in order to punish the individual judged to have committed the injury. Compensatory damages recompense for the injury itself. See Damages.

PURE CUT: See Cutting current.

PURKINJE FIBERS: See Heart, conduction system of.

PYLORIC STENOSIS: A severe congenital anomaly which occurs once in every 300-900 live births with a 4:1 male predominance. The pathophysiology of the disease is that the pylorus, or outlet of the stomach, becomes progressively more hypertrophic and obstructive. The condition appears to be self-limiting and if nutritional support can be maintained long enough it disappears without surgical intervention. If nutritional support cannot be maintained, however, the operation of choice is called a pyloromyotomy. An anesthetic consideration for this procedure is patient dehydration due to the prolonged vomiting. Also, full stomach precautions are necessary.

PYREXIA: See Hyperpyrexia.

PYRIDOSTIGMINE (MESTINON): An anticholinesterase agent closely related to neostigmine but with fewer side effects. It is used for the treatment of myasthenia gravis and as a reversal agent for neuromuscular blockade. See Neuromuscular blockade, assessment of.

PYROMETER: An instrument for measuring high temperatures.

QRS COMPLEX: The electrocardiogram representation of the electric impulses through the ventricles. A Q wave is the first negative (downward) deflection. An R wave is the first upward deflection whether or not it is preceded by a Q wave. An S wave is a negative deflection following an R wave. See Electrocardiogram.

QUATERNARY AMMONIUM COMPOUND: A molecule containing a nitrogen atom which is bonded to four other atoms. In the charged quarternary binding, the nitrogen atom is relatively deficient in electrons and therefore behaves as if it is positively charged. These compounds are relatively incapable of passing through biologic membranes which reject charged molecules. Neostigmine is a quarternary ammonium compound which does not readily cross the blood-brain barrier. See Hofmann elimination.

QUECKENSTEDT SIGN: A test for intact cerebrospinal fluid (CSF) pathways in the central nervous system. It is based on the fact that unilateral or bilateral compression of the internal jugular vein(s) in the neck causes a rise in cerebral venous pressure and an increase in cerebral blood volume. This leads to a rise in intracranial and CSF pressures. This elevation of pressure decreases on release of the compression on the neck. No CSF pressure rise indicates a blockage of the path of egress of the CSF (the Queckenstedt sign is positive). This blockage may be due to tumor, blood clot, or cord transection. The test is very dangerous in cases of raised intracranial pressure as it can precipitate cerebral herniation. See Cerebrospinal fluid.

QUICK CONNECTOR: A device which allows a rapid, often one-handed connection between a gas line and a wall receptacle.

QUINIDINE: An isomer of quinine used for its antifibrillatory and antiarrhythmic effects on cardiac musculature. It decreases automaticity and conduction velocity in the heart. Quinidine depresses all muscle tissue. If administered to a patient with myasthenia gravis, it produces extreme weakness. It is given either orally or intramuscularly. As with many antiarrhythmic drugs, toxic effects include arrhythmias; these effects may be additive to other antiarrhythmic drugs being given.

RAD: An acronym for Radiation Absorbed Dose. It is the unit of absorbed dose of ionizing radiation. One rad is equal in energy to 100 ergs/g of irradiated material and is approximately equal to the energy absorbed by soft tissue when it is exposed to 1 R (roentgen) of medium voltage x-rays. Total body irradiation with as little as 50-100 rads can cause injury. See Roentgen-equivalent-man.

RADFORD NOMOGRAM: See Nomogram.

RADIOACTIVITY: A spontaneous change in the nucleus of certain atoms resulting in the formation of an element with different chemical properties. This change also results in a change of the element's atomic number when accompanied by emission of either alpha or beta particles. The atomic number does not change when only a gamma ray is emitted, but the nucleus drops to a lower energy state. For any given number of molecules of a radioactive element, half of these molecules will decay in a period of time that is constant and characteristic of that element (half-life) ranging from millionths of a second to thousands of years.

RADIOFREQUENCY (RF) CHOKE: A small electric component consisting of a tuned coil which offers extremely high resistance to frequencies in the radio band of the electromagnetic spectrum. In medical equipment the purpose of the RF choke is to prevent RF energy from following pathways which can lead to patient injury. The RF chokes are often used in the inputs of electrocardiograph (ECG) machines to prevent electrosurgical instruments from establishing an energy return path using the ECG leads.

RADIOSENSITIVITY: The relative destructibility of a tissue exposed to ionizing radiation. A concept used both in treating neoplastic disease and in calculating the exposure limits of those individuals who must work around sources of radiation.

RADIOTHERAPY: The utilization of ionizing radiation including gamma rays, electron beams, and x-rays to treat disease.

RANDOM ACCESS: A specific type of memory device that allows immediate access to a piece of information without having to review all the data contained in the memory. Each piece of information has a particular address or physical location in the memory.

RANDOM NUMBERS: A list of numbers in which one particular number has no discernible relationship to any other number in the list. The concept of random numbers has its greatest usefulness in statistics.

RANGE, STATISTICAL: The difference between the largest and smallest numbers in a set. With the following set of serum potassium values, 3.5, 4.0, 4.5, 5.0, 5.5, 6.0, the range is 2.5.

RAPID EYE MOVEMENT (REM): See REM.

RAPID SEQUENCE INDUCTION: See Induction, Sellick maneuver.

RARE GASES: A collective name given to five elements: helium, neon, argon, krypton, and xenon. These gases are rare because they have very low partial pressures at ordinary temperatures and are found in minute quantities in the atmosphere. Under normal circumstances these gases are not bound chemically to any other element. They are also referred to as inert gases.

RASHKIND PROCEDURE: The deliberate creation of an atrial septal defect via the passing of a balloon-tipped catheter across the foramen ovale, inflating the baloon, and then forcibly withdrawing the catheter so as to rupture the atrial septum. It is a palliative procedure used in pediatric patients with congenital defects such as transposition of the great vessels, tricuspid or mitral valve atresia, hypoplastic right heart syndrome, or total anomalous pulmonary drainage.

RATE-PRESSURE PRODUCT (RPP): An index of cardiac O_2 consumption. It is obtained by multiplying the systolic blood pressure by the heart rate. A product of over 12,000 is considered a sign of possible ischemia in patients with coronary artery disease.

RATIO OF A TRANSFORMER: See Transformer.

RAUWOLFIA ALKALOID: The generalized name for preparations, e.g., reserpine, obtained from a climbing shrub indigenous to India. See Reserpine.

RAY: A moving photon or particle of ionizing radiation.

REACTIVE HYPEREMIA: See Tourniquet.

READILY RELEASABLE VERSUS DEPOT ACETYLCHOLINE: The two forms in which acetylcholine is believed to exist in a nerve terminal. The readily releasable fraction is immediately available for use as a transmitter, whereas the large depot store serves to replenish the readily releasable stock as required. The readily releasable portion appears to be contained in vesicles close to or attached to the portion of the nerve terminal membrane which borders the synaptic cleft. The depot store would be contained in vesicles further back. There appears to be some delay in the conversion of depot acetylcholine to readily releasable acetylcholine. The readily releasable fraction then becomes partially exhausted by frequently repeated action potentials as seen in tetanic nerve stimulation. This partial exhaustion appears to be responsible for the fade seen during tetanic stimulation when a nondepolarizing block exists. See Neuromuscular blockade, assessment of; Neuromuscular transmitter, quantal release of.

READ ONLY MEMORY (ROM): See Memory, computer.

READ/WRITE HEAD: An electromagnetic device which can sense (read) and/or change (write) magnetic fields on a magnetic recording disc or tape.

REAL-TIME ANALYSIS: An examination which takes place concurrently with the process being analyzed. The implication is that real-time analysis can be used to guide the process. For example, arterial CO_2 analysis using the Van Slyke-Cullen method takes many hours and is of no use for regulating respiration by ventilator. However, continuous arterial blood sampling via a mass spectrometer gives values second by second in real time.

REBREATHING BAG: See Breathing bag.

RECEPTOR OCCLUSION TECHNIQUE: A technique for determining the quality of neuromuscular blockade. This technique estimates the fraction of receptors blocked by a nondepolarizing relaxant. The procedure involves the administration of succinylcholine with graded doses of a nondepolarizing blocker such as d-tubocurarine or pancuronium starting from zero.

RECEPTOR/RECEPTOR SITE: A cellular phenomenon which allows a small quantity of drug or hormone to produce large changes in a tissue or organ. A receptor site is a specialized area on a cell's surface having a three-dimensional configuration and/or electric charge capable of interacting with specific substances to cause a change in the entire cell. Receptor sites allow for economy and efficiency by acting as tiny switches that control the function of the cell as a whole. An example of a receptor site is the specialized portion of a motor endplate which interacts with acetylcholine to trigger an action potential. Acetylcholine acts only at this special area, and does not affect the remainder of the cell. Receptors for the neurotransmitters released by the adrenergic (norepinephrine-releasing) fibers of the sympathetic nervous system have been extensively classified. Alpha receptors mediate vasoconstriction, mydriasis, and intestinal relaxation. $Beta_1$ receptors are responsible for cardiac stimulation and also lipolysis. $Beta_2$ receptors are involved with adrenergic bronchodilatation and vasorelaxation. Dopaminergic receptors seem to be present in only certain vascular networks. Dopamine produces vasoconstriction in the intracerebral, renal mesenteric, and coronary arteries. Cholinergic (acetylcholine-releasing) fibers interact with specific receptors to mediate the function of the parasympathetic nervous system. Neurons of the central nervous system have receptors for the enkephalins and endorphins and are stimulated by narcotics. Many hormones achieve their results by mating with a cell receptor. The combination of hormone and receptor causes the intracellular formation of a "second messenger" which then alters cytoplasmic function. Identified second messengers are cyclic 3',5'-adenosine monophosphate (cAMP) and cyclic 3',5'-guanosine monophosphate (cGMP). Within the context of the nervous system, a receptor is the specialized ending of a sensory nerve fiber which converts a stimulus into a nerve impulse. An example of this type of receptor is the stretch receptor or muscle spindle which responds to elongation of the muscle and informs the central nervous system continuously of the muscle's degree of contraction. Specific receptors also exist for such entities as pain and temperature sensation. See Fig.

RECIRCULATION CURVE: See Cardiac output.

RECORD: A documentation of an event or process on paper, tape, film, etc. For example, in operating room practice the anesthesia record is the real-time recording and, in fact, often the only evidence of the conduct of an anesthetic.

RECOVERY/RECOVERY ROOM: The time period between emergence from anesthesia and the stabilization of the patient's vital signs and state of consciousness. The patient typically spends this time in the postanesthetic recovery room (PAR),

Receptor/Receptor Site: Major systemic sites of receptors for adrenergic amines and their effects.

Effector Organ or Function	Receptor	Response	Comments
Cardiovascular system			
Heart rate	β_1	Increase	May be masked by vagal reflexes
Contractile force	β_1	Increase	
Coronary blood flow	β_1	Increase	Flow largely controlled by local factors
	α	Decrease	
Peripheral resistance	α	Increase	
	β_2	Decrease	
Pulmonary system			
Bronchial muscle	β_2	Relaxation	
Vasculature	α	Constriction	Redistribution to pulmonary circulation increases pressure
	β_2	Dilatation	
Gastrointestinal system			
Motility and tone	$\beta_1\ \alpha$	Decrease	Gastrointestinal effects depend on existing tone
Sphincters	α	Contraction	
Metabolism			
Insulin secretion	α	Decrease	
	β	Increase	
Glycogenolysis gluconeogenesis	β	Increase	
Lipolysis	β_1	Increase	
Salivary glands			
Secretion	$\alpha\ \beta_1$	Increase	
Vasculature	α	Constriction	

a way station between the intense monitoring of the anesthetic period and the more casual monitoring of the patient's ward. The PAR was not typical of operating technique until the 1940s. Prior to that time, the patient would have been transported directly from the operating room to the ward bed. Because recovery rooms are now the standard of practice, emergence from anesthesia blends into the recovery perior and postoperative patient safety is much improved.

RECTAL ANESTHESIA: The method of inducing anesthesia via the rectum. Dosage of the anesthetic agent is calculated according to the patient's weight. Rectal anesthesia is believed to provide a smoother, less psychologically traumatizing method of induction, particularly for children. However, speed of onset and total absorption are unpredictable. The method has become less popular since the introduction of the nonirritating inhalation anesthetics. Bromethol (Avertin, Tribromethanol) was a popular agent for this technique but became obsolete due to a tendency for liver and kidney damage.

RECTAL TEMPERATURE MEASUREMENT: A means of temperature measurement which is advantageous because the monitoring site (rectum) is usually undisturbed during surgery. A disadvantage of this method is that it is slow to reflect the actual core temperature.

RECTIFIER: A device found in electric circuitry that permits current to flow in only one direction. It can thus change alternating current (AC) into direct current (DC) since it suppresses or attenuates alternate half-cycles of the current waveform. In order to generate a steady DC, rectifiers must contain mirror image components, each of which operates on only half of the current cycle.

REDUNDANCY: The part of the total amount of information which can be eliminated without destroying the essential message. In a broader sense, it refers to the number and effectiveness of backup systems of a particular process.

REFERENCE ELECTRODE: An electrode with electric potential difference from a second electrode. This difference is constant due to the chemical makeup of the reference electrode. See Half-cell.

REFERENCE, EXTERNAL OR INTERNAL: A known or given value or quantity which is used to determine the accuracy of a particular piece of equipment. For example, in the calibration of a blood-gas analyzer, an external reference would be a fluid of known gas values fed into the machine to check the machine's performance. An internal reference is a known constant already "on board." Most modern scintillation counters contain a precisely known quantity of radioactive material which can be used to check the accuracy of the instrument at any time.

REFERRED PAIN: A general term for pain which is not localized at the site of its cause, but rather in an area which may be adjacent to or at some distance from this site. Usually the distribution of referred pain falls within the segmental distribution of the nerves which supply the afferent fibers. For example, the pain incurred due to air trapped under the diaphragm is often referred to the shoulder because the innervation of the diaphragm comes from the cervical area.

REFLECTION COEFFICIENT: See Staverman reflection coefficient.

REFLUX: See Esophageal reflux.

REFRACTORY: A term meaning highly resistant to therapy. Refractory also means the ability to withstand very high temperatures (at least 1580 degrees Celsius) without physical change. The most common and oldest refractory material is clay.

REFRACTORY PERIOD: The time when a membrane is relatively incapable of depolarization. During the shorter absolute refractory period no amount of stimulation will depolarize the membrane.

REFRIGERANT: A gas or liquid with an extremely low boiling point which is used to absorb heat in refrigerating machines. The most common refrigerants used today are from the group of fluorinated hydrocarbons called freons. See Fluorocarbon, Freon.

REGENERATIVE DEPOLARIZATION: A description of the effect of sodium pores on the nerve action potential. The sodium pores amplify or regenerate the action potential which would be attenuated because of continuous diffusion of ions away from the nerve through the conducting fluid which surrounds the nerve membrane. Sodium pores, however, increase the ionic current as the action potential passes them. Two other physiologic entities allow the action potential to travel a greater distance before requiring amplification. One is an increase in the diameter of the axon which reduces the internal resistance to current flow, and the other is the myelin sheath, which surrounds and insulates the axon, thereby reducing the loss of current through direct and capacitive leakage. See Action potential, Depolarization, Sodium channel.

REGISTER: A high-speed but usually temporary storage device where an intermediate value can be stored until called for by the master program of a computer. See Shift register.

REGITINE: See Phentolamine.

REGURGITATION: See Esophageal reflux.

RELAXANT: See Neuromuscular blocking agent.

RELAY: An electric device in which one current controls the switching on or off of an independent current. Relays, for example, isolate strong power currents from weak control currents.

RELIABILITY: An estimate of the trustworthiness of the output of a device. In reference to medical equipment, such as patient-monitoring instruments, reliability implies both repeatability under similar circumstances and the capability to tolerate gross malmanipulation by the maladroit.

REM: An acronym for Rapid Eye Movement. It is used to describe a stage of sleep during which dreaming is associated with muscle jerks and rapid eye movement.

REMAK FIBER: See Nerve fiber, anatomy and physiology of.

REMOTE ACCESS: The ability to receive or handle information at a distance from the place where it is generated or stored. A computer terminal on the ward that communicates with the main hospital computer which stores laboratory values is an example of remote access.

RENAL TOXICITY, ANESTHESIA: The deleterious effects of anesthesia on the kidney. With the exception of methoxyflurane (Penthrane), anesthetics in general do not damage the kidney. Decreased renal blood flow usually accompanies the anesthetic state, however, and this can exacerbate preexisting renal disease. See Methoxyflurane.

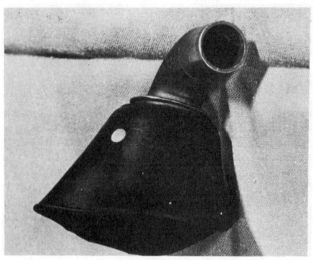

Rendell-Baker-Soucek Mask: Cuffless mask.

RENDELL-BAKER-SOUCEK MASK: A type of mask used in pediatric anesthesia and characterized by low dead space between the surface of the mask and the patient's face. See Fig.

RENIN: An enzyme manufactured in the kidney which activates an angiotensin precursor in the blood. Angiotensin, in turn, is an extremely potent vasoconstrictor which raises systemic blood pressure. See Angiotensin.

REPRODUCIBILITY: The ability of a piece of equipment to reliably reach the same determination when presented with the same specimen on multiple occasions. Reproducibility does not imply accuracy, as a piece of equipment can make the same mistake again and again if, for example, it is improperly calibrated. See Reliability.

RESERPINE (SERPASIL): A naturally occurring plant product of the climbing shrub Rauwolfia serpentina (hence the name rauwolfia alkaloid) used for thousands of years in Hindu medicine. Introduced to modern clinical medicine for its antipsychotic properties, it is currently used only as an antihypertensive agent. When reserpine is combined with a hypotensive anesthetic agent such as halothane, cardiovascular failure is a distinct possibility. Its greatest common drawback, however, appears to be related to its central nervous system actions causing depression, drowsiness, and lethargy.

RESERVOIR BAG: A rubber bag ranging in size from 500 ml to 5 L which is used in a patient breathing circuit to pressurize the circuit when squeezed and to buffer changes in gas concentrations.

RESIDUAL VOLUME (RV): The amount of gas remaining in the lung after maximal expiration. See Lung volumes and capacities.

RESIN: A group of substances originally obtained from tree gum. Resins have been used from earliest times for such things as pharmaceuticals, lacquers, varnishes, adhesives, inks, and building materials. Synthetic resins are a huge class of similar, usually polymerized, chemicals such as polyvinyl, polyethylene, polystyrene, and polyester that can be either thermoplastic or thermosetting.

RES IPSA LOQUITUR DOCTRINE: A legal doctrine, first delineated over a hundred years ago in England, stating "the thing speaks for itself." In malpractice cases, it means that the negative outcome of a particular doctor-patient relationship was so obviously caused by negligent behavior (as understood by the average individual) that no proof of negligence is required. An obvious case in which the doctrine of res ipsa loquitur could be applied is when a forceps is left in a patient after surgery.

RESISTANCE, AIRWAY: A measurement of the pressure differential necessary to move air from the nose and mouth to the alveoli. It is expressed in centimeters of water per liter per second. Airway resistance rises with obstruction. Measured by body plethysmograph, airway resistance is 0.05-1.5 cm H_2O/L/sec in adults. An indirect clinical evaluation of airway resistance is measurement of the timed vital capacity. See Pulmonary physiology symbols.

RESISTANCE, ELECTRIC: The ratio of the potential difference (voltage) across a conductor to the current flowing through the conductor. Resistance is measured in ohms. See Impedance, Ohm law.

RESISTANCE TO AIR IN LUNG: See Lung volumes and capacities.

RESISTANCE VESSELS: The vessels mainly comprising the arterioles which, by means of sympathetic stimulation, can change their lumen size and thereby alter the resistance offered to blood flow. In contrast to the resistance vessels are the capacitance vessels, which are composed of the medium and large veins and can, by means of sympathetic stimulation, change their cross-sectional dimensions to act as reservoirs for part of the circulating volume. They can therefore actively alter blood volume returned to the heart. See Central venous pressure.

RESISTANCE WIRE: A wire which is heated when an electric current is passed through it. Usually these wires are made of nickel and chromium and are not oxidized at high temperatures.

RESOLVING POWER: The ability of a microscope or telescope to separate two objects that are positioned close together.

RESPIRATION: The chemical and physical process by which either a single cell or an entire organism utilizes O_2 and disposes of CO_2. The terms respiration and respirators are often used interchangeably with the terms ventilation and ventilators. Strictly speaking, ventilation refers to the movement of gas in and out of the lungs. Therefore, it is appropriate to speak of cellular respiration but not of cellular ventilation.

RESPIRATORY ACIDOSIS: A rise in $PaCO_2$ above the normal range of 36-44 torr which does not compensate for metabolic alkalemia. Respiratory acidosis augments neuromuscular block by d-tubocurarine and limits and opposes reversal of the block by neostigmine.

RESPIRATORY ALKALOSIS: A fall in $PaCO_2$ below the normal range of 36-44 torr which does not compensate for metabolic acidemia.

RESPIRATORY CARE: The activities which, taken as a whole, aid in patient respiration, including such modalities as intermittent positive pressure breathing, humidification of inspired gases, and chest physiotherapy. Other techniques in respiratory care include incentive spirometry, in which the patient breathes from or into a device designed to demonstrate and encourage maximal effort. Respiratory care can also involve the administration of drugs by inhalation therapy, such as mucolytic agents which are designed to increase fluidity and decrease the viscosity of secretions. Examples of mucolytic agents include acetylcysteine (Mucomyst) and the pancreatic enzyme dornase (Dornavac). See Postural drainage.

RESPIRATORY DISTRESS SYNDROME (RDS): See Adult respiratory distress syndrome, Infant respiratory distress syndrome.

RESPIRATORY EFFORT: See Work of breathing.

RESPIRATORY EXCHANGE RATIO; RESPIRATORY QUOTIENT (RQ): The ratio of the minute production of CO_2 to the minute consumption of O_2. Both are determined by tissue metabolism and are normally measured in a steady state. In the 70-kg man at rest, 200 ml CO_2 is exhaled/min while 250 ml O_2 is consumed for an RQ of 0.8.

RESPIRATORY FAILURE: The inability of a patient to maintain appropriate lung ventilation to prevent hypoxia and/or hypercapnia without mechanical assistance. For practical purposes in acute situations, active intervention to assist respiration is done when the $PaCO_2$ rises above 50 torr and arterial oxygenation falls below 60 torr. This is called the partial pressure crossover point.

RESPIRATORY GAS EXCHANGE, ALTITUDE EFFECTS ON: The consequences of altitude changes on oxygenation. The barometric pressure of air decreases as the distance from the earth's surface increases. At 18,000 ft, the barometric pressure is approximately one-half the normal 760 mmHg. Among the body processes which adapt to high altitudes are (1) hyperventilation based on hypoxic stimulation of the peripheral chemoreceptors; (2) polycythemia, in which the hemoglobin concentration is increased by 3-5 g/100 ml; (3) a shift to the right of the O_2-hemoglobin dissociation curve; (4) and the increase in maximum breathing capacity when the air is less dense. See Oxygen-hemoglobin dissociation curve.

RESPIRATORY LOBULE: See Secondary lobule.

RESPIRATORY QUOTIENT: See Respiratory exchange ratio.

RESPIRATORY RATE: The number of complete respirations (inspirations and expirations) per minute.

RESPIRATORY RESISTANCE: See Forced expiratory volume.

RESPIRATORY SPARING EFFECT: See Tubocurarine chloride.

RESPIRATORY TREE: See Conducting airways.

RESPIRATORY ZONE: The zone of the lung beyond the connecting pathways which contains alveoli for gas exchange.

RESPIROMETER: See Spirometer.

RESPIROMETER, HOT WIRE: See Anemometer, hot wire.

RESTING MEMBRANE POTENTIAL: See Action potential.

RESUSCITATION: See Cardiopulmonary resuscitation.

RETRIEVAL, DATA: The ability to call back data by search, retransmission, or, in some cases, recreation from a file, data bank, or other storage unit.

RETROFIT: The ability to add new capabilities or modes of action to an already existing piece of equipment, usually implying that no major function is lost in the process. A digital display added to an electrocardiograph (ECG) machine so that it can simultaneously display pulse rates and ECG is an example of retrofit.

RETROLENTAL FIBROPLASIA (RLF): The formation of a fibrovascular membrane behind the lens of the eye, leading to blindness. It is almost exclusively confined to premature infants who have been exposed to high concentrations of O_2 and is one of the most feared outcomes of supportive O_2 therapy for these infants.

RETURN TO FLOW METHOD: A technique for determining the accuracy of blood pressure recorded from an arterial line. The technique involves inflating a blood pressure cuff above the point of entry of the arterial line until the trace is abolished, then slowly deflating the cuff until the beginning of the trace is just detected. This is systolic pressure and the cuff pressure can now be read to determine the calibration and accuracy of the arterial tracing.

REVELL CIRCULATION: See Circulator, Revell.

REVERBERATION: The persistence of sound (after its source has ceased) in a series of closely spaced echoes so that the listener perceives a continuous sound of diminishing intensity.

REVERSE POLISH NOTATION (RPN): A streamlined system for performing arithmetic operations by calculator, derived from the system developed by Polish mathematician Jan Lukasiewicz in 1949. In brief, the mathematic operation to be performed is entered into the machine after the numbers to be operated upon are entered.

REVERSIBLE INHIBITION: See Competitive antagonism.

REYE SYNDROME (ACUTE TOXIC ENCEPHALOPATHY): A recently identified disease which occurs in an extemely small number of patients following an otherwise uneventful respiratory or varicella (chickenpox) infection. The mortality rate of Reye syndrome is at least 15-20%. The disease is characterized by recurrent vomiting, stupor, and coma, with continually deepening depression terminating in death. The key to treatment of Reye syndrome appears to be monitoring for an acute elevation in intracranial pressure and then taking appropriate measures to reduce it. See Fig. See Cerebral blood flow.

Reye Syndrome: Signs, symptoms, and stages of severity of Reye syndrome. *

Stage 1:	1) vomiting, lethargy**, sleepiness 2) liver dysfunction 3) type I EEG
Stage 2:	1) disorientation** 2) delirium, combativeness 3) hyperventilation 4) hyperactive DTR's 5) type II EEG
Stage 3:	1) obtunded, coma** 2) decorticate rigidity**
Stage 4:	1) decerebrate rigidity** 2) loss of oculocephalic reflexes 3) large, fixed pupils 4) type III or IV EEG
Stage 5:	1) seizures, loss of DTR's 2) respiratory arrest** 3) flaccidity** 4) type IV or V EEG 5) hepatic function often normal

* Lovejoy, 1974
** Best clinical signposts delineating stage of encephalopathy.

REYNOLDS NUMBER: A measurement of the tendency for turbulence to occur in a vessel or container. The Reynolds number relates the change in fluid flow pattern from laminar to turbulent. This change is related to velocity, viscosity, and length and diameter of the conducting tube or vessel. See Critical velocity, Laminar flow, Poiseuille law, Turbulent flow.

Rh FACTOR: See Blood types.

RHEOLOGY: The branch of science which studies the deformation and flow of matter.

RHEOMACRODEX: See Dextran.

RHEOSTAT: A type of potentiometer used for large electric currents.

RHIZOTOMY: The technique of sectioning nerve roots for the treatment of intractable pain.

RIGHT, LEGAL: The legally enforceable expectation on the part of an individual owed a duty that the duty will be carried out. For example, if a patient enters into a contract with a physician for an operative procedure, the physician has a duty to perform the operation and the patient has a right to expect the physician to do so.

RMS VALUE: See Root mean square.

ROBERT SHAW TUBE: See Double-lumen tube.

ROBIN HOOD SYNDROME: See Intracerebral steal syndrome.

ROBINUL: See Glycopyrrolate.

ROCKING BOAT MOVEMENT: A paradoxic depression of the chest wall during inspiration coupled with a flaring of the lower chest margins and a bulging of the abdomen. This is seen when diaphragmatic action is unopposed by normal intercostal contraction. It can occur in upper airway obstruction, partial muscle paralysis, or deep general anesthesia.

ROENTGEN: The international unit of x-radiation/gamma radiation. The quantity of radiation which, when absorbed completely, produces in 1 cc dry air at 0 degrees Celsius and standard pressure ions carrying 2.58×10^{-4} coulomb of electric charge of either sign. See Rad, Roentgen-equivalent-man.

ROENTGEN-EQUIVALENT-MAN (rem): A unit of exposure to ionizing radiation which has the same biologic effectiveness as 1 rad of x-rays.

ROOT MEAN SQUARE (RMS VALUE; EFFECTIVE VALUE): The effective current or voltage is a function of the peak current or voltage divided by the square root of 2 in any situation where current or voltage alternates in magnitude. By convention, the root mean square value is used when speaking about supplied current or voltage. Therefore, when one speaks of a wall supply being 115 V, one is actually speaking of a wall voltage which peaks at approximately 145 V.

ROTAMETER: A common float used in flowmeter tubes which looks like a skirted, upside-down cone. The grooves cut in the skirt cause the rotameter to turn when it is freely suspended in the gas stream of a flowmeter tube. If the rotameter is suspended in the gas stream but not turning, it is an indication that it may be jammed in the flowmeter tube. The rotameter is read at the rim.

ROTATING DISC OXYGENATOR: A device for gas exchange used in the early years of extracorporeal circulation. Such a device consisted of a row of metal disks threaded on a common shaft which rotated in a cylinder half-filled with the patient's venous blood. The gas over the blood was O_2. This technique was relatively atraumatic to blood, but it did require gas and metal contact with the blood, therefore traumatizing it somewhat.

ROULEAU FORMATION: The arrangement of red blood cells piled one on top of another like a stack of coins. If present to any great extent in the circulation, it causes clogging and cessation of flow in the microcirculation. The red blood cells of patients with sickle cell disease are particularly prone to rouleau formation.

ROUTINE (SUBROUTINE): A circumscribed set of instructions that allows a machine to carry out a well-defined function. For example, in determining patient charges, a hospital computer in a cashier's office might have a routine or subroutine as part of its master program which would query the hospital's laboratory computer for laboratory charges to the particular account in question.

RUBBER/GAS COEFFICIENT: The concentration of a gaseous agent, particularly an anesthetic agent, in contact with rubber materials at equilibrium. Rubber gas coefficients range from 1.2 for N_2O to 120 for halothane, and to over 600 for methoxyflurane. Therefore, these rubber items are a significant source of gas cross contamination when they are used for more than one patient. See Partition coefficient.

RUBEN VALVE: See Nonrebreathing valve.

RULE OF NINES: A method of rapidly estimating the extent of body burns. According to this rule, the head and each arm are figured to have 9% of the body surface area. Each leg has 18%, as does the front and the back of the torso, respectively. The perineal area is credited with the remaining 1%.

S

SACRAL-EPIDURAL ANESTHESIA: See Caudal anesthesia.

SAFETY RELEASE DEVICE: The part of a gas cylinder valve designed to release the contents of the tank to the atmosphere when internal pressure conditions rise to explosive levels. The device consists of three operating segments: (1) frangible disc assembly (frangible disc and safety caps), which blocks the path to the outside atmosphere and bursts whenever a minimum pressure behind it is exceeded, (2) fusible plug, a low melting point alloy that occludes a discharge channel and melts at a predetermined temperature, and (3) safety relief valve, which contains a spring that holds the valve against a seat until the pressure within the tank exceeds that for which the spring is set. The valve then opens and gas escapes through the safety valve vents until the pressure is lowered causing the valve to close again. These three segments are often used in combination.

SALICYLATE: See Acetylsalicylic acid.

SALTATORY CONDUCTION: See Myelin sheath.

SALTING OUT EFFECT: The observation that increased electrolytes in the blood decrease the aqueous solubility of an anesthetic agent. This effect is normally outweighed by the increased solubility associated with elevation in protein and lipid components of the blood.

SANDERS JET (JET ANESTHESIA): A device used to ventilate patients during bronchoscopy. A jet injector is attached to the bronchoscope and a thin stream of high-pressure O_2 is delivered down the trachea alongside the bronchoscope. This high-pressure jet draws air down the trachea or through the lumen of the bronchoscope by the principle of entrainment. The jet is pulsed to initiate inspiration and then stopped so that passive expiration can take place. See Fig.

SA NODE: See Heart, conduction system of; Sinoatrial node.

SARCOMERE: See Actomyosin.

SATURATED VAPOR: See Vapor, saturated.

SCALER: A circuit which produces an output pulse when a specified number of input pulses have been received.

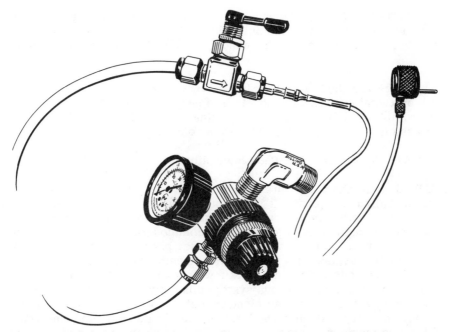

Sanders Injector: Sanders injector showing the pressure regulating
valve, triggering valve, and the gas jet which is aimed down the trachea.

SCANNING: A process by which a particular area is searched or explored in a me-
thodic manner to peruse or examine displayed or stored information. There are two
general types of scanning. In the first, a beam from a sensor, which could be made
up of particles such as electrons or waves from the electromagnetic spectrum,
sweeps across the area to be scanned. The other method of scanning has a receiver
tracking across a field or body in a preconceived pattern sensitive, for example, to
radiation emitted from various parts of the body. This technique is utilized in medicine for liver, spleen, and lung scans. Radioisotopes are administered to the patient and the detector then searches for alterations in density and concentration of
the radioisotope.

SCATTERING: The random deflection of electromagnetic energy. For example, an
x-ray beam is both absorbed and deflected (scattered) by shielding.

SCAVENGER SYSTEM: A device used to remove waste anesthetic gases from the
immediate operative environment. (Before the advent of scavengers, excess gases
were freely released into the operating room.) Waste gas is collected into a reservoir bag or tube and continuously exhausted into the centralized suction system of
the hospital. Paradoxically, this improvement in the operating room atmosphere
has lead to a deterioration of the atmosphere in and around the central suction
pumps.

SCIATIC NERVE BLOCK: The injection of a local anesthetic solution around the sciatic nerve for relief of chronic pain or as part of a series of nerve blocks prior to
surgery on the leg.

SCIATIC NERVE PALSY: A neuropathy of the sciatic nerve resulting from trauma
due to improper injection technique. It may be seen as an iatrogenic injury. See
Nerve palsy.

SCIENTIFIC NOTATION: A shorthand expression of quantities denoted as a value times ten to the nth power. It is particularly useful for extremely large or extremely small numbers. For example, the number 0.005678 is 5.678×10^{-3} in scientific notation.

SCINTILLATION: The flash of light exhibited by certain materials (scintillators) when struck by radiation. Light production is proportional to the original radiation. Radioactive samples can be quantified by mixing them with a scintillation solution and counting the light flashes in a scintillation counter.

SCINTILLATION COUNTER: See Photomultiplier.

SCOPOLAMINE; L-HYOSCINE: An antimuscarinic agent similar to atropine and obtained from the belladonna plant. It is a competitive antagonist of acetylcholine at receptor sites in smooth muscle, cardiac muscle, and exocrine glands. Scopolamine produces mydriasis and paralysis of ocular accommodation. It inhibits secretions of the respiratory tract including the mouth, nose, pharynx, and bronchi, and is therefore frequently used as a premedicant for anesthesia (in conjunction with a narcotic). Scopolamine causes drowsiness at low doses because it penetrates the blood-brain barrier into the central nervous system much more readily than atropine. In the past, however, it was often used alone in higher doses for sedation, a technique known as "twilight sleep," during which the patient would be somnolent, responsive, and would have no memory of the procedure. Delirium, an adverse side effect caused by scopolamine, may be reversed by physostigmine (Antilirium). See Atropine, Physostigmine.

SCREEN OXYGENATOR (MAYO GIBBON PUMP OXYGENATOR): A type of pump oxygenator used for exchange of gases during cardiopulmonary bypass. Gas exchange takes place as the patient's blood flows down a fine-mesh screen which is contained in a high-O_2 atmosphere. See Cardiopulmonary bypass.

SECOBARBITAL (SECONAL): A short-acting sedative-hypnotic agent. See Barbiturate.

SECOND: The standard international unit of time determined by the duration of a specific number of periods of radiation emitted by a cesium-133 atom decaying between two known states. It was formerly defined as 1/86,400 of the mean solar day.

SECONDARY EMISSION: The liberation of electrons from a material which has been struck by a high-velocity electron. Secondary electrons can be accelerated by an electromagnetic field and go on to strike another metal surface, causing further secondary emission, thereby leading to an electron avalanche or cascade. See Photomultiplier.

SECONDARY FIBRINOLYSIS: See Primary fibrinolysis.

SECONDARY LOBULE (RESPIRATORY LOBULE): An anatomic unit of the lung surrounded by connective tissue septa and consisting of a small cluster of terminal bronchioles together with the respiratory tissue it supplies. See Conducting airways.

SECONDARY WINDING: See Transformer.

SECOND GAS EFFECT: A phenomenon seen in inhalation anesthesia, particularly during induction, when a high concentration of a primary gas (soluble agent) is given in conjunction with a second gas (anesthetic vapor). The rapid uptake of the primary gas accelerates the rate of rise of alveolar concentration of the second gas, i.e., the constituents of the alveolar gas which do not leave the alveoli and enter the blood quite as rapidly as the primary gas form a larger percentage of the remaining alveolar gas volume. The second gas effect is best illustrated by the administration of 75% N_2O, 1% halothane, and 24% O_2. Since N_2O crosses the alveolar membrane much more rapidly than halothane, the gas remaining in the alveoli has a higher concentration of halothane. If the second gas is also extremely soluble, the second gas effect is negligible; however, a rapid transfer of both agents to the blood creates an increase in inspired volume. Gas is drawn down the trachea to replace alveolar gas which has crossed into the lung. See Concentration effect.

SEDATION: A drowsy state of consciousness which allows an individual to respond to commands appropriately. The patient may fall asleep spontaneously unless stimulated. See Conscious sedation.

SEDIMENTATION: The tendency of free particles in a liquid to clump together under the influence of gravity or centrifugal force.

SEEBECK EFFECT: See Thermocouple.

SEGMENTAL ATELECTASIS: See Atelectasis.

SEGMENTAL BLOCK(S): An imprecise term usually used to mean an epidural block of levels T10-L1. It is imprecise because "segmental block" has also been used to mean either a unilateral or bilateral paravertebral block of one or more levels of the sympathetic chain.

SEIZURE: A state of excessive, uncontrolled overactivity affecting part or all of the central nervous system. See Epilepsy.

SELDINGER TECHNIQUE: A method of placing a catheter (of the same size as the needle) into a vessel via a puncture needle and stylet (guidewire). The Seldinger technique was originally designed for arterial catheterization with the injection of contrast medium. This method has since been used to insert an endotracheal tube following the placement of the guidewire through the cricothyroid membrane and upward into the mouth. The wire is then used to guide the tube for proper placement. A variation of the Seldinger guidewire, the J-wire, has a curved tip which is able to bypass a partial obstruction in a vessel.

SELECTIVITY: The ability of a device, such as an electric circuit, to discriminate among specific frequencies.

SELF-INFLATING BAG: See Breathing bag.

SELF-PROPAGATING FLAME: A combustion process in which fuel is mixed with air at a rapid rate so that a flame will travel from the point of ignition. The flame will continue to burn after the original point of ignition has cooled.

SELF-TAMING OF SUCCINYLCHOLINE: A technique of administering succinylcholine to attenuate muscle fasciculation. A small dose is administered (1/5-1/10 the total dose) and the patient is observed for fasciculation before the remainder is given. Controversy exists as to whether or not fasciculation is decreased with this technique.

SELF-TEST CAPABILITY (SELF-CALIBRATION; CALIBRATION SIGNAL): A built-in feature of many sophisticated electronic monitors whereby the monitor is able to generate a signal internally (cal signal) which acts precisely like the signal it is meant to acquire, display, and/or record. The unit can therefore be checked without being attached to a patient.

SELLICK MANEUVER: A procedure used to block regurgitation of stomach contents into the esophagus during a rapid sequence intubation technique. It involves pressing on the cricoid cartilage of the trachea to compress the esophagus. See Induction.

SEMICONDUCTOR: A material which resists the flow of an electric current more than a conductor but less than an insulator. Unlike most materials, semiconductors also have a negative temperature coefficient of resistance, i.e., as the temperature rises, the relative resistance of the material decreases. The rare elements germanium and selenium are examples of a semiconductor. Semiconductors are important in solid state electronics. In certain semiconductors, there is an absence of an electron (a "hole") in the orbit of an atom. This hole functions as a positive charge carrier. Since some semiconductors have a relative overabundance of holes (p-type material) and others have a relative overabundance of electrons (n-type material), differences of potential can be set up by layering wafers of these different materials. The interface of the two materials, the pn junction, functions as a rectifier of alternating current as electrons will only flow across the junction when the polarity is in the same direction as the junction (negative source attached to n-material, etc.).

SEMIPERMEABLE MEMBRANE: A membrane which allows certain particles and solvents to pass through but excludes other particles and solvents. See Osmotic pressure.

SENSITIVITY: A criterion for evaluating diagnostic tests. It is the number of true-positives (TP) detected by the test ÷ TP + the number of false-negatives (FN) missed by the test X 100 to give a percentage (TP/TP + FN X 100). See Specificity.

SENSOR: A device used to detect changes in physically measurable parameters, such as temperature, pulse, and air flow.

SEPTICEMIA: A condition caused by the persistent presence of pathogenic micro-organisms and their toxins in the blood. Regional anesthesia is contraindicated in the presence of septicemia as any bleeding at the injection site would be contaminated by the offending microbes and would therefore be an immediate threat to the nerve trunks in the area.

SEPTIC SHOCK: See Shock.

SEQUENTIAL MULTIPLE ANALYZER (SMA 1260; SMA 660): See Automated analysis instrument.

SERIES: A type of electric connection in which the same current flows in all elements of the circuit providing a single path; however, the voltage drop is different across each element depending on its individual resistance.

SEROTONIN (5-HYDROXYTRYPTAMINE, 5-HT): A vasoactive substance distributed throughout the central nervous system in nerve endings, hypothalamus, and enterochromaffin cells of the gastrointestinal tract. High concentrations of serotonin are found in the platelets. Excessive amounts of serotonin are secreted by metabolic carcinoid tumor cells. See Carcinoid syndrome.

SERPASIL: See Reserpine.

SERUM, BLOOD: The clear fluid part of the blood plasma with fibrinogen removed.

SERUM OSMOTIC PRESSURE: See Osmotic pressure.

SERVOMECHANISM: A device which automatically corrects the performance of a system by a feedback mechanism.

SEVOFLURANE: A nonflammable inhalation anesthetic which is not in current clinical use because it is not compatible with CO_2 absorbents. Its chemical formula is $C_4H_3F_7O$.

SHERIFF OF NOTTINGHAM SYNDROME: See Intracerebral steal syndrome.

SHIFT REGISTER: A discrete circuit for storing digital data. A typical shift register has 1024 locations, each one capable of storing one word (usually a byte of 8 bits). In the recirculate mode, the shift register can provide a "freeze" (unchang-

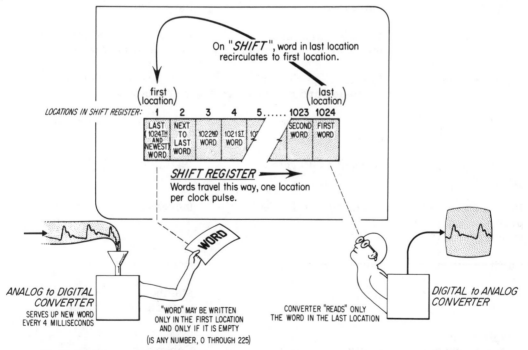

Shift Register: Shift register operating in the recirculate mode, in which the word in the 1024 slot is recycled to the number 1 slot and the word sequence is reread. Only if there is no word in the first slot (the shift register is in the write and recirculate mode) can the analog-to-digital converter add a new word to the first slot.

ing) trace of a particular few seconds of an electrocardiogram (ECG). (The pattern stored is constantly fed back to the electron beam.) In the unit mode, a continuous real-time ECG can be displayed. With two shift registers, a continuous ECG can be compared on the screen with a desired portion of a previous ECG. See Fig.

SHOCK: A condition in which there is a decrease in the function of vital organs due to an inadequate blood supply or vascular perfusion. Although it may be the result of many different causes, this decreased blood supply ultimately leads to tissue hypoxia, metabolic acidosis, and cellular death. Shock may be classified on the basis of primary cause or on the type of functional disturbance produced. Types of shock include hypovolemic, cardiogenic, septic, vasogenic, and neurogenic. Hypovolemic shock is characterized by fluid loss of either blood, plasma, or extracellular fluid,

Shock: Clinical signs and symptoms of early and late shock (not all may be present at all times).

Parameters	Early	Late
Blood pressure	Mildly decreased	Markedly hypotensive to unobtainable
Pulse	Mildly tachycardic	Markedly tachycardic, peripherally weak and thready
Respiration	Increased	Increased
Skin	Usually warm and dry but may be cool and clammy	Usually cold and moist but may be warm and dry
Mental status	Restless, periods of confusion and disorientation	Markedly disoriented to unconscious
Renal	Output normal to mildly decreased	Output mildly decreased to oliguric
Central venous pressure	Normal to elevated	Variable
Pulmonary artery pressure/pulmonary wedge pressure	Normal to increased	Increased
Cardiac output	Normal to increased	Decreased
Acid-base balance	Respiratory alkalosis	Metabolic acidosis and respiratory acidosis

Respirations
  breath sounds
  PO_2
  PCO_2
	Clear
	Normal
	Normal to decreased
		Congested
		Decreased
		Increased

Serum K^+	Mildly decreased	Mildly increased

e.g., due to hemorrhage, burns, diarrhea, or dehydration. The body attempts to compensate for this loss by shifting fluid from the intracellular space to the extracellular and intravascular spaces. This is mediated by increased sympathetic activity causing a heightened vasomotor tone. The body also attempts to compensate hormonally by releasing aldosterone, which leads to the retention of sodium. These responses are attenuated by the administration of a general anesthetic. Cardiogenic shock is characterized by an inadequate cardiac output although a normal blood volume exists. This is most commonly seen after myocardial infarction, although other causes exist such as dysrhythmia, acute valvular failure, or cardiac tamponade. Septic shock appears to be due to pathogenic microorganisms or circulating bacterial endotoxins and exotoxins. Although blood volume is usually normal, O_2 is not efficiently utilized by the cells. Vasogenic shock occurs when vasodilatation causes the normal blood volume to be inadequate in supplying the vessels. This may be evident following an anaphylactic reaction which releases excessive histamine into the blood and produces a strong antigen-antibody reaction. Neurogenic shock is associated with syncopic episodes during which the functions of the sympathetic autonomic system are altered and vasodilation results. All types of shock may be involved concurrently. The key element in any type of shock appears to be the loss of effectiveness of the normal mechanisms which control the intravascular space. The clinical signs are instability of pulse, blood pressure, and cardiac function, and increasing metabolic acidosis. Treatment of shock involves the restoration of adequate circulatory volume, adequate pumping action of the heart (with inotropic drugs or digitalis), and adequate peripheral resistance. In addition, metabolic acidosis must be reversed (by appropriate drug administration), maintenance of organ function (particularly urine output) must be attained, and sepsis must be treated with appropriate antibiotics. See Fig.

SHOCK THERAPY: See Electroconvulsive therapy.

SHOCK WAVE: See Explosion.

SHORT CIRCUIT: An electronic connection of low resistance between two points in a circuit in which the resistance is usually higher.

SHRADER FITTING: A type of quick disconnect joint in gas lines which allows hoses to be quickly attached and detached from a central gas outlet. Various shapes and diameters are used to prevent cross-connection between different gases.

SHUNT: The blood which enters the arterial system without undergoing gas exchange in the lungs. Sources of this blood include bronchial artery blood (collected by the pulmonary veins following perfusion of the bronchi and depletion of O_2) and coronary venous blood (which drains directly into the left ventricle via the thebesian veins). The combination of thebesian and bronchial flow is called physiologic shunt or venous admixture and measures 1-2% of the cardiac output of the healthy individual. Anatomic shunt refers to a transfer of mixed venous blood from right to left without passing a ventilated area in the lung (cardiac septal defect or patent ductus arteriosus). Atelectatic shunt refers to mixed venous blood which returns to the left side of the heart after passing closed (atelectatic) alveoli, and therefore does not come into contact with respiratory gas. Physiologic shunt and ventilation/perfusion abnormalities contribute to alveolar-arterial O_2 difference. See Fig. See Alveolar-arterial oxygen difference.

SHUNT EQUATION: An equation for estimating the amount of physiologic shunt flow in the lungs. See Shunt.

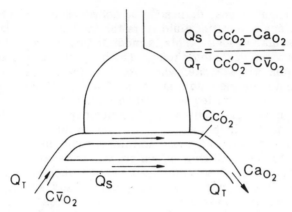

$$\frac{Q_S}{Q_T} = \frac{Cc'_{O_2} - Ca_{O_2}}{Cc'_{O_2} - C\bar{v}_{O_2}}$$

Shunt: Measurements of shunt flow with the shunt equation; QT = total blood flow, Q_s = amount of shunted blood/time, Cc'_{O_2} = amount of O_2 in pulmonary capillary blood, $C\bar{v}_{O_2}$ = amount of O_2 in venous blood, Ca_{O_2} = amount of O_2 in arterial blood.

SIALAGOGUE: See Antisialagogue.

SIDE EFFECT: A consequence (possibly adverse) which occurs as a result of a drug or procedure which differs from the desired result.

SIGGAARD-ANDERSEN ALIGNMENT NOMOGRAM: A mathematic device for inter-relating base excess, total CO_2, and HCO_3^- when pH and PCO_2 are known in an arterial sample. See Fig.

SIGH: A deep, audible, semivoluntary breath usually in response to a strong emotion. Alternately, in the control of respiration, a sigh is a deliberate, stepwise change in inspiratory volume of 2-3 times normal tidal volume, repeated on a fairly vigorous basis each hour. The purpose of the sigh is to open terminal airways which have a tendency to collapse during stereotypic ventilation (when respiration delivers exactly the same tidal volume at exactly the same flow rate and flow pattern, breath after breath).

SIGHT GLASS: A vertical glass tube attached to a chamber of liquid so that the height of the liquid in the chamber is duplicated in the glass tube. This allows the volume of liquid in the chamber to be determined without actually looking into the large chamber. The sight glass was used on older anesthetic vaporizers.

SIGN: The objective evidence perceptible to an examiner and indicative of disease. Signs are, to some extent, measurable and quantifiable. See Symptom.

SIGNAL: A variable parameter used to convey information.

SIGNAL AVERAGING: A technique for extracting a signal from random background noise thereby improving the signal-to-noise ratio. Random noise will cancel itself out when averaged over an increasing number of trials, whereas a steady strength signal will be unaffected by the number of trials averaged. This signal-averaging technique is used in electroencephalogram (EEG) analysis to identify an evoked potential "lost" in the regular EEG activity. The stimulus for the evoked potential is presented repeatedly, and gradually the evoked potential emerges out of the background noise. See Fig.

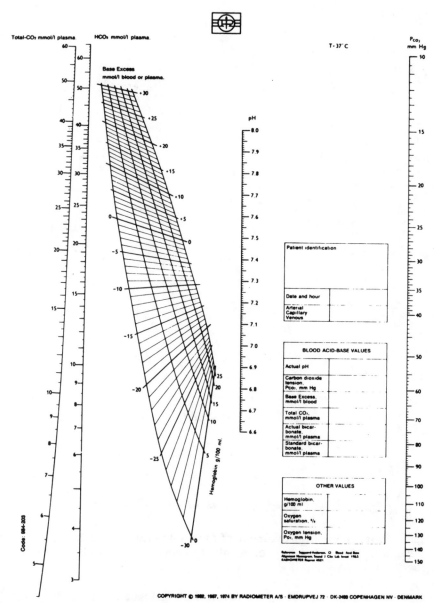

Siggaard-Andersen Alignment Nomogram.

SIGNAL-TO-NOISE RATIO: The ratio of the strength of the desired information (signal) in a communication to that of unwanted random sounds (noise). The purpose of most signal-processing equipment is to enhance the signal-to-noise ratio. For example, while using a stethoscope to listen to blood pressure sounds (signal), sounds generated by body movement and the environment (noise) are also heard.

SIGNIFICANCE LEVEL: The maximum probability of arriving at a type I or type II error in evaluating observations. In practice, a level of significance of 0.05 or 0.01 is common. At 0.05 or 5% level of significance, one is 95% certain of reaching the

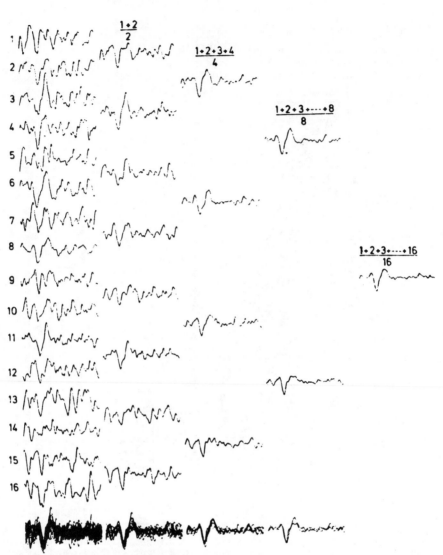

Signal Averaging: Improvement of signal-to-noise ratio by signal averaging. The noise is progressively reduced left to right with the repetition of the signal.

correct interpretation; at 0.01 or 1% level of significance, one is 99% certain. See Type I error, Type II error.

SIKER MIRROR LARYNGOSCOPE BLADE: A modification of the curved laryngoscope blade which incorporates a mirror to allow vision around an obstruction.

SILENT GENE: See Dibucaine number.

SILENT ZONE OF LUNG: The area of the lung comprising the small peripheral airways. In healthy individuals, this zone contributes only 20% of total peripheral resistance and therefore remains "silent" until significantly diseased.

SILICON-CONTROLLED RECTIFIER (SCR): A semiconductor device which permits current flow in one direction when an appropriate signal is applied to one of its electrodes (gate). SCRs are used in many devices as precision switches.

SILICONE: A polymeric organic compound containing silicon. Silicones are heat-resistant, have a high dielectric strength, and are highly water-resistant.

SINGLE-BREATH TEST: A test to measure the inequality of lung ventilation. A patient takes a single breath of 100% O_2 and then exhales slowly and evenly into a N_2 meter, which rapidly measures the concentration of expired N_2. The expiratory volume is recorded simultaneously. After the first 750 ml are expired (assuming this volume clears the dead space), the N_2 concentration is measured throughout the next 500 ml. Nitrogen concentration does not increase by more than 1.5% (the alveolar plateau) in healthy individuals. In patients with pulmonary disorders such as emphysema, bronchiectasis, or cancer, the N_2 concentration rises more rapidly. In these patients, there is an uneven dilution of lung N_2 by inhaled O_2. In addition, poorly ventilated regions of the lung, i.e., damaged by disease, receive little or no O_2 from a single breath and empty toward the end of expiration. The single-breath test can be modified to determine closing volume and anatomic dead space. See Closing capacity, Multibreath test, Infrared analyzer.

SINOATRIAL NODE (SA NODE): The normal pacemaker or determinant of the pulse rate in the heart. From the SA node a wave of depolarization spreads across the atria to the atrioventricular node (AV node). The normal pacemaker action of the SA node is dependent on the fact that it is the fastest cardiac tissue to depolarize spontaneously. The vagus nerve acts to decrease this spontaneous discharge; higher body temperature increases this rate and lower temperature decreases it. The rate of discharge is also depressed by digitalis and is increased by sympathetic stimulation or circulating catecholamines. See Heart, conduction system of.

SI UNIT: A standard international unit (from the French Système International d'Unites) which is the agreed on system of measurement or quantification for all

SI Unit: Prefixes used with SI units.

Name of Factor	Prefix	Symbol	Name of Factor	Prefix	Symbol
10	deca-	da	10^{-1}	deci-	d
10^2	hecto-	h	10^{-2}	centi-	c
10^3	kilo-	k	10^{-3}	milli-	m
10^6	mega-	M	10^{-6}	micro-	μ
10^9	giga-	G	10^{-9}	nano-	n
10^{12}	tera-	T	10^{-12}	pico-	p
			10^{-15}	femto-	f
			10^{-18}	atto-	a

scientific and most technical needs. SI units are based on the meter-kilogram-second system (MKS) and replace the centimeter-gram-second system (CGS). See Fig.

SKIN PREPARATION: The procedure for reducing the bacterial count on the skin by applying an iodine solution or alcohol prior to puncture or incision. This technique does not sterilize the skin. The effectiveness of the reduction of the bacterial count depends not so much on the individual agent, but on the vigor and length of time of its application. Although the method has been used for nearly 100 years, the parameters of skin preparation are still controversial.

SLANDER: A verbal statement which defames or misrepresents another person. See Defamation.

SLEEP: A normal physiologic state which is associated with relaxation, reduced environmental awareness, mild hypotension, mild bradycardia, and a definite reduction of metabolic state. Different levels of sleep can be distinguished by the ease with which the subject is awakened and by specific changes in the electroencephalogram. Sleep appears to be a required bodily function without which severe and progressive mental disability occurs.

SLEEVE: A form of adaptor used to alter the external diameter of a system component.

SMA 1260: See Automated analysis instrument.

SNOW, JOHN: The English physician who is credited with being the first specialist in anesthesia. His administration of chloroform to Queen Victoria for childbirth in 1853 was a key element in counteracting the fundamentalist arguments, biblically based, that women must bring forth children in pain. He died in 1858 at the age of 45.

SODA LIME: A widely used absorbent to remove CO_2 from anesthesia rebreathing systems. Soda lime consists of small amounts of sodium hydroxide and potassium hydroxide mixed with a large amount of calcium hydroxide. Inert silica and a color indicator are also added. Because the mixture of sodium and calcium hydroxide was protected by a patent, competitors used other metal hydroxides, e.g., barium hydroxide, in manufacturing absorbents. This led to production of Baralyme, a major competitor of soda lime. Baralyme (barium hydroxide lime) is a mixture of 20% barium hydroxide octahydrate and 80% calcium hydroxide. It may also contain some potassium hydroxide and a color indicator. Price and handling characteristics usually determine choice of absorbent.

SODA LIME CANISTER: See Carbon dioxide absorption canister.

SODIUM (Na): An alkaline metallic element with an atomic number of 11 and an atomic weight of 23. It provides the principle cation of the extracellular body fluids. The normal range of serum Na is 135-145 mEq/L. Since Na has a valence (charge) of 1, the osmotic pressure of serum Na has the same value, i.e., 135-145 mOsm/L of water. The total body content of exchangeable Na in a normal 70-kg man is 2700-3800 mEq. A large proportion of Na (at least 2000 mEq) is extracellular. Intracellular Na is in the range of 10 mEq/L of intracellular water. Excess Na can be easily excreted in the urine (in a normal urine volume), whereas Na balance can be maintained (during Na deprivation) by intake of as little as 10-15 mEq/day. Aldosterone, a mineralocorticoid secreted by the adrenal cortex, helps to

Sodium: Factors affecting sodium levels.

Elevated Serum Na	Decreased Serum Na
Dehydration	Diuresis
Primary Aldosteronism	Dilutional
Diabetes Insipidus	Cirrhosis
	Inappropriate ADH syndrome
	Na-losing nephropathy
	Addison disease

regulate Na metabolism in the body. In addition, antidiuretic hormone (ADH) controls the Na concentration of extracellular fluids. See Fig. See Action potential.

SODIUM CHANNEL: The passageway, or pore, in a nerve membrane which allows a rapid influx of sodium (Na) ions (necessary for depolarization). The "gateway" to the pore appears to maintain the positive charges of calcium. In the resting state this "gate" remains nearly closed to Na ion diffusion. When the gate opens, the permeability of the Na channels increases approximately 5000-fold. See Potassium channel.

SODIUM NITROPRUSSIDE (NIPRIDE): A rapid-acting, short-term vasodilator administered by intravenous (IV) infusion. (A freshly prepared solution must be used.) Nitroprusside is used to produce deliberate hypotension for surgical procedures and to relieve hypertensive crisis. Nitroprusside dilates both arteriolar and venous smooth muscles. The drug is extremely sensitive to light and precautions must therefore be taken to ensure that the IV tubing and bottle are covered. Although cyanide is an intermediate breakdown product of nitroprusside, cyanide toxicity is rare. Toxic effects of nitroprusside are related to excessive vasodilation and hypotension. Symptoms include nausea, vomiting, palpitation, and headache.

SOFTWARE: The written programs, values, information bits, data, equations, etc. which direct functioning of the computer electromechanics (hardware).

SOLENOID: An electromagnetic switch that usually consists of a coil of wire with a length greater than its diameter. A metal rod slides on the track inside the coil and extends beyond the end of the coil. When current flows through the coil, a magnetic field is created which attracts the rod. The rod moves into the coil or, if the rod is a permanent magnet and polarities are arranged properly, it can be made to extend outside of the coil. The rod contains a contact for making and breaking a circuit.

SOLID STATE: See Semiconductor.

SOLUBILITY: The relative ability of a given substance (gas, liquid, or solid) to dissolve when mixed with another substance. Solubility is dependent on temperature, pressure, and polarity.

SOLUTE: The substance dissolved in a solvent.

SOLUTION: The homogeneous mixture of a solute (liquid, gas, or solid) with a solvent (usually liquid, but may be gas or solid).

SOLVENT: A substance which dissolves another substance and forms a homogeneous solution.

SOMATIC: A term which pertains to the nonreproductive parts of the body.

SOUND: The audible vibrations transmitted through fluids and solids and measured in decibels. Under most ordinary circumstances, sound is transmitted to the human ear by means of vibrations of the air in the range of 20-20,000 Hz/sec. Infrasound is the vibrations below the frequency range of the waves usually perceived as sound (<16 Hz). The speed of sound varies depending on the density of the material through which it is moving, temperature, pressure, and altitude. Sound cannot travel through a vacuum. Ultrasound is the vibrations above the audible frequency of 20,000 Hz/sec and may extend to 10 or 12 MHz. Ultrasound is used as a valuable diagnostic technique in the detection of abnormalities in various body organs and in the evaluation of fetal development. See Ultrasound.

SPACE BLANKET: An extremely lightweight nylon sheet with one reflective surface that maintains a high percentage of body heat. Since it is lightweight, the space blanket does not interfere with the patient's movement and is an effective passive technique for raising body temperature.

SPARK: The visible evidence of an electric current between two electrodes separated by an air gap. Sparks are generated when the potential difference between the electrodes is raised high enough that the charged particles present are accelerated to the point at which they strike neutrally charged gas molecules, thereby dislodging electrons. The gas molecules themselves become charged and move in an electric field. This becomes a self-propagating process depending on the magnitude of the potential difference, the length of time it is maintained, and the molecular composition of the gas mixture. The potential difference which is just adequate to cause a minimum spark discharge is called the breakdown voltage. The spark discharge is an economic source of ignition, since a large amount of energy is focused in a very small volume of gas, heating that portion of the gas very rapidly before heat dissipation into the surrounding gas can drop the temperature.

SPARK GAP: An arrangement of electrodes between which a disruptive discharge occurs when a voltage is applied that exceeds a specific predetermined value. A spark gap generator is a type of electrosurgical unit, useful in coagulation, which uses a spark gap to generate radiofrequency waves. See Cauterization, Coagulation current.

SPARKOVER: See Flashover.

SPECIFIC HEAT CAPACITY: The heat needed to raise the temperature of the unit mass of a substance by 1 degree. In SI units, this measurement is in joules per kilogram kelvin. Each substance has a specific heat capacity.

SPECIFICITY: A criterion for evaluating diagnostic tests. It is the number of true-negatives (TN) detected by the test ÷ TN + the number of false-positives (FP) detected X 100 to give a percentage: $TN/(TN + FP) \times 100$. See Sensitivity.

SPECTRAL EDGE FREQUENCY: See Leading edge analysis.

SPECTROMETER: An instrument used to determine the index of refraction of a prism and the wavelength of light rays. An unknown substance can be heated until it begins to emit light by incandescence. The specific substance can then be identified because each substance has its own wavelength. Alternately, a light of known frequency can be passed through an unknown liquid or gas and the absorption of part of that known spectrum can be used to analyze and determine the unknown substance. Spectrometers are commonly used in the laboratory to detect and quantify the hemoglobin molecule by its absorption of a particular frequency of light.

SPECTROPHOTOMETER: An instrument for measuring the relative intensity of various light rays in the spectrum. This measurement aids in identifying unknown substances.

SPHYGMOMANOMETER: An instrument used to determine arterial blood pressure.

SPINA BIFIDA: A congenital anomaly in which the bony encasement of the spinal cord is not complete. The cord and meninges may or may not protrude through the defect.

SPINAL ANESTHESIA (SUBDURAL BLOCK, SUBARACHNOID BLOCK): A form of regional anesthesia in which a local anesthetic solution is deposited into the cerebrospinal fluid in the area of the lumbar vertebrae. The interspace of choice for needle placement is L4-L5. Spinal anesthesia may be used for most surgical procedures done below the level of the diaphragm but may be inadequate for extensive bowel surgery, as it does not block parasympathetic cranial outflow to the intestines. Spinal anesthesia can produce adequate sensory and motor blockade. Even when the blockade is inadequate, the sympathetic trunks are completely blocked, causing vasodilation and hypotension. See Epidural anesthesia; Epidural patch; Hyperbaric solution; Nerve fiber, anatomy and physiology of; Total spinal, accidental.

SPINAL HEADACHE: A known complication of spinal anesthesia ascribed to leakage of cerebrospinal fluid through the hole made in the dura by the spinal needle. Incidence is partially dependent on the patient's age and size of the needle. (Larger needles and younger individuals have a higher incidence.) Conservative treatment includes bedrest, increased fluid intake, and analgesics. Severely affected patients may require an epidural blood patch. See Epidural patch, Spinal anesthesia.

SPINAL NEEDLE: A needle usually measuring 20-25 gauge X 3-1/2 in used to deposit a regional anesthetic under the dura or to withdraw cerebrospinal fluid by lumbar puncture. The bevel-ended and diamond-point needles are examples of spinal needles. See Fig. See Epidural needle, Hustead epidural needle.

SPINAL SEGMENT: The portion of the spinal cord which contains a dorsal and ventral nerve root. The segment's name refers to the surrounding vertebra. There are a total of 31 segments in the human (C1-C8, T1-T12, L1-L5, S1-S5, and Co1).

SPINAL SHOCK: A condition which follows injury or partial transection of the spinal cord, characterized by flaccid paralysis and loss of visceral and somatic sensations below the level of the lesion or transection. Tendon and abdominal reflexes are absent as is the plantar response. Bladder and bowel functions are not under voluntary control. A zone of enhanced sensation may be evident above the level of the lesion. The clinical presentation of spinal shock (areflexia) persists from a few days to several weeks when there is a slow return of reflex activity.

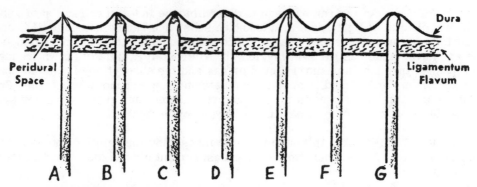

Spinal and Epidural Needles: (A) Standard spinal needle with a sharp point which readily punctures the dura. (B) Needle with a solid end and a side opening. (C) Needle with a rounded solid point and a side opening close to its distal end. The Lutz needle has this type of point. (D) Needle with a short, blunt beveled point with rounded edges such as is found on the standard Crawford peridural needles. (E) Needle with a modified huber point as is present on the various Tuohy or Hustead needles. (F) Needle with a directional huber point bent at an acute angle such as is present on the Wagner needle. (G) Needle with an extremely blunt, rounded point and an opening near its end such as is found on the Cheng needle.

SPIROMETER: A device used to measure the quantity of air taken into and exhaled from the lungs. With the early mechanical spirometers, the patient's nose was clamped closed and he or she breathed through a mouthpiece into a bell inverted in a cylinder of water. Movement of the bell was recorded as the air volume inside of the cylinder rose and fell with respiration. This apparatus was quite accurate but it was also cumbersome and bulky. It has since been replaced by other less accurate mechanical or electric means of determining respiratory volumes. See Anemometer, hot wire.

SPIRONOLACTONE (ALDACTONE): A diuretic agent used with other diuretics to reverse hypokalemia and antagonize the effects of aldosterone. Aldosterone acts to conserve sodium and enhances potassium excretion, whereas spironolactone favors sodium excretion and potassium retention. To prevent hyperkalemia, potassium supplements should not be administered in conjunction with spironolactone.

SPLANCHNIC: A term which pertains to the viscera. Splanchnic circulation comprises the blood flow to the gastrointestinal tract, pancreas, liver, and spleen. Various anesthetic agents (cyclopropane, methoxyflurane, halothane, and isoflurane) reduce this circulation.

SPONTANEOUS RESPIRATION: See Ventilation, spontaneous.

STAGES AND PLANES OF ANESTHESIA: A system, codified by Guedel, of evaluating a patient's response to anesthesia. This system relates specifically to unpremedicated patients during ether anesthesia and is no longer clinically applicable because most patients are premedicated and ether is no longer used. Guedel believed that depth of anesthesia progressed in recognizable increments from consciousness to death by generalized depression. Each increment is identified by

Stages and Planes of Anesthesia: Outline.

	Respiration			Pupils		Reflex Depression
	Rhythm	Volume	Pattern	Size	Position	
STAGE I (Analgesia) Analgesia to loss of consciousness	Irregular	Small	∿	Small	Divergent	Nil
STAGE II (Excitement) Loss of consciousness to rhythmical respiration	Irregular	Large	∿	Large	Divergent	Eyelash Eyelid
STAGE III (Surgical anaesthesia) PLANE 1 Rhythmical respiration to cessation of eye movement	Regular	Large	∿	Small	Divergent	Skin Vomiting Conjunctival Pharyngeal Stretch from limb-muscles
PLANE 2 Cessation of eye movement to start of respiratory muscle paresis (excl. diaphragm)	Regular	Medium	∿	1/2 dilated	Fixed centrally	Corneal
PLANE 3 Respiratory muscle paresis to paralysis	Regular Pause after expiration	Small	∿	3/4 dilated	Fixed centrally	Laryngeal Peritoneal
PLANE 4 Diaphragmatic paresis to paralysis	Jerky Irregular Quick inspiration Prolonged expiration, i.e., "see-saw"	Small	∿	Fully dilated	Fixed centrally	Anal sphincter Carinal
STAGE IV Apnoea						

*If the respiration is slow, an expiratory pause may be seen in plane 2.

changes in the eyes, respiration, muscle tone, response to incision, and pharyngeal and laryngeal reflexes. Stage I (amnesia and analgesia) lasts from onset of anesthesia to loss of consciousness. The pupils are small, the patient's response to pain is altered, muscle tone is normal, and pharyngeal reflexes are unaffected. Stage II (delerium or excitement) lasts from the loss of consciousness to the beginning of rhythmic breathing. The pupils are large and the eyelid reflex is depressed, muscles are tense, and breathing may be irregular. The patient may cough, struggle, swallow, or vomit. Pharyngeal and laryngeal reflexes are depressed toward the end of this stage. Stage III (surgical anesthesia) is composed of four planes and lasts from the onset of regular breathing to respiratory arrest. Plane 1 includes the time from the onset of rhythmic respiration and absent lid reflex to the cessation of eye movement. During plane 1 the eye may oscillate or may be eccentrically fixed, and pupillary size changes from dilated to constricted. The vomiting reflex is lost as is lacrimation. Plane 2 includes the time from absence of eye movement to the beginning of respiratory muscle (intercostal) paralysis. The pupils begin to dilate and become centrally fixed, and muscle tone is decreased. Plane 3 includes the time from the beginning to the completion of respiratory paralysis. Tidal volume is decreased since respiration is accomplished only by the diaphragm. Toward the end of plane 3 the pupils are nonreactive to light. Plane 4 includes the time from complete intercostal paralysis to diaphragmatic paralysis and, therefore, to cessation of spontaneous respiration. Pupils are dilated and nonreactive. Stage IV (overdosage, apnea) lasts from the onset of diaphragmatic paralysis to cardiac arrest. Most reflexes are absent. Prompt measures must be taken to lighten this inadvertent stage of anesthesia. See Fig.

STAINLESS STEEL: An alloy of iron and chromium which resists corrosion because of a surface coating of chromium oxide that forms on exposure to the atmosphere. This coating is insoluble, self-healing, and nonporous.

STANDARD BICARBONATE OF THE BLOOD: The amount of bicarbonate in the plasma when the blood sample is in equilibration at a $PaCO_2$ of 40 mmHg, 37 degrees Celsius, and pH of 7.4. The bicarbonate is measured in millimoles per liter. It is indicative of the degree of metabolic acidosis or alkalosis present. Although the test quantifies the contribution of $PaCO_2$ to a change in pH, it is not as popular as previously because of difficulty with testing procedures.

STANDARD DEVIATION (SD): A measure of the dispersion of a series of numbers around their arithmetic mean. It is the square root of the sum of the squared deviation (variance) of each value from the arithmetic mean. (It may also be derived by dividing by one less than the number of squares in the sum of squares rather than taking the arithmetic mean.) A large SD indicates a wide dispersion about the mean, whereas a small SD indicates a distribution close to the mean. For a normal distribution, 68.2770 of all observations will lie ±1 SD from the arithmetic mean, 95.4570 will lie ±2 SD from the arithmetic mean, and 99.7370 will lie ±3 SD from the arithmetic mean.

STANDARD ERROR OF THE MEAN (SEM): A measurement of data dispersion calculated as the standard deviation (SD) of the sample observations divided by the square root of the number of observations. Large standard errors of the mean imply that there is a good chance that the mean of the sample is not close to the real mean. The SEM approaches the SD as the number of samples increases.

STANDARD OF DISEASES AND OPERATIONS (SNDO): A six-digit system for coding diagnoses and surgical procedures formulated by the American Medical Association.

STANDARD TEMPERATURE AND PRESSURE (STP): A formal set of conditions to standardize determinants of the physical characteristics of liquids and gases. The conditions correspond to a standard temperature of 0 degrees Celsius (273.15 degrees Kelvin) and a standard pressure of 1 atmosphere (approximately 760 torr).

STAT: An abbreviation for the Latin word statim used to indicate that something must be done immediately and without delay.

STATIC: A random, unwanted noise present in electric circuits. See Signal-to-noise ratio.

STATIC FLAME: A combustion process in which fuel is combined with O_2 at such a slow rate that the position of the visible flame does not move. A burning candle is an example of a static flame. Even though plenty of wax is available, it melts and burns at such a slow pace that the flame does not consume the entire candle at once. Static flames can ignite explosive gas mixtures such as ether/O_2 when brought into contact with them.

STATISTICS: A branch of mathematics which deals with collecting, organizing, analyzing, summarizing, and presenting numeric data.

STATUS EPILEPTICUS: A rapid succession of seizures, during which the patient does not regain uninterrupted consciousness or respond to external stimuli.

STAVERMAN REFLECTION COEFFICIENT: A mathematic term expressing the permeability of a membrane to a particular substance. A value of 1 indicates impermeability and 0 indicates total permeability. This coefficient becomes important when dealing with effects of an oncotic pressure gradient.

STEAL SYNDROME: See Intracerebral steal syndrome.

STEEL: An alloy which contains iron and up to 1.7% carbon. Low-carbon steels are malleable whereas high-carbon steels are brittle. The high-carbon steels are used for tools and high-strength materials even though they are difficult to machine.

STEINERT DISEASE: See Myotonia atrophica.

STELAZINE: See Phenothiazine, Trifluoperazine hydrochloride.

STELLATE GANGLION: A star-shaped cluster of nerve cell bodies on the sympathetic trunk formed by the fusion of the inferior cervical and first thoracic sympathetic ganglia. It is located on the transverse process of the seventh cervical vertebra and the neck of the first rib. The postganglionic fibers of the stellate ganglion supply blood vessels, sweat glands, salivary glands, retro-orbital fat, and, heart and provide pilomotor fibers to the skin of the head, arm, hand, and upper chest. See Autonomic nervous system.

STELLATE GANGLION BLOCK: An anesthetic block used to diagnose and/or treat sympathetic dystrophies of the upper limb and peripheral vascular disease. The landmark for locating the stellate ganglion is the enlarged tubercle of the sixth cervical vertebra (Chassaignac tubercle). Stellate ganglion block dilates the blood vessels of the upper limb and therefore may be performed to aid in some surgical procedures. The block disrupts the sympathetic nerve supply to the head, upper extremities, and thorax. A successful block is demonstrated on the anesthesized side by Horner syndrome or Horner triad, stuffy nostril, absence of sweating, blushing of the skin, increased lacrimation, and increased temperature of the face and arm. See Autonomic nervous system, Horner syndrome.

STEPHEN-SLATER VALVE: See Nonrebreathing valve.

STERILIZATION: The total destruction and elimination of microorganisms, e.g., bacteria, virus, fungi. Sterilization may be accomplished by different methods, e.g., moist or dry heat, liquid chemical, gas, or gamma radiation depending on the objects to be sterilized. Moist heat in the form of autoclaving is the most dependable method of destroying pathogens. The moisture increases cellular permeability and the heat (>100 degrees Celsius) coagulates protein. Autoclaving, however, may corrode some equipment, deteriorate plastic and rubber, and prevent penetration of oils, grease, or powder. Dry heat (160 degrees Celsius for 1 hr) may be useful for powder, oil, grease, and glass syringes. Liquid chemical (cold) sterilization is useful for heat-sensitive equipment; however, it is questionable whether a liquid agent can completely sterilize. The gas ethylene oxide (ETO) is used to sterilize the anesthetic and respiratory therapy equipment which is heat- or moisture-sensitive. ETO must be allowed to diffuse out of material such as rubber, however, before tissue contact because it is a strong irritant. Gamma radiation is bactericidal and viricidal. Heat-sensitive objects may be sterilized by this technique. The radioisotope cobalt-60 is commonly used in this method. The items to be sterilized may be prepackaged and will remain sterile indefinitely (as long as the package is sealed). Gamma radiation, however, does produce changes in plastics such as polyvinylchloride (PVC). Irradiated PVC articles must not be resterilized with ethylene oxide or tissue-toxic ethylene chlorohydrin will be released. See Ethylene oxide sterilization.

STEROID: See Corticosteroid.

STETHOSCOPE: A device, invented by Laennec, used during auscultation of sounds in the body. The original stethoscope consisted of a simple wooden tube. The current standard is binaural with the earpieces connected by appropriate tubing to a chest piece which should include both a diaphragm and bell regulated by a valve. The diaphragm is used for high-frequency vibrations whereas the bell is used for low-pitched sounds and murmurs. The earpieces must fit the ear canal snugly, and the tubing should be as short as possible for efficiency, long enough for comfort, and double walled to lessen sound distortion. The monaural or single-ear stethoscope is used extensively in anesthesia to listen to heart and breath sounds while leaving the other ear free for monitoring alarms. A Ploss valve is used to connect the chest stethoscope and blood pressure stethoscope, automatically switching from one to the other as the cuff is inflated and deflated.

STOICHIOMETRIC MIXTURE: A chemical mixture in which fuel molecules react completely with O_2 molecules (complete combustion) until no unreacted molecules remain.

STOPCOCK: A rotary valve used to redirect or stop flow.

STORAGE: The retention of data for later retrieval.

STORAGE CAPACITY: The maximum amount of data or information that a memory device is able to retain at one time. See Shift register.

STORED BLOOD: See Blood storage.

STOVAINE: An obsolete local anesthetic agent synthesized in 1905 (one year before procaine). It was abandoned because it was much more irritating than procaine.

STRAIN GAUGE: An instrument for measuring distortions in an object caused by tension, compression, or twisting. This distortion produces a change in the electronic resistance, capacitance, or inductance which can be quantified to determine the original pressure producing the distortion. (A strain gauge may also be called an extensometer.) See Transducer.

STRAY CAPACITANCE: The collection of electric charges of opposing polarity on the two sides of an insulator. This occurs randomly due to the physical arrangement of components in an electric circuit. Most stray capacitance is undesirable as it both dissipates energy and produces unwanted feedback of signals throughout an electric circuit. Stray capacitance can be avoided by heavily insulating conductors and by proper planning of electric design.

STRAY INDUCTANCE: The casual, unplanned creation of an electromagnetic field around a coiled conductor. Stray inductance can cause unwanted signal transfer and energy loss as in stray capacitance.

STREPTOMYCIN: An antibiotic of the aminoglycoside class. Introduced in 1944, it was used against tuberculosis and certain gram-negative microorganisms. Resistance to streptomycin developed rapidly, however, thereby limiting its clinical usefulness in the long-term treatment of bacterial disease. In addition, streptomycin is ototoxic and nephrotoxic. Currently, the use of this agent is limited to unusual infections such as tularemia, bubonic plague, and bacterial endocarditis. Other members of the aminoglycoside class include neomycin, kanamycin, gentamicin, tobramycin, and amikacin, and all produce similar adverse side effects. See Aminoglycosides, Antibiotic.

STRIDOR: A marked, high-pitched, harsh respiratory sound usually heard during inspiration and caused by acute laryngeal obstruction.

STUDENT t TEST: A statistical measurement which compares two means in an attempt to determine the amount of departure from the standard error of these means. The student t test was developed in 1908 by the statistician Gosset, who published under the pseudonym "Student." The t test is useful for small samples which do not approximate a normal distribution. See Standard error of the mean.

STUMP PRESSURE: An invasive procedure used to measure internal carotid artery stump pressure (ICASP) in the surgically exposed carotid artery. The resulting value provides a relative indication of the adequacy of the collateral circulation to the brain. Stump pressure is normally measured by inserting a small needle immediately distal to a clamp which occludes the internal carotid artery. The needle is attached to a transducer which directly records pressure. This pressure reading is believed to represent the cerebral perfusion pressure delivered to the cerebral hemisphere on the same side as the clamped vessel. Blood flow is supplied by the internal carotid on the other side and by the vertebral arteries via the circle of Willis. It was believed that a stump pressure of 50 mmHg or more was a sign of adequate cerebral circulation (collateral flow). It has been shown, however, that this is not consistently true. In surgical repair of internal carotid artery occlusion, stump pressures aid in deciding whether or not to shunt a large-bore cannula around the surgical incision site. This technique is known as internal carotid shunt.

STYLET: A wire which is inserted into the lumen of a tube or catheter to stiffen it in order to facilitate its proper placement. The stylet may also be used to remove foreign material from a catheter, tube, or needle. It may remain inside a needle or catheter to maintain patency.

STYLUS: A penlike light source which modifies the display on a computer terminal when it touches the screen.

SUBARACHNOID SCREW (INTRACRANIAL PRESSURE BOLT; SUBARACHNOID BOLT): A device for measuring or monitoring intracranial pressure (ICP). A hollow bolt is threaded into a hole in the skull and then through a small dural opening onto the brain surface. The bolt is then attached to a transducer to directly measure pressure. This technique has the advantage over the ventriculostomy catheter because the screw is easy to insert and does not penetrate brain tissue; however, this technique cannot be used to withdraw or sample cerebrospinal fluid. Clinical indications for ICP monitoring include head injuries, hypoxic brain damage, subarachnoid hemorrhage, metabolic coma, stroke, and hydrocephalus. See Intracranial pressure measurement, Ventriculostomy catheter.

SUBDURAL ANESTHESIA: See Epidural anesthesia.

SUBLIMATION: The direct conversion of a solid to a vapor or vice versa with no intervening liquid phase. Dry Ice (solid CO_2) is an example of this physical phenomenon.

SUBLIMAZE: See Fentanyl.

SUBROUTINE: See Routine.

SUBSTANTIA GELATINOSA: See Gate theory of pain.

SUCCINIC ACID: A breakdown product of succinylmonocholine, one of the final products in the degradation of succinylcholine (succinyldicholine).

SUCCINYLCHOLINE HYPERSENSITIVITY: A phenomenon seen in skeletal muscle which has sustained damage causing it to be in a catabolic state. This includes direct trauma to the muscle, denervation, burn injury, or simply prolonged forced rest. The hypersensitivity to succinylcholine appears to occur within 5-7 days after the injury or trauma and has been reported to last up to a year. In those individuals with catabolizing muscle, the administration of succinylcholine causes a huge outpouring of potassium through the muscle membrane into the circulation. Potassium concentration in the serum can increase 2-3 times the normal level. The effect on the heart is catastrophic: intractable fibrillation often leading to death.

SUCCINYLCHOLINE, SUCCINYLDICHOLINE, SUXAMENTHONIUM (ANECTINE): A depolarizing neuromuscular blocking agent. Its onset of activity is very rapid and its duration of action is very short due to the rapid enzymatic inactivation by plasma pseudocholinesterase. Succinylcholine may be administered both as a single intravenous dose or as a continuous infusion for prolonged procedures to obtain skeletal muscle relaxation. Adverse side effects consist mostly of an extension of the pharmacologic actions of the drug and include bradycardia, increased salivation, and profound or prolonged muscle relaxation leading eventually to respiratory depression and apnea. Some individuals may be sensitive to succinylcholine by virtue of a genetically determined enzyme, atypical plasma cholinesterase. They exhibit prolonged apnea due to a low level of normal cholinesterase. Predisposition to this may be determined by the "dibucaine number." Other individuals may possess an abnormal fluoride-resistant enzyme or a "silent gene." Patients with a familial history of malignant hyperthermia should be tested for this disorder prior to use of succinylcholine. In addition, since this neuromuscular blocker tends to increase intraocular pressure, it is contraindicated in patients with penetrating eye injuries or acute glaucoma. Lastly, succinylcholine causes a spikelike rise in serum potassium, which pours out of recently damaged or denervated muscle (burns, cord transection). This response can occur within as little as 7 days after injury and last up to a year. See Dibucaine number, Malignant hyperthermia, Neuromuscular blocking agent, Phase I block, Phase II block.

SUCCINYLMONOCHOLINE: The primary breakdown product of enzymatic hydrolysis (via pseudocholinesterase) of succinylcholine. It is a very weak depolarizing agent and is subsequently hydrolyzed to succinic acid and choline by pseudocholinesterase and a liver enzyme. See Acetylcholinesterase.

SUDOMOTOR PATHWAY: The pathway which innervates sweat glands.

SUFENTANYL: See Fentanyl.

SUGGESTIBILITY: See Hypnosis.

SUMMATION: The combined pharmacologic effect in which the total effect of two or more drugs equals the sum of their individual actions. See Antagonism, Synergism.

SUNSTROKE: See Heatstroke.

SUPERCONDUCTIVITY: A physical phenomenon occurring in many metals and alloys during which there is virtually a complete disappearance of the electric resistance when the metals are cooled to temperatures approaching absolute zero. Electric equipment operating at or near absolute zero can perform an enormous amount of work and yet remain small in size.

SUPERCOOLING (PROFOUND HYPOTHERMIA): See Hypothermia.

SUPERHEATING: The careful heating of a liquid under specific pressure conditions so that it remains a liquid beyond its normal boiling point.

SUPERSATURATED VAPOR: The phenomenon seen when a vapor under a pressure which exceeds the normal amount needed for condensation to a liquid remains vaporous.

SUPINE HYPOTENSIVE SYNDROME: See artocaval syndrome.

SUPRAMAXIMAL STIMULATION: See Neuromuscular blockade, assessment of.

SUPRASPINOUS LIGAMENT: See Lumbar puncture.

SURFACE-ACTIVE AGENT: A substance which is used to reduce surface tension between two liquids or a liquid and solid. Surface-active agents are classified into three categories: emulsifier, wetting agent, and detergent. An emulsifier stabilizes a mixture of two or more liquids which would otherwise be immiscible. Wet-ing agents are added to water to facilitate penetration into or flow over another surface by reducing the surface tension of water. Detergents concentrate at oil-water interfaces, thereby emulsifying oil. The terms detergent, wetting agent, and emulsifier are often used interchangeably. See Surface tension.

SURFACE TENSION: A physical phenomenon occurring at the interface between two liquids or between a liquid and a gas. The interior molecules of the liquid are attracted by other molecules equally in all directions. At the surface molecules are attracted toward the interior of the liquid. This uneven pull deforms the surface of the liquid, which acts as if it is covered by an elastic membrane. Surface tension is measured in newtons per meter. See Surface-active agent.

SURFACTANT: A phospholipid (lecithin and sphingomyelin) produced by type II (septal) alveolar cells. Surfactant helps prevent the collapse of alveoli by decreasing surface tension in the lungs. It forms a thin coating over the alveoli so they will not be pulled in on themselves following expiration. Inadequate amounts of surfactant at birth result in hyaline membrane disease (infant respiratory distress syndrome). See Infant respiratory distress syndrome.

SURITAL: See Thiamylal.

SUXAMETHONIUM: The British term for succinylcholine. See Succinylcholine.

SWAN-GANZ CATHETER (Pulmonary artery catheter): A device used for hemodynamic monitoring, usually in cardiac patients. The catheter can be introduced into the venous system through the subclavian, femoral, or internal jugular vein. It is then advanced to the level of the superior vena cava, then to the right ventricle, and ultimately into the pulmonary artery. The tip of the catheter is flow-directed by an inflatable balloon. The catheter is left in place for continuous monitoring of pulmonary arterial pressure (PAP), cardiac output (CO), and, indirectly, mean left atrial pressure. The Swan-Ganz catheter is available in sizes 5- and 7-French (Fr)

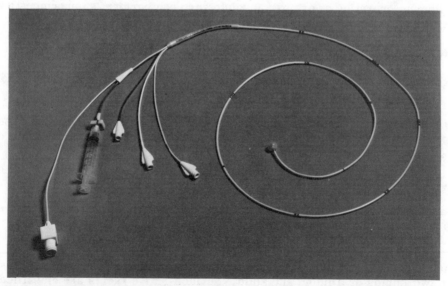

Swan-Ganz Catheter: Multilumen Swan-Ganz catheter with a thermistor channel for calculation of cardiac output. Note the inflated guide balloon at the tip.

for adults (smaller sizes are available for children). The 5-Fr catheter has one pressure lumen at its tip to record PAP, whereas the 7-Fr has two pressure lumens: one at the tip for measuring PAP and one more distally located for measuring central venous pressure (CVP). The catheters come with or without a thermistor which measures CO by the thermal dilution technique. See Fig. See Cardiac output.

SWEATING: See Diaphoresis.

SYMPATHETIC NERVE BLOCK: A class of regional anesthetic injections which interrupt transmission in sympathetic fibers and produce vasodilation, increased blood flow, and a rise in skin temperature. Since sympathetic fibers are blocked by a very low concentration of local anesthetic, sympathetic block can often be done without affecting sensory or motor nerve fibers. Examples of sympathetic blocks include paravertebral lumbar, celiac, and stellate ganglion. These regional blocks may be performed for diagnostic, therapeutic, or prognostic reasons in the first stage of labor, and are indicated for use in patients with causalgia, peripheral vascular disease, vasospasm, and abdominal pain due to acute or chronic pancreatitis or pancreatic carcinoma. See Autonomic nervous system, Causalgia, Celiac plexus block, Paravertebral lumbar sympathetic block.

SYMPATHETIC NERVOUS SYSTEM: See Autonomic nervous system.

SYMPATHETIC TONE; PARASYMPATHETIC TONE: The basal rates of the activity of the sympathetic and parasympathetic systems, the two components of the autonomic nervous system. Under circumstances which increase or decrease the degree of stimulation of either segment, this tone can be enhanced or decreased. Diethyl ether and cyclopropane are two general anesthetics which maintain or increase sympathetic tone. In addition, the basal level of activity of the sympathetic nervous system is partially regulated by the secretion of epinephrine and norepinephrine.

SYMPATHOLYTIC AGENT: A drug which blocks or reverses the actions of the sympathetic nervous system or sympathomimetic (adrenergic) agents. Phentolamine (Regitine), for example, blocks alpha receptors, thereby counteracting vasoconstriction. See Receptor/receptor site.

SYMPATHOMIMETIC DRUG (ADRENERGIC DRUG): An agent which mimics the pharmacologic effects of adrenergic nerve or adrenal medulla stimulation. Some sympathomimetic drugs interact directly with adrenergic receptors, e.g., epinephrine, norepinephrine, isoproterenol. Other agents act indirectly by stimulating the release of norepinephrine from nerve endings, e.g., amphetamine, ephedrine. Sympathomimetic drugs produce mainly vasoconstriction with some vasodilation and generally increase heart rate and blood pressure. See Epinephrine, Norepinephrine.

SYMPTOM: A subjective sensation reported by a patient and not observable by an examiner. See Sign.

SYNAPSE: The junction between two neurons. Impulses are conducted or transmitted from one nerve cell to another at the synapse. Neurons proximal to the synapse are known as presynaptic whereas those distal to the synapse are postsynaptic. At the synapse there is no direct physical contact between the pre- and postsynaptic neurons. These are separated by a gap of approximately 200-300 angstroms. Axons of the presynaptic neurons release chemical mediators (neurotransmitters) which either block or facilitate impulse transmission. The action of the neurotransmitter is rapidly terminated by either reuptake by the presynaptic membrane or degradation by enzymes in the gap. In the central nervous system two classes of synapses exist: excitatory and inhibitory. Excitatory synapse transmitters, e.g., acetylcholine, cause depolarization in the postsynaptic membrane and thus facilitate impulse transmission, whereas inhibitory synapse transmitters, e.g., gamma-aminobutyric acid (GABA), hyperpolarize the postsynaptic membrane and thus block neurotransmission. See Neuromuscular blockade, assessment of.

SYNCHRONIZATION MODE (SYNCH MODE; CARDIOVERSION SYNCHRONIZATION): An electric modality found on defibrillators used for cardioversion. When activated, the patient's electrocardiogram is constantly monitored and the pulse discharge is synchronized with the electrocardiogram to avoid the peak of the T wave. Synchronization is done to prevent inadvertent ventricular fibrillation. See Cardioversion.

SYNCURINE: See Decamethonium.

SYNDROME: A group of signs and symptoms that consistently appear together to characterize a specific disease entity or abnormality.

SYNERGISM: The combined action of two or more drugs in which the total effect produced is more than the sum of their individual effects. For example, if antibiotic A kills 10,000 bacteria/hr and antibiotic B kills 15,000 bacteria/hr, synergism exists if the concurrent administration of A and B kills more than 25,000 bacteria/hr. See Potentiation, Summation.

SYRINGE: A cylinder with a plunger and a narrow opening at one end to accept the hub of a needle. A syringe may be plastic or glass and is used for injection, withdrawal, or irrigation. The injecting syringe has been used in medicine for about 120 years.

SYROSINGOPINE (SINGOSERP): A drug, closely related to reserpine, which is used as an antihypertensive agent.

SYSTEM, REAL-TIME: See Real-time analysis.

SYSTEMS ANALYSIS: The study of any activity, procedure, or technique to improve the flow of information and increase the rapidity of the operation.

SYSTOLIC PRESSURE: The peak pressure reached in the large arteries due to the contraction of the ventricle.

SYSTOLIC TIME INTERVALS (STI): The breakdown of left ventricular systole into different time phases. These measurements are a noninvasive method to evaluate myocardial ventricular function. The time intervals are defined as follows. (1) The pre-ejection period (PEP) is the time from the onset of electric activity in the ventricle (Q wave) until the beginning ejection of blood. (2) The isovolumic contraction time (ICT) is the time between the start of the ventricular pressure rise to the start of ejection. (3) The left ventricular ejection time (LVET) includes the period from the beginning to the end of ejection. The entire period, from the onset of the Q wave through the end of ejection, is called electromechanical systole (EMS). PEP appears to be an indication of myocardial contractility. The weaker the heart, the longer it takes the ventricle to develop enough pressure to open the aortic valve and begin ejection. PEP encompasses the first derivative of left ventricular pressure measurement (dP/dt), which is a continuous record of the slope of the left ventricular pressure curve and is by itself an index of left heart function. When the contraction is strong, pressure rises quickly, the slope becomes very steep, and the dP/dt is very short. Indirect measurement of STI requires three simultaneous recordings: electrocardiogram, heart sounds, and peripheral pulse wave.

TACHYCARDIA: An abnormally fast heart rate.

TACHYPNEA: An abnormally fast breathing rate.

TALWIN: See Narcotic, Pentazocine.

TANK VENTILATOR: See Iron lung.

TECHNETIUM (^{99}Tc): A radioactive element (gamma-ray emitter) tagged onto another molecule which has an affinity for a particular body site. When injected intravenously, the ^{99}Tc travels to the target organ, e.g., heart, thyroid, liver, and outlines it to a gamma-ray detector placed over the organ. It has been used to outline tumors and differential blood flow patterns.

TEFLURANE: A fluorinated hydrocarbon which has physicochemical properties (except flammability) similar to those of cyclopropane. After limited clinical trials, interest in its use as a general anesthetic ceased due to the high incidence of cardiac arrhythmias seen.

TEGRETOL: See Carbamazepine, Trigeminal neuralgia.

TELEMETRY: The remote recording or evaluation of information. This usually involves an acquisition system at the measurement site which sends data by automatic sensors to a central location. The most typical application in medicine is the electrocardiographic (ECG) portable telemetry unit which converts the ECG signal into a radio signal and broadcasts it to a receiver at a remote location. The patient can actually wear this unit and free movement is possible without physical attachment to an ECG machine.

TEMPERATURE: The amount or degree of hotness or coldness. The temperature of an object determines the direction of heat flow when it is brought into contact with another substance, since heat flows from regions of higher to lower temperatures. Temperature can also be considered as the relative amount of vibration of the individual atoms of a substance; the vibration decreases as the temperature drops. Theoretically, all motion ceases at absolute zero. The concept that relative molecular vibrations account for temperature differentials explains the phenomenom of evaporative cooling. The faster atoms escape into the vapor phase decreasing the average vibration of the remaining atoms. See Celsius scale, Hypothermia.

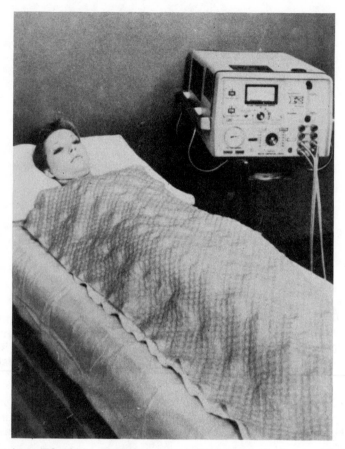

Temperature Blanket: Heating and cooling blanket along with its appropriate control unit.

TEMPERATURE BLANKET (HEATING OR COOLING BLANKET): A device for heating or cooling the body by means of surface application of hot or cold temperatures. A typical temperature blanket is composed of two layers of rubberized material which contain coils for the passage of water or a mixture of alcohol and water. Hoses lead from the blanket back to the heating and cooling machine, which usually has both manual and automatic modes of operation. In the manual mode, the device will either heat or cool the fluid running through the blanket, cycling on and off depending on a preset temperature. In the automatic mode, a probe placed on or in a patient is used to sense body temperature and cycles the device as required. See Fig.

TEMPERATURE COEFFICIENT OF RESISTANCE: A specific physical property of a material which is the amount of electric resistance change per unit temperature change. In general, most materials have a positive coefficient of resistance; as they become hotter, their resistance increases. Semiconductors, however, have a negative coefficient of resistance; their resistance decreases as they become hotter.

TENS: See Transcutaneous electrical nerve stimulation.

TENSILE STRENGTH: The greatest resistance a material can withstand before it is torn.

TENSILON: See Edrophonium.

TENSION: The condition of being taut, strained, stretched, or under pressure.

TENSION OF A GAS: See Partial pressure.

TENSION PNEUMOTHORAX: See Pneumothorax.

TENSION TIME INDEX (TTI): A means for evaluating cardiac function. It is the measurement of the area under the systolic portion of the aortic pressure curve, and is calculated as the mean systolic pressure X duration of systole. This index correlates relatively well with myocardial O_2 consumption. The correlation becomes poorer during exercise, epinephrine administration, or sympathetic activation.

TERATOGENESIS: The formation of a defect, either anatomic, biochemical, or behavioral, initiated in utero and detected at birth or later.

TETANIC CONTRACTION (TETANIZATION): A state in which muscle stimulation occurs so frequently that successive contractions fuse together and cannot be distinguished from one another. Critical frequency is the lowest frequency of stimulation at which tetanization occurs. See Neuromuscular blockade, assessment of.

TETANIC STIMULATION: See Neuromuscular blockade, assessment of.

TETANUS (LOCKJAW): An acute infectious disease characterized by tonic muscular spasms of the jaws and neck. It is caused by the toxin of Clostridium tetani, an anaerobic bacillus. Tetanus has a high mortality rate when untreated. Severe tetanus is one of the few conditions which may be treated primarily by an anesthesiologist because of his or her expertise in the areas of muscle relaxants and ventilatory care.

TETRACAINE HYDROCHLORIDE (AMETHOCAINE; PONTOCAINE): A local anesthetic of the ester series. It can be injected or applied topically. Tetracaine is a highly potent drug (10 times more toxic and active than procaine after intravenous injection) which has a long duration of action. It has a slow onset of action when administered as a caudal anesthetic, but its effects are long-lasting. It is commonly used as a spinal anesthetic and as a topical anesthetic for the eyes, pharynx, and tracheobronchial tree. It is rapidly absorbed through mucous membranes and therefore its use should be limited to small areas. There is a great potential for systemic toxicity. See Local anesthetic.

TETRACYCLINES: A class of broad-spectrum antibiotics which has been used clinically since the late 1940s. The closely related tetracycline derivatives include tetracycline (Tetracyn), chlortetracycline (Aureomycin), oxytetracycline (Terramycin), and doxycycline (Vibramycin). Absorption of tetracyclines is incomplete in the gastrointestinal tract and is impaired by milk and milk products, antacids containing aluminum, and oral iron preparations. Administration of tetracyclines is not recommended for pregnant patients or children under 8 years of age because the drug is specifically stored in the growing bones and teeth. This results in a brown discoloration of teeth as they become calcified. See Fig. See Antibiotic.

TETRAETHYLAMMONIUM (TEA): A ganglionic blocking agent currently of no clinical interest.

TETRALOGY OF FALLOT: A group of congenital cardiac defects including ventricular septal defect, pulmonary artery stenosis, right ventricular hypertrophy, and

Tetracyclines.

Generic Name (Trade Name)	Spectrum of Activity	Comments
Tetracycline (Tetracyn) PO IM IV	Broad spectrum, including G^- and G^+ microbes, Mycoplasma, Treponema, Borrelia, Leptospira, Rickettsia, Chlamydia, and some protozoa, including amebas.	Tetracycline is bacteriostatic except in high concentrations. Its oral absorption is impaired by calcium, oral iron preparations, magnesium, and antacids containing aluminum. All of the tetracyclines are stored in the body in growing bones and teeth, thus should not be given to pregnant women or children under 8 yrs of age. Side effects include hypersensitivity reactions, GI disturbances, photosensitivity, and superinfections that can lead to staphylococcal enterocolitis. Hepatotoxicity can occur with larger doses, as can nephrotoxicity.
Chlortetracycline (Aureomycin)	Similar to tetracycline.	Similar to tetracycline.
Oxytetracycline (Terramycin) PO IM	Similar to tetracycline. It is used in the treatment of amebiasis.	Oxytetracycline shows a high incidence of GI disturbances.
Demeclocycline (Declomycin) PO	Similar to tetracycline.	Demeclocycline shows a high incidence of photosensitivity reactions. It has a longer half-life than tetracycline and is more potent.
Methacycline (Rondomycin) PO	Similar to tetracycline.	Methacycline has a longer half-life.

Drug		
Doxycycline (Vibramycin) PO IV	Similar to tetracycline.	Doxycycline is the best absorbed of the tetracyclines. It has greater potency as well as a longer half-life and duration of action. It does not accumulate in the blood in conditions of renal failure and it has less impact on intestinal flora than the other tetracyclines.
Minocycline (Minocin) PO IV	Similar to tetracycline.	Minocycline has greater potency and a longer half-life than tetracycline. It can cause vestibular toxicity. It appears to be metabolized almost completely in vivo.
Chloramphenicol (Chloromycetin) PO IV	Broad spectrum. It is the drug of choice for treating salmonella infections such as typhoid fever.	Chloramphenicol is primarily bacteriostatic though it can be bactericidal against some species. It easily passes the blood-brain barrier. Of considerable importance is its ability to cause bone marrow depression leading to anemia, pancytopenia, thrombocytopenia, and aplastic anemia. This reaction is not dose-related. Chloramphenicol should not be given to infants under 4 wks old as they lack the enzymes required to metabolize the drug and may develop the "gray syndrome."

Note: Tetracyclines are rarely used intravenously or topically.

overriding aorta. These anomalies are all associated with obstruction of pulmonary outflow to some degree; if severe, the infant may be markedly cyanotic at birth. Most children with this disorder, however, appear cyanotic by 6 months of age.

TETRODOTOXIN (TTX): A marine toxin derived from the Japanese puffer fish, investigated as a possible local anesthetic as it is a highly selective blocker of sodium channels on the exterior of cell membranes. TTX and its derivatives are currently considered too toxic for clinical use.

THALAMUS: A large oval structure located within the diencephalon on either side of the third ventricle. It serves as a relay center for sensory impulses that reach the cerebral cortex from the spinal cord, brain stem, cerebellum, and parts of the cerebrum. The thalamus also aids in the perception of some types of sensation, such as pain and temperature. See Limbic system.

THALASSEMIA: See Anemia.

THALLIUM-201 (^{201}Tl) IMAGING: A nuclear scanning procedure to detect exercise-induced decreased coronary perfusion. The radioisotope ^{201}Tl is injected intravenously at the time of maximum treadmill exercise. Areas of ischemia or scarring of the myocardium appear as defects in the scintigram of the myocardium. After a rest of 4 hr, another image is made of the myocardium. Previous areas of poor perfusion will appear normal, whereas infarcted areas still appear poorly perfused at rest.

THAM: See Tromethamine.

THEBAINE: A natural alkaloid found with morphine and codeine in the poppy plant. It has no current clinical use.

THERAPEUTIC INDEX (THERAPEUTIC RATIO): The ratio of LD_{50} to ED_{50} in animal experiments. The safety of the drug increases as the ratio increases. In clinical situations, however, the therapeutic ratio is the ratio of the TD_{50} (toxic dose 50%) to the ED_{50}. The estimated TD_{50} is used because a precise determination is both hazardous and unethical and therefore experimentally impossible. See ED_{50}, LD_{50}.

THERAPEUTIC NERVE BLOCK: The injection of a local anesthetic around a nerve in order to treat disease or alleviate pain. An example of a therapeutic nerve block would be the injection of a local anesthetic into the chest wall to relieve the pain from fractured ribs. See Sympathetic nerve block.

THERAPEUTIC RANGE: The plasma concentration of a drug with which a satisfactory pharmacologic response (minimal or absent toxicity) is achieved.

THERMISTOR: A semiconductor that has a large negative coefficient of resistance. As it is warmed, more current flows through it. A thermistor can be used for temperature measurement or as a controlling unit in electronic circuits. See Swan-Ganz catheter, Temperature coefficient of resistance.

THERMOCOUPLE (THERMAL JUNCTION): A junction of two dissimilar metals across which an electric potential is produced when the metals are kept at different temperatures. The potential difference is proportional to the temperature difference, and thermocouples can therefore be used to quantify this difference. If a voltage is applied across the junction of two metals, heat is discharged or absorbed (the Peltier effect). Reversing the direction of the voltage reverses this effect. The Seebeck effect is an electromotive force produced when two junctions of dissimilar metals are at varying temperatures in the same circuit. A thermopile is a number of junctions connected together to increase sensitivity of the thermocouple.

THERMODILUTION: A technique used to measure ventricular blood volume and cardiac output in which a cold solution is injected and temperature sampled by a thermistor. See Cardiac output, Swan-Ganz catheter.

THERMOMETER, CLINICAL: An instrument used to determine body temperature. It operates by the expansion of a mercury column along a scale. It is calibrated between 94 and 108 degrees Fahrenheit or between 35 and 42 degrees Celsius.

THERMOPILE: See Thermocouple.

THIAMYLAL (SURITAL): An ultrashort-acting barbiturate with pharmacologic properties similar to thiopental. See Barbiturate, Thiopental sodium.

THIAZIDES: A group of diuretic agents useful in the control of hypertension and edema. These agents are to be used with caution in the diabetic patient. In addition, they tend to increase uric acid levels and induce hypokalemia. Serum potassium levels should be monitored closely and potassium supplementation may be necessary.

THIETHYLPERAZINE (TORECAN): A phenothiazine derivative currently useful as an antiemetic agent. See Phenothiazine.

THIOPENTAL SODIUM (PENTOTHAL): An oxybarbiturate used primarily as an intravenous anesthetic agent. Currently considered the standard induction agent to which other agents are compared, its action on the brain is enhanced because it is highly lipid-soluble and readily crosses the blood-brain barrier. Thiopental depresses both brain metabolism and O_2 consumption and it appears to protect the brain against anoxic insult. Its central nervous system action is thought to terminate mainly by redistribution out of the brain rather than by metabolism. See Barbiturate.

THIOXANTHENE: A group of antipsychotic drugs similar to the phenothiazine derivatives. Chlorprothixene (Taractan) and thiothixene (Navane) are examples of thioxanthene derivatives. See Antipsychotic agent.

THIRD SPACE: The body fluid volume that is not intracellular fluid (first space) or extracellular fluid (second space) but rather is sequestered to some degree so that it cannot easily interact with either. Significant third space fluid is seen in massive ascites, crush injuries, and burns. It is also present in the peritoneum, bowel wall, and lumen of the gastrointestinal tract during abdominal surgery. Third space volume is extremely variable and depends on the extent and duration of surgery or trauma. Significant third space volume causes difficulty in the fluid and electrolyte management of patients. As this fluid is within the body, it ultimately must be mobilized and returned to the circulation so that it can be suitably redistributed or excreted. In acute situations, however, since it is not available to the circulation, this fluid may have to be replaced immediately.

THOMSEN DISEASE: See Myotonia congenita.

THOROUGHFARE CHANNEL: See Microcirculation.

THORPE TUBE: See Flowmeter.

THRESHOLD: The point at which a stimulus just begins to elicit a response. For example, a nerve membrane threshold is the state of membrane polarization just prior to depolarization.

THRESHOLD BLOCK: See Wedensky effect.

THROMBOCYTOPENIA: A condition in which there is a decrease in the number of platelets. Thrombocytopenia can be the result of decreased production (from cytotoxic chemotherapeutic agents), increased destruction (disseminated intravascular coagulation), defective maturation (vitamin B_{12} or folate deficiency; myeloproliferative disorders; Wiskott-Aldrich syndrome), altered distribution (massive splenomegaly), or antibody-mediated thrombocytopenia (autoantibodies; alloantibodies). See Platelet.

THROMBOPHLEBITIS: An inflammation of the wall of a vein associated with the formation of a thrombus. In the practice of anesthesia, thrombophlebitis is most commonly seen in veins which have been used for the infusion of drugs with irritating qualities, such as thiopental and diazepam. Thrombophlebitis may also be due to blood stasis in the veins of the lower extremities when the patient has been immobile for an extended period of time.

THYROID STEAL: An obsolete anesthesia induction technique for patients with hyperthyroidism. Tribromoethanol (Avertin) was administered to allow the patient to be quietly "stolen" away to the operating room, thereby preventing anxiety which would trigger catecholamine release and the thyroid storm. See Thyroid storm, Tribromoethanol.

THYROID STORM: A complication of hyperthyroid disease characterized by a sudden massive increase in metabolism, leading to an increased O_2 demand, hyperpyrexia, and life-threatening arrhythmias. Treatment includes correction of fluid and electrolyte imbalance and administration of propranolol and possibly a short-acting barbiturate (thiopental sodium). See Thyroid steal.

TIBIAL NERVE PALSY: An iatrogenic injury seen in patients who have been poorly or carelessly positioned on the operating table. The tibial nerve may be compressed against the head of the fibula by stirrups.

TIC DOULOUREUX: See Trigeminal neuralgia.

TIDAL VOLUME (TV): The amount of air which moves into and out of the lungs during each respiratory cycle. See Lung volumes and capacities.

TIME CONSTANT: The time necessary for a physical characteristic to increase by approximately 63% of its full value or to decrease by 37% of its initial value. In respiratory physiology, the time constant is the time required for a 63% washin or washout of a new gas from the lungs.

TIME SHARING: An efficient method of using a computer facility in which several operators have the advantages of a high-speed system without each individual having to own his or her own system. Time sharing often requires the use of data processing buffers. See Data processing buffer.

TIME TENSION INDEX: See Tension time index.

TIME WEIGHTED AVERAGE (TWA) GAS SAMPLING: A method used to determine an average level of trace anesthetic contamination. Ambient atmospheric gas is continuously pumped into an inert bag at a constant low flow rate. The average contamination is determined by analyzing the trace anesthetic concentration in the bag.

TISSUE SOLUBILITY: The quantity of a drug or anesthetic in a tissue at an equilibrium point. The term is often used interchangeably with blood-tissue solubility coefficient.

T_{max}: The time when maximum plasma levels of an administered drug are seen. T_{max} is a composite of rate of absorption and rate of elimination.

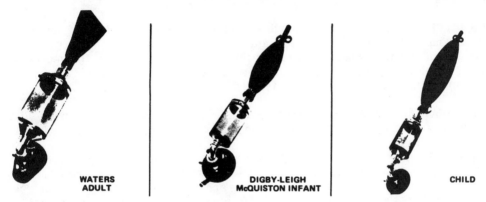

WATERS ADULT   DIGBY-LEIGH McQUISTON INFANT   CHILD

To-and-Fro Carbon Dioxide Absorption: Various modifications of the to-and-fro CO_2 absorber.

TO-AND-FRO CARBON DIOXIDE ABSORPTION: An anesthesia system for the rebreathing of expired gas during which nearly all the CO_2 is absorbed. The absorption canister is placed very close to the anesthesia mask or endotracheal tube. Carbon dioxide absorption produces a large amount of heat which does not dissipate well due to the limited space between the canister and the patient. This heat may elevate the patient's temperature. Other disadvantages of the to-and-fro system include the possibility of absorber dust entering the patient's respiratory tract and the system's inadequacy for use in head and neck surgery due to the proximity of the surgical field. Advantages of the system include its low resistance and its simplicity. See Fig.

TOBRAMYCIN (NEBCIN): An antibiotic of the aminoglycoside series useful in treating infections caused by gram-negative organisms. It is closely related to gentamicin, is nephrotoxic and ototoxic, and may enhance neuromuscular blockade. See Aminoglycoside, Antibiotic.

TOCOLYTIC: A class of drugs which slow down or stop labor.

TOKODYNAMOMETER: A device applied to the abdominal wall of the pregnant patient to measure the force of uterine contractions during labor. This force is detected by a variable resistance strain gauge or similar device, and the resultant pressure is converted into an electric signal.

TOLAZOLINE HYDROCHLORIDE (PRISCOLINE): A weak alpha-blocking agent with a direct relaxant effect on vascular smooth muscles. It is a cardiac stimulant and produces tachycardia.

TOLBUTAMIDE (ORINASE): An oral sulfonylurea hypoglycemic agent used to treat adult onset diabetes of the insulin-independent type in patients uncontrolled by diet and unable or unwilling to take insulin. Its use is now controversial as it may have long-term deleterious cardiovascular effects. Tolbutamide may produce an intolerance to alcoholic beverages and various gastrointestinal complaints (less appetite, cramps, nausea, diarrhea). Its use is contraindicated in patients with hepatic or renal insufficiency.

TOLERANCE: The need for increasing amounts of a drug to produce the same therapeutic effect as previously possible with lower doses.

TOMOGRAPHY: A radiologic technique for forming an x-ray picture of one plane or section through a body part. The technique involves moving both the x-ray tube and the film simultaneously with the theoretic pivot being at the level of the section desired. This blurs all other structures above and below the section while leaving the plane of interest in focus. See Computerized axial tomography.

TOMOMANIA: A morbid and unnatural desire to be operated on or, alternately, the tendency for a surgeon to perform an unnecessary operation for a minor ailment.

TONOMETER: A device used to measure pressure or tension. Tonometers may be used to bring a blood specimen into equilibrium with a known concentration of gas. This is usually done in a vibrating or rotating spherical glass cylinder. The resultant sample of blood can then be used to calibrate or check the accuracy of an instrument. Mechanical tonometers are also used to determine intraocular pressure.

TOOTH: A hard, bony projection located in the maxillary and mandibular alveolar ridges of the oral cavity. Teeth are necessary for mastication and proper speech. Enamel, an extremely hard inorganic substance, covers the dentin of the tooth crown. Teeth can be damaged by endotracheal tubes during instrumentation for anesthesia. Claims of tooth injury are one of the leading causes of malpractice actions against anesthetists and anesthesiologists. See Fig.

TOPICAL ANESTHESIA: The application of an anesthetic agent directly on the surface to produce numbness or loss of sensation. A local anesthetic spray is used to anesthetize the hypopharynx prior to intubation. Uncontrolled absorption of a systemically active drug is a rare complication of topical anesthetic application.

TORECAN: See Thiethylperazine.

TORQUEMETER: See Dynamometer.

TORR: A unit of measurement for pressure equal to 1/760 normal atmospheric pressure. One torr is equal to the pressure needed to support a column of mercury 1 mm high at 0 degrees Celsius and standard gravity on earth (1 torr = 1 mmHg). On other planets torr would be different.

TORT: A wrong done by one individual to another individual which may be addressed in a civil action.

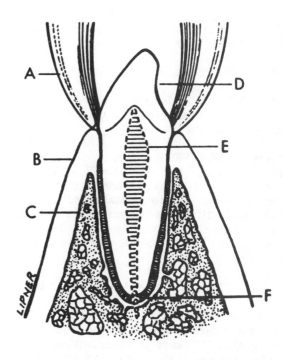

Tooth: Tooth about to be extracted showing the anatomic relationship with the bony structures of the alveolus. (A) Forceps; (B) gingiva; (C) alveolar process; (D) tooth crown; (E) root canal; and (F) root apex.

TOTAL PERIPHERAL RESISTANCE (TPR): A derived value representing the resistance to flow in the cardiovascular system. In a normal cardiovascular system, arteriolar tone accounts for 60% of the TPR. Clinically, TPR = mean arterial pressure - central venous pressure ÷ cardiac output X 80 (TPR = MAP - CVP/CO X 80).

TOTAL SPINAL, ACCIDENTAL: A feared complication of a spinal anesthetic in which all or nearly all nerve trunks from the spinal cord are blocked. The direct effects can include massive peripheral blood pooling (due to sympathetic blockade), loss of circulating catecholamines (denervation of the adrenals), loss of the sympathetic nerves affecting cardiac rate (sympathetic blockade of T3-T5), and loss of intercostal and diaphragm motion (block of thoracic motor nerves and the cervical plexus). A total spinal can present as respiratory and circulatory collapse. The patient should survive if appropriate cardiopulmonary resuscitation is performed.

TOURNIQUET: A device which provides circumferential pressure around a limb to prevent bleeding to or from a distal area. The tourniquet is used during the procedure of exsanguinating a limb (starting at the distal end, progressively wrapping a constrictive band further and further up the limb until the tourniquet site is reached). The current operating room tourniquet is a stiff rubber bladder which is inflated by O_2 or N_2 to a pressure considerably above arterial blood pressure so that the transmission of pressure through muscle mass will block even the deeper vessels. Tourniquets are dangerous if left on too long (>1-2 hr) because nerve trunk compression impedes nerve blood supply and, depending on time and degree, can lead to permanent destruction. Muscles, bones, ligaments, and tendons tolerate hypoxia better than large nerves. Upon the release of the tourniquet, a phenomenon known as reactive hyperemia (the opening and filling of all the vascular beds in the limb), which results in tissue swelling, is frequently seen. Patients with sickle cell disease or sickle cell trait, whose limbs may not be totally exsanguinated before application of the tourniquet, pose a functional problem. Any red blood cells remaining in the limb may sickle with red cell clumping. These acidotic red cell masses return to the central circulation when the tourniquet is released and can cause severe cardiac arrhythmias.

TOXICITY: The quality of being poisonous.

TOXIFERINE: A derivative of curare and a potent neuromuscular blocking agent not used in clinical practice. It may have been an active ingredient in the original South American arrow poisons.

TRACE ANESTHETIC: The level of anesthetic gas too low to produce overt effects. However, these levels are implicated in the decreased performance in operating room (OR) and dental personnel and the observed increase in stillbirths, spontaneous abortions, and congenital defects of offspring in these individuals as well. The National Institute for Occupational Safety and Health (NIOSH) has proposed a standard for trace anesthetics in ORs of less than 25 parts per million (ppm) for N_2O, 0.5 ppm for halogenated agents, and 2 ppm for halogenated agents when used with O_2 alone.

TRACE FREEZE CAPABILITY (FREEZE TRACE): See Oscilloscope, Shift register.

TRACHEOESOPHAGEAL FISTULA WITH ESOPHAGEAL ATRESIA: A combination of two serious congenital anomalies which usually occur together (although each may occur alone). There is a discontinuation of the esophagus (a blind proximal pouch) and an opening from near the carina to the lower esophageal segment. In the normal fetus, the tracheobronchial tree separates from the primitive foregut during the third to sixth week of life in utero. Interference with the vascular supply of the esophagus occurring during this time apparently results in atresia of the esophagus, whereas failure of a complete separation results in a fistula between the trachea and esophagus. The neonate exhibits excessive salivation and nasal secretions. Coughing and cyanosis are evident when these secretions enter the trachea. In addition hydrochloric acid from the gastric contents may enter the lungs causing a chemical

CONGENITAL ESOPHAGEAL ANOMALIES

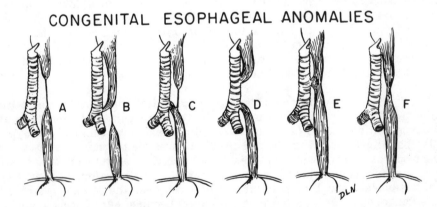

Tracheoesophageal Fistula: Types of congenital esophageal anomalies. (A) Esophageal atresia; (B) esophageal atresia with a proximal segment communicating with the trachea; (C) esophageal atresia with a distal segment communicating with the trachea (approximately 90% of the anomaly occurs with this configuration); (D) esophageal atresia with both segments communicating with the trachea; (E) esophagus has no atresia, but a fistula does exist through the trachea; and (F) esophageal stenosis but no communication with the trachea.

pneumonia, the most severe complication of this disorder. A 30% incidence of other abnormalities, particularly imperforate anus, other gastrointestinal atresias, and heart disease, occur in infants with tracheoesophageal fistula and esophageal atresia. Treatment begins at birth with the correction of fluid and electrolyte imbalances and respiratory and acid-base abnormalities, followed by the surgical repair of the fistula. The presence of aspiration or chemical pneumonia renders surgery extremely hazardous or impossible. See Fig.

TRACHEOSTOMY: An exterior opening into the trachea created therapeutically to bypass an obstructed airway. Under controlled circumstances, the opening is usually made below the level of the first tracheal ring. For emergencies, it is recommended that the opening be created in the membrane between the thyroid and cricoid cartilages in the neck (a surgical procedure known as cricothyrotomy). See Larynx.

TRACKING: The ability of a device to precisely reflect changes in the parameter it is monitoring. For example, an electrocardiograph machine may not track very rapid atrial fibrillations. The changes are made too quickly and are of such low magnitude that they are ignored by the device.

TRACTION REFLEX: The phenomenon of hypotension following traction on intra-abdominal structures such as the gallbladder, appendix, uterus, or stomach. It appears to be mediated by the autonomic nervous system.

TRADEMARK (TRADE NAME): A name or symbol identifying a product. It is registered by the government and legally restricted to use by its owner. For example, Fluothane is the trademark for halothane produced by Ayerst laboratories. No other firm may call its halothane Fluothane.

TRAIN OF FOUR: See Neuromuscular blockade, assessment of.

TRANQUILIZER: A pharmacologic agent used to promote peace of mind or a more placid outlook on life. The mechanism of action remains obscure. Tranquilizers may be classified as major (antipsychotic) or minor (antianxiety) agents. See Antipsychotic agents, Anxiety, Benzodiazepine, Phenothiazine.

TRANSCUTANEOUS ELECTRICAL NERVE STIMULATION (TENS): A technique used for the control of pain in which the skin associated with an injured area or its nerve supply is stimulated by an electric current of various frequencies, waveforms, current densities, or pulse widths. This treatment has been shown to be beneficial to 15-50% of patients. It is considered an empiric form of therapy and is believed to have an extremely low complication rate. It is relatively inexpensive and enables the patient to be in control of his or her own therapy. The basis for the use of TENS is the gate theory of pain, which hypothesizes that the transmission of pain impulses can be interrupted and the perception of pain altered by appropriate stimulation of sites other than the site of origin of the pain. See Gate theory of pain.

TRANSCUTANEOUS MONITORING: A noninvasive technique in which a sensor is attached to the skin surface containing a heating element and an O_2 or CO_2 electrode. The heating element is precisely controlled to warm the skin surface under the sensor, thereby dilating blood vessels and causing gas to diffuse through the skin and underlying tissue. This gas is measured by the electrode. Under the best circumstances (good peripheral circulation, no hypothermia, normal hematocrit, normal systolic pressure, and PaO_2 in the range of 60-100 torr), there is good correlation between the transcutaneous PO_2 measurement and the PaO_2 measurement. Transcutaneous measurement of PCO_2 has a poor correlation to $PaCO_2$. See Noninvasive monitor.

TRANSDUCER: A device which converts a nonelectric parameter such as light, pressure, or sound into an electric signal. See Fig.

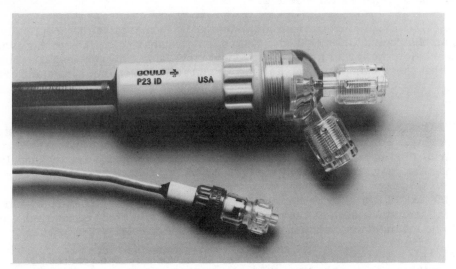

Transducer: Conventional and miniature transducers.

TRANSFILLING: The extremely hazardous practice of refilling gas cylinders from other cylinders. The danger involves the rapid recompression of any gas which may remain in the emptied cylinder, causing a dramatic increase in temperature and resulting in an explosion. All modern anesthesia systems contain check valves which prevent crossfilling (a type of transfilling) between small cylinders which are otherwise connected. See Adiabatic.

TRANSFORMER: An electric device for changing voltage in an alternating current circuit. The input side (primary coil) and the output side (secondary coil) are coupled by the magnetic fields produced when current flows through a coil of wire. The voltage change is proportional to the number of turns in the coils. A primary with 10 turns and a secondary with 100 turns will charge 20-200 V. For both sides, however, the product of voltage times current will remain the same. Some losses will occur due to the inefficiency of magnetic transfer so that the current times the voltage of the secondary side will be slightly less.

TRANSFUSION FILTER: A particulate filter added to transfusion lines to prevent small debris from entering the circulation. The standard in-line filter has a pore size of 170 μm whereas add-on types can filter particles down to 20 μm in size; however, the latter tend to slow transfusion rates.

TRANSFUSION REACTION: See Blood types.

TRANSFUSION THERAPY: The direct introduction of fluids into the circulation to restore the volume and functional elements of the blood. Transfusion therapy is divided into three categories: (1) restoration of circulatory volume to maintain adequate cardiac output, (2) restoration of O_2-carrying capacity, and (3) restoration of

Transfusion Therapy: Parenteral infusion solutions.

Solutions	Electrolyte Content (mEq/L)								Glucose (g/L)
	Na^+	K^+	Ca^{2+}	Mg^{2+}	NH_4^+	Cl^-	HCO_3^- equiv*	PO_4^{2-}	
Glucose (5%) in water									50
Glucose (10%) in water									100
Isotonic saline (0.9%)	155					155			
Sodium chloride (5%)	855					855			
Ringer solution	147	4	4			155			
Ringer lactate (Hartmann)	130	4	3			109	28		
Dorrow solution (KNL)	121	35				103	53		
Potassium chloride									
0.2% in 5% dextrose		27				27			50
0.3% in 5% dextrose		40				40			50
Modified duodenal solution with 10% dextrose	80	36	5	3		64	60		100
Gastric solution with 10% dextrose	63	17			70	150			100
Ammonium chloride (0.9%)					170	170			
Sodium lactate (1/6 molar)	167						167		
Sodium bicarbonate (1/6 molar)	167						167		
Examples of "maintenance solutions":									
Pediatric electrolyte									
"No 48" with 5% dextrose	25	20		3		22	23	3	50
Maintenance electrolyte									
"No 75" with 5% dextrose	40	35				40	20	15	50
Levulose and dextrose with electrolyte (Butler II)	58	25		6		51	25	13	100
Dextrose (5%) in 0.2% saline	34					34			50
Dextrose (10%) in 0.45% saline	77					77			100

* HCO_3^- equivalent may be lactate, acetate, gluconate, citrate, or a combination.

clotting factors. Volume replacement can consist of crystalloid or colloid solutions. Crystalloids, e.g., lactated Ringer solution or 0.9% sodium chloride solution, are clear fluids containing dissolved inorganic salts which diffuse easily across semipermeable membranes. Ringer solution is considered a balanced salt solution because its inorganic salts are similar to the normal ratios of those found within the body. Colloids, e.g., albumin, plasma protein precipitate, dextrans, or hetastarch, contain large molecules that are not freely diffusible across semipermeable membranes. Crystalloids distribute themselves out of the circulating volume in a short period of time and attain a distribution ratio between extracellular fluid and intravascular fluid of approximately 2:1 or 3:1. In contrast, colloids remain in the circulation until metabolic degradation or further hemorrhage occurs. Therefore, the practical consideration in volume expansion of the circulation is that crystalloids must be given in a volume 2-3 times that required to return the circulating volume to normal, whereas colloids may be given on a 1:1 replacement basis. The O_2-carrying capacity is restored with packed red blood cells. (Currently, artificial solutions are being studied as substitutes for red blood cells.) The functioning red cell increases the O_2-carrying capacity of the blood 10-fold compared with simple O_2 dissolution in serum. If volume is replaced, the otherwise normal individual can withstand an acute loss of at least 20% of his circulating red cell mass before significant compromise is evident. Restoration of clotting factor is possible by administering platelet concentrates, fresh whole blood, or fresh frozen plasma. Usually clotting factors are in such abundance in normal blood that serious bleeding or dilution by massive transfusion must take place before clotting factors drop to such low concentrations as to cause a loss of clotting ability. See Fig. See Albumin, Blood storage, Dextran, Hetastarch, Third space.

TRANSILLUMINATION: The technique of passing a very bright light source through body tissues to allow visualization of subcutaneous structures. Transillumination has been used for many years in viewing air-fluid levels in the sinuses and has recently been used to identify blood vessels lying deep beneath the skin in the limbs of infants and young children in order to expedite percutaneous puncture.

TRANSMISSION: The movement of transfer of an impulse, disease, genetic trait(s), or signal from one location or individual to another.

TRANSMURAL PRESSURE: The pressure difference between the inside and outside of a vessel. See Laplace law.

TRANSPLANTATION: The transfer or grafting of tissue from one location to another. Organ transplantation involves removing a donor organ and transferring it to a recipient. Inherent in the procedure is the removal of the diseased organ from the recipient and the assurance of an adequate vascular connection to the donor organ. Transplantation may involve genetically dissimilar tissue from the same species (allogeneic) or genetically identical tissue (autologous or syngeneic). A xenograft or heterograft is a graft of tissue involving individuals of two different species.

TRANSPORT: The movement of biochemical substances across cell membranes. Passive transport occurs in response to concentration gradients. Active transport occurs when a substance is aided in its passage through a membrane, at times in the face of a reverse concentration gradient. For example, the "sodium pump" of the nerve cell membrane actively moves sodium from the inside to the outside of the membrane in direct opposition to a charge gradient that favors sodium remaining on the inside of the cell.

TRANSTRACHEAL ANESTHESIA: The injection of local anesthetic into the lumen of the trachea via the cricothyroid membrane to produce a cough which will effectively spread the anesthetic. This technique provides excellent topical anesthesia of the larynx and trachea; however, it may initiate bronchospasm.

TRANSURETHRAL RESECTION OF PROSTATE (TURP): A surgical procedure, performed through a cystoscope, for the treatment of benign prostatic hypertrophy. The adenomatous tissue of the prostate is removed up to the false capsule with an electrosurgery loop under direct vision. (The entire prostate is not removed.) The TURP poses unique anesthetic problems in that continuous irrigation to keep the surgical field clear is necessary. This irrigating fluid enters the circulation via the many blood vessels opened and then sealed by the electrosurgery loop, and may cause acute circulatory overload. There is, therefore, a strict time limit of 1 hr for the entire surgical procedure. Another complication is the possibility of perforation of the bladder, causing air and fluid to enter the abdominal cavity. This causes a great deal of pain (often referred to the shoulder) in the patient who has received a spinal anesthetic. In the patient who has received a general anesthetic for the procedure, a bladder perforation is difficult to detect and significant abdominal distention may occur before the problem is recognized. See Referred pain.

TREND ANALYSIS: A technique for evaluating accumulated data, in an effort to determine whether or not a patient is improving or is remaining stable. A single observation of a patient's condition may not be sufficient for accurate evaluation.

TRIAMTERENE (DYRENIUM): An oral diuretic agent usually used in combination with the thiazide diuretics. It causes mild sodium excretion and mild potassium retention.

TRIBROMOETHANOL (AVERTIN): A rectally administered general anesthetic used clinically in the 1920s. Drug dose is calculated according to the patient's weight and is given by enema. Respiratory depression occurs in approximate proportion to dose. Tribromoethanol is reported to aggravate liver and renal disease. It is not used routinely at the present time.

TRICHLOROETHANOL: See Chloral hydrate.

TRICHLOROETHYLENE (TRILENE; TRIMAR): A nonflammable, colorless (coloring is sometimes added to distinguish it from chloroform), liquid general anesthetic which is extremely potent due to its very high gas/oil solubility coefficient. It has a low vapor pressure and is unstable. It decomposes into phosgene and hydrochloric acid when exposed to light or heat and therefore should not be used in systems containing soda lime absorbers. Impure trichloroethylene has been associated with cranial nerve palsies, particularly affecting the fifth cranial nerve. It is currently used to produce analgesia in obstetrics and in dentistry, but its use appears to be decreasing in the United States.

TRICHLOROFLUOROMETHANE: See Freon.

TRICYCLIC ANTIDEPRESSANT: A drug used to treat depression. Examples of tricyclic antidepressants include imipramine (Tofranil), amitriptyline (Amitril, Elavil), doxepin (Adapin, Sinequan), desipramine (Norpramin), nortriptyline (Aventyl, Pamelor), and protriptyline (Vivactil). These drugs can cause cardiovascular abnormalities such as tachycardia, some arrhythmias, prolongation of conduction time, and alpha blockade. They can also add to the central sedation effect of central nervous system depressants. Severe arrhythmias can result from the combination of halothane pancuronium and the tricyclics. See Fig.

402

Tricyclic Antidepressant.

Generic Name (Trade Name)	Structure	Comments
A. Tricyclic Antidepressants		The tricyclic antidepressants have an onset of action of 1-3 wks and their side effects include atropine-like effects due to their anticholinergic action, orthostatic hypotension, sedation, tachycardia, arrhythmias, and prolongation of AV conduction time. They also may block the antihypertensive action of guanethidine.
Amitriptyline HCl (Elavil)	$CHCH_2CH_2N(CH_3)_2$	Amitryptyline has significant sedative properties while having lower incidence of atropine-like effects than other tricyclics.
Nortriptyline HCl (Aventyl)	$CHCH_2CH_2NHCH_3$	Nortriptyline demonstrates moderate sedation while still possessing some sedative properties.
Doxepin HCl (Adapin)	$CHCH_2CH_2N(CH_3)_2$	Doxepin has a moderate sedative effect and is used as both an antianxiety and antidepressant agent.
Protriptyline HCl (Vivactil)	$CH_2CH_2CH_2NHCH_3$	Protriptyline lacks sedative and tranquilizing properties. It has a more rapid onset of action than the other tricyclics and is particularly suited for withdrawn, lethargic, and depressed patients. There are more cardiovascular effects than with the other tricyclics.

Trimipramine HCL (Surmontil)

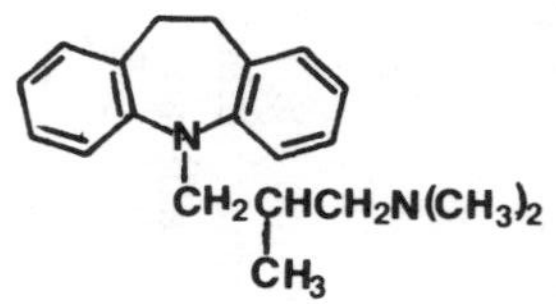

Imipramine HCl (Tofranil)

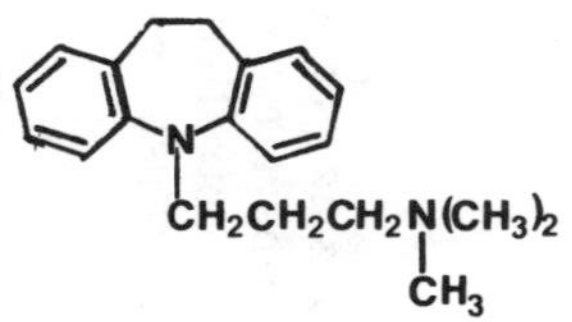

Desipramine HCl (Norpramin)

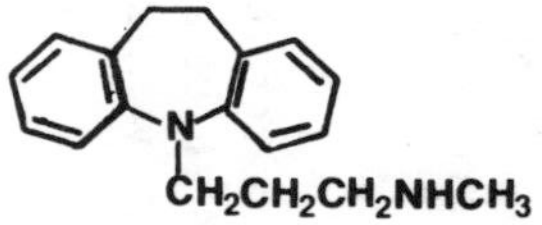

B. MAO Inhibitors

1. Hydrazine MAO Inhibitors

   Isocarboxazid (Marplan)
   Phenelzine (Nardil)

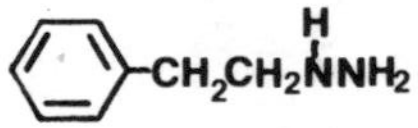

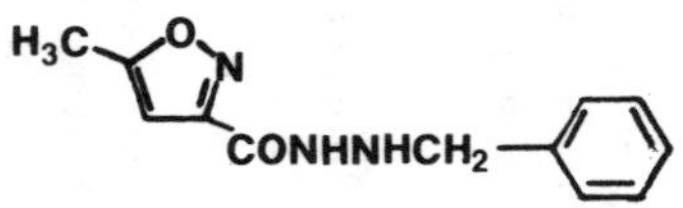

2. Non-Hydrazine MAO Inhibitors

   Tranylcypromine (Parnate)

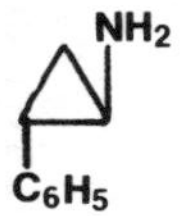

Trimipramine is used for the treatment of mild depression.

Imipramine is less sedative than amitryptiline and doxepin. It is used for the treatment of bed-wetting in children.

Desipramine has sedative properties like nortriptyline.

The hydrazine MAO inhibitors have a slow onset of action (2–4 wks) and may cause hepatotoxicity. The non-hydrazine MAO inhibitors have a direct amphetamine-like stimulant action, a faster onset of action than the hydrazine.

MAO inhibitors may or may not cause hepatotoxicity. MAO inhibitors as a class can cause excessive central stimulation, orthostatic hypotension, insomnia, constipation, and paradoxical behavior. They are contraindicated in patients taking meperidine as cardiovascular collapse can occur. Severe hypertension reactions can occur when cheese or other tyramine-containing foods are ingested during tranylcypromine therapy.

TRIFLUOPERAZINE HYDROCHLORIDE (STELAZINE): A tranquilizer of the phenothiazine group. See Phenothiazine.

TRIFLUOROETHYL VINYL ETHER: See Fluroxene.

TRIGEMINAL NERVE: The fifth cranial nerve. See Cranial nerves.

TRIGEMINAL NEURALGIA (TIC DOULOUREUX): A painful disturbance (usually without organic cause) in the function of the fifth cranial nerve. It can occur in any of the three divisions of the nerve, and is frequently described as the worst possible human pain. Carbamazepine (Tegretol) is used to treat this condition but frequent adverse reactions limit its usefulness. The only definitive treatment is surgical de-afferentation of the affected nerve root. This technique may be implemented as a last resort in a patient disabled by pain due to the permanent sensory loss and, depending on the root involved, the motor complications it produces. See Carbamazepine.

TRIGGER CIRCUIT: A specific electric circuit which has the characteristic of having no output until its input waveform exceeds a specific parameter. When this occurs, the trigger "fires" a constant output. This circuit is often used to initiate an oscilloscope sweep when the QRS complex is detected across the screen.

TRIGGER POINT: See Myofascial syndrome.

TRIGGERED VENTILATION: The mode of operation of a ventilator in which the initial negative pressure generated in the air passageways at the start of patient inhalation activates ventilator function. The sensitivity of the ventilator is usually adjustable.

TRILENE: See Dichloroacetylene, Trichloroethylene.

TRIMAR: See Trichloroethylene.

TRIMETHAPHAN (ARFONAD): A very short-acting, nondepolarizing ganglionic blocking agent which is administered intravenously to produce deliberate controlled hypotension during some surgical procedures. It is not as easily controlled as nitroprusside which has replaced it. In addition, trimethaphan may cause respiratory depression and tachycardia.

TRIPLE POINT OF WATER: The point on a pressure-temperature plot where the lines representing the solid, liquid, and vapor phases of water intersect.

TRIS: See Tromethamine.

TROCAR: See Cannula.

TROMETHAMINE (THAM, TRIS): A synthetic buffer solution useful as an alternative drug to sodium bicarbonate in the treatment of metabolic acidosis. Its use is advocated when an acute sodium load is inappropriate. Tromethamine, also known as TRIS [tris(hydroxymethyl)aminomethane], is contraindicated during pregnancy or for patients with uremic or chronic respiratory acidosis. It is also available in powder form (THAM-E).

TRUE CAPILLARY: See Microcirculation.

t TEST: See Student t test.

TUBOCURARINE CHLORIDE; D-TUBOCURARINE (TUBARINE): The class leader of the nondepolarizing neuromuscular blocking drugs. Tubocurarine is the active ingredient in curare. Introduced into the clinical practice of anesthesia during the 1940s, it rapidly became popular as an adjunct to anesthesia for the production of muscle flaccidity. The diaphragm is thought to be partially resistant to curare, this being the so-called respiratory sparing effect of the drug. The drug appears to cause some ganglionic blockade and histamine release. It can therefore produce profound hypotension. Moderate hypothermia diminishes the effect of curare (and other nondepolarizing muscle relaxants), whereas profound hypothermia greatly intensifies it. Equipment for artificial ventilation must be available whenever the drug is used. See Neuromuscular blockade, assessment of.

TUOHY NEEDLE: A large-bore (12- to 19-gauge) needle with a curved tip used in epidural blocks. See Epidural needle.

TURBULENT FLOW: A type of disorderly fluid flow through a vessel or container in which all the molecules tend to move at approximately the same velocity. Turbulence increases when fluid flow velocity and/or vessel lumen increase. It decreases as fluid viscosity increases. These relationships are used to calculate the Reynolds number. See Laminar flow, Reynolds number.

TURP: See Transurethral resection of prostate.

TWEEN 20; TWEEN 80: The nonionic chemical agents of low molecular weight which markedly decrease surface tension.

TWILIGHT SLEEP: See Scopolamine.

TWITCH RESPONSE: See Neuromuscular blockade, assessment of.

TWO-TAILED TEST: An evaluation of a hypothesis that is concerned with values above and below the mean. This evaluation is in contrast to the one-tailed test, which is concerned with values either above or below the mean. Both one- and two-tailed tests are only valid for large samples.

TYMPANIC MEMBRANE TEMPERATURE: A monitoring technique for temperature in which a small thermocouple is placed in the ear near the tympanic membrane. The temperature of the tympanic membrane is thought to be closely associated with the temperature of the brain. Difficulties associated with the technique involve possible puncture of the membrane and excessive ear wax which can preclude proper measurement.

TYPE I ERROR: The type of error that occurs when one rejects a null hypothesis although it is true. See Null hypothesis.

TYPE II ERROR: The type of error that occurs when one accepts a null hypothesis although it is false. See Null hypothesis.

U

ULTRASONIC FETAL HEART RATE DETERMINATION: See Fetal monitor.

ULTRASONIC FLOWMETER: See Blood flow, methods for measuring.

ULTRASONIC NEBULIZER: See Nebulizer.

ULTRASOUND: The sounds above the human hearing range in frequency. See Doppler effect, Sound.

ULTRASOUND, DIAGNOSTIC: A noninvasive method to evaluate tissue density differences associated with certain disorders. Diagnostic ultrasound is valuable in assessing the size and location of cysts, effusions, and tumors. It can also be used to evaluate fetal development. Its efficacy is based on the patterns of sound reflection caused by different layers of tissue. See Sound.

UNDERWRITER LABORATORY (UL): An organization which investigates products for safety at the expense of the requesting manufacturers. Departments of UL include Burglary Protection, Casualty and Chemical Hazard, Electrical, Fire Protection, Heating, Air Conditioning and Refrigeration, and Marine. The UL was organized by William Merrill, called the Underwriter's Electrical Bureau, and incorporated in 1901. Its headquarters are in Northbrook, Illinois.

UNITARY HYPOTHESIS OF ANESTHESIA: The theory which states that the mechanism of action at the molecular level is the same for all inhalation anesthetics.

UNIVERSAL VAPORIZER: See Vaporizer.

UNIVERSAL VAPORIZER OUTPUT CALCULATION (MEASURED FLOW VAPORIZER CALCULATION): The technique for determining the anesthetic concentration in a fresh gas supply to which the output of a measured flow vaporizer has been added. The computation requires the amount of O_2 flowing to the vaporizer, the vapor pressure of the liquid anesthetic at the temperature of the vaporizer, and the total of all other flows.

UPTAKE: The process by which a drug is combined with the blood. The drug may be administered by an intravenous, intramuscular, oral, or inhalation route. Uptake is primarily concerned, however, with the speed of transfer of gaseous anesthetics from the alveolar gas into the alveolar capillary blood.

URECHOLINE: See Bethanechol chloride.

UREMIA: A condition caused by the presence of waste products in the blood which should normally be excreted in the urine. Signs and symptoms include lethargy, weight loss, vomiting, anemia, pruritis, and an unpleasant taste in the mouth. Uremia is seen in the end-stages of kidney disease or in urinary obstruction.

URETHAN: See Ethyl carbamate.

URTICARIA (HIVES): An allergic manifestation marked by raised, itchy, patchy areas on the skin. It is due to contact with a specific etiologic agent (food, drug, insect, or environmental factor).

UTERINE CONTRACTILITY: The rhythmic movements of uterine smooth muscle which become more pronounced and more frequent as labor progresses. Uterine contractions may be initiated by any of the smooth muscle cells comprising its musculature. No true pacemaker for the uterus exists. When cells of the uterus contract in a tetanic manner, a contracture occurs. This is a rare condition usually resulting from hyperstimulation of the uterus or from excessive administration of oxytocin. It leads to a profound loss of mechanical efficiency and a reduction in uterine blood flow. The halogenated anesthetics are potent depressants of uterine activity, whereas routine doses of morphine and meperidine produce no change in contractility. Nitrous oxide, depending on dose, appears to have no effect or a depressant effect. In general, uterine contractility is independent of direct innervation, but contractions may decrease or stop when afferent impulses to the uterus are blocked early in labor. In the active phase of labor these same doses cause little or no effect on uterine contractility. See Montevideo unit, Oxytocin.

UTEROSACRAL BLOCK: See Paracervical block.

VACUUM TUBE CIRCUITRY: See Circuit, solid state.

VALIDITY: The ability of a test used for screening to demonstrate which individuals of a class of individuals have a particular characteristic and which do not. The two components of validity are sensitivity and specificity. See Sensitivity, Specificity.

VALIUM: The trade name for diazepam. See Benzodiazepine.

VALMID: See Ethinamate.

VALSALVA MANEUVER: Forced expiration against an obstruction such as a closed glottis. The physiologic consequences of the Valsalva maneuver are dramatic. Initially, stimulation of the vagus nerve causes bradycardia, and the increased pressure in the chest prevents cardiac filling. This is followed by a decrease in stroke volume and cardiac output. Tachycardia and elevated blood pressure due to peripheral constriction are present as well. The momentary venous stasis may lead to dramatic increases in intracranial pressure which is deleterious, especially to postoperative neurosurgery patients.

VALVE: A device which regulates flow of liquids or gases in a pipe or duct system.

VALVULAR HEART DISEASE: A condition affecting (singly or together) the aortic, mitral, pulmonic, and/or tricuspid valves of the heart. Valvular heart disease is commonly due to stenosis, in which the valve becomes less pliable resulting in blood flow obstruction and/or regurgitation, i.e., the valve is incapable of closing completely and therefore backflow occurs. Both conditions can occur simultaneously and not to the same extent in any particular valve.

VAPOR: A substance in gaseous form at a temperature below its critical temperature. A vapor can be liquefied by pressure changes without lowering the temperature.

VAPORIZER: A device which converts liquid into vapor. A vaporizer is a necessary component of anesthesia machines in order to convert volatile liquids into anesthetic vapors. A vaporizer can be specific for one agent (precision) or used for any liquid anesthetic agent (universal). Its temperature may be automatically (variable bypass), manually (controlled by anesthetist), or passively compensated. A vaporizer may be located outside the breathing system (out-of-circle) on the back bar in series with the flow column or inside the breathing system (in-circle) in series with the CO_2 absorber. It can bubble gas through a volume of liquid, move gas over the surface of the liquid and/or a wick, or use a combination of both techniques. With a variable bypass vaporizer only a portion of the gas flow to the vaporizer contacts the anesthetic agent. Vaporizers without a variable bypass allow all the gas to contact the anesthetic agent, picking up an unknown amount of anesthetic vapor (determined by temperature, gas flow, and agent partial pressure). See Boyle bottle; Copper kettle; Draw-over vaporizer; EMO inhaler; Goldman vaporizer; Vaporizer, draw-over; flow-over; bubble-through.

VAPORIZER CAPABILITY: The maximal concentration of anesthetic vapor which can be delivered by a vaporizer. In practice, out-of-system or in-system vaporizers used in a nonrebreathing circuit must have a high capability because no additional anesthetic will be added to the gas to be inhaled by the patient.

VAPORIZER CIRCUIT CONTROL VALVE (VCCV): A device used on anesthesia machines containing a built-in vaporizer and requiring a measured O_2 flow (copper kettle, Vernitrol). The VCCV directs O_2 through the vaporizer to the machine outlet.

VAPORIZER CONCENTRATION: See Vaporizer output.

VAPORIZER, DRAW-OVER; FLOW-OVER; BUBBLE-THROUGH: The types of vaporizers which bring fresh gas (the atmosphere or anesthesia machine) into contact with the surface of a volatile liquid anesthetic. The draw-over vaporizer obtains its fresh gas supply from the negative pressure created when the patient inhales, thereby drawing or pulling gas over the surface of the anesthetic. A flow-over vaporizer obtains its fresh gas supply from the positive pressure caused by its in-series attachment to a continuous flow anesthesia machine. The terms draw-over and flow-over are often used interchangeably. In the bubble-through type of vaporizer, the fresh gas flow is placed under the liquid surface. Therefore, equilibration between the liquid and gas is more rapid due to the creation of many bubble/liquid interfaces. See Vaporizer.

VAPORIZER, FLUOMATIC: An agent-specific vaporizer for halothane (Fluothane). It is a variable bypass, flow-over with wick, out-of-system, temperature-compensating vaporizer manufactured by Foregger Company. A similar vaporizer, the Fluotec Mark II (or Mark III), is manufactured by Cyprane Limited. See Fig.

VAPORIZER, IN-CIRCLE: See Vaporizer.

VAPORIZER, OHIO NO.8: A flow-over, variable bypass vaporizer which contains a wick but has no temperature compensation. It is used inside the circle system. The quantity of vapor put out by the unit must be controlled by monitoring the clinical signs.

VAPORIZER, OUT-OF-CIRCLE: See Vaporizer.

VAPORIZER OUTPUT: The concentration of anesthetic vapor at the outlet of a vaporizer. Vaporizer output usually refers to an in-circle vaporizer, in which gas entering the vaporizer already contains a significant percentage of anesthetic vapor. Vaporizer concentration, which refers specifically to vaporizers out of the breathing circuit, is the concentration of vapor delivered by the vaporizer when the fresh

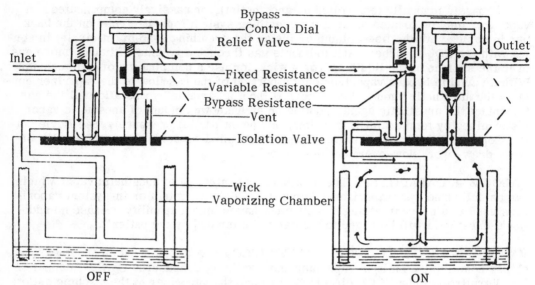

Vaporizer, Fluomatic: Diagrammatic representation of the internal
construction of the Fluomatic Foregger vaporizer.

gas (having no vapor) passes through it. Therefore, vaporizer output is equal to vaporizer concentration in an out-of-circuit system. See Pumping effect; pressure effect.

VAPORIZER, PRECISION (AGENT-SPECIFIC VAPORIZER): See Vaporizer, Fluomatic.

VAPORIZERS, "TEC" SERIES: The precision vaporizers named according to the
specific agent they are designed to vaporize, i.e., Fluotec, Pentec, Ethrec. They
are out-of-system, flow-over with wick, variable bypass, and temperature-compensating. Three model series have been manufactured thus far: Mark I, II, and III.

VAPORIZERS, "VAPOR" SERIES: A group of out-of-circuit, variable bypass, flow-
over with wick, precision vaporizers. The "Vapors" are distributed by North American Drager. They are unique in their manual method of temperature compensation.
The anesthetist can adjust the concentration of the vaporizer and thereby increase
the gas flow as the vaporizing chamber is cooled.

VAPORIZER TEMPERATURE COMPENSATION: The appropriate adjustments or
modifications needed to counterbalance the heat lost during vaporization of an anesthetic liquid. A constant vapor pressure, with a concomitant constant temperature,
is necessary to preserve a stable vapor output. The temperature can be maintained
by passive or active compensation. In passive compensation, a good thermal conductor such as copper is used in the body of a vaporizer to aid in maintaining a stable temperature. These copper vaporizers can be mounted to the copper top of an
anesthesia machine to efficiently transfer heat. In active compensation, a mechanism such as a variable bypass is used to change the amount of gas exposed to the
liquid (useful in out-of-system vaporizers). Only a portion of fresh gas is exposed
to the anesthetic liquid; this portion is increased either by a bimetallic spring-oper-
ated valve or by a manual control as the temperature of the liquid decreases during
vaporization. In active compensation, the vaporizer can also be heated by means of
a water bath or heating coil.

VAPORIZER, UNIVERSAL: See Vaporizer.

VAPOR PRESSURE: The pressure constant exerted by a vapor, at a given temperature, which is in equilibrium with its solid or liquid form. The vapor pressure of a volatile anesthetic agent must be known to determine the inspired concentration of the agent via a bubble-through vaporizer. At room temperature (20 degrees Celsius) the vapor pressure of halothane is 242 mmHg. When a substance is at its boiling point, its vapor pressure equals the atmospheric pressure. See Boiling point, Partial pressure.

VAPOR, SATURATED: The equilibrium point between a liquid and its vapor. Additional liquid can be vaporized only if the temperature is raised.

VARIABLE: A value which is subject to change. For example, in the Henderson-Hasselbalch equation for determining pH, the pK_a is the constant whereas the concentration of bicarbonate is the variable, i.e., it can fluctuate over a wide range and must be directly sampled.

VARIABLE, DEPENDENT: A unit of information or data which changes in relation to another value.

VARIABLE, INDEPENDENT (EXPERIMENTAL VARIABLE): A unit of information which is directly manipulated and controlled by an investigator.

VARIABLE PATTERNS OF FETAL HEART RATE: See Fetal heart rate terminology.

VARIANCE: The square root of the standard deviation (SD). It is a measure of the dispersion of values in a normal distribution. See Standard deviation.

VASCULAR RING: A type of aortic arch malformation in which the trachea and/or the esophagus are compressed within a ringlike vascular (aortic) anomaly. The most common vascular ring is caused by a double aortic arch.

VASOCONSTRICTION: A narrowing of the lumen of a blood vessel. Vasoconstriction may be precipitated by an increased sympathetic nervous system tone, serotonin release by platelets, local metabolic factors (elevated PCO_2, decreased pH), and circulating hormones (epinephrine and norepinephrine). See Autonomic nervous system, Epinephrine, Norepinephrine, Receptor/receptor site.

VASODILATION: A widening of the lumen of a blood vessel. Vasodilation can be produced by central sympathetic blockade (spinal, epidural), by peripheral sympathetic blockade (with ganglionic blocking agents), or by direct action on the vessels by drugs (halothane, nitroprusside). The total effect is to decrease peripheral resistance, decrease blood pressure, and store blood in the peripheral capacitance vessels, thereby causing a decrease in blood return to the heart and a decrease in stroke volume.

VASOMOTOR CENTER: A large, diffuse area, located in the medulla oblongata, which controls the extent of dilatation of the arterial resistance vessels and the venous capacitance vessels by regulating sympathetic tone.

VASOPRESSIN: See Antidiuretic hormone, Diabetes insipidus.

VASOSPASM: The constriction of a blood vessel (caused by smooth muscle contraction), thereby reducing its diameter and blood flow. Vasospasm appears to be the end point of an intrinsic mechanism for regulating local tissue blood flow. (An extrinsic mechanism also exists that is mediated by the sympathetic nervous system.) Vasospasm can occur in both cerebral and cardiac arteries and is apparently precipitated by only a slight insult or no insult at all. In these circumstances, vasospasm can initiate or worsen infarcts.

VASOXYL: See Methoxamine.

VECURONIUM: A new, nondepolarizing muscle relaxant related to pancuronium.

VENIPUNCTURE: The introduction of a cannula or needle into a vein, usually by piercing rather than incising the skin. A venipuncture unit composed of a Teflon cannula over a stainless steel needle is available. The needle penetrates the skin and vein wall, and blood flow back through the needle (flashback) indicates that the vein has been punctured. The cannula is pushed over the needle and threaded into the vein. The needle is then withdrawn and the cannula end is attached to a fluid line. Other types of venipuncture units include a "through the needle" cannula and a "butterfly." The butterfly is composed of a short stainless steel needle with plastic wings and is applicable for short-term use.

VENOUS AIR EMBOLISM: See Embolism.

VENOUS PRESSURE: The blood pressure measured in the veins. The peripheral venous pressure is variable and is dependent on the central venous pressure. See Central venous pressure.

VENOUS RETURN: The amount of blood returning to the right atrium from the venous circulation.

VENTILATED LUNG VOLUME: The lung area in communication with air passageways. Its gas composition can therefore be altered by ventilation.

VENTILATION AND PERFUSION, REGIONAL DIFFERENCES IN: The variations in the amount of ventilation per unit volume that different segments of the normal lung receive. When a patient is upright, ventilation to the base of each lung is enhanced; in the supine position, ventilation to the posterior segments is improved. An analysis of diseased lung ventilation has led to the two-compartment analysis in which the lung is considered to have two types of alveoli: fast-ventilated or slow-ventilated. Perfusion studies indicate that the dependent lung is perfused better than the nondependent lung; however, perfusion differences are much more pronounced than ventilation differences. Both are caused by gravitational and hydrostatic effects. See Pulmonary perfusion, zones of; Ventilation/perfusion abnormality.

VENTILATION, ASSISTED: The introduction of positive pressure to the upper airways after normal, patient-initiated inspiration has begun. By this technique, flow is increased and tidal volumes are enhanced when the patient has depressed respiration but is still breathing spontaneously. See Ventilation, controlled.

VENTILATION, CONTROLLED: A type of respiration which requires neither patient cooperation nor initiation. The patient's tidal volume, respiratory rate, and flow characteristics are all determined by the anesthetist and are usually machine settings on the ventilator. Patient acquiescence is usually secured by anesthesia and/or muscle relaxants. See Ventilation, assisted.

VENTILATION/PERFUSION ABNORMALITY (V/Q RATIO; VENTILATION/PERFU-
SION RATIO): An imbalance in the alveolar ventilation/pulmonary capillary blood
flow (V/Q) which occurs when either an excessive amount of blood flows through an
alveolus for the volume of alveolar gas that can diffuse into it (decreased V/Q ratio)
or when excessive alveolar gas is available for an inadequate blood flow (increased
V/Q ratio). The concept is most easily understood at its extremes. When an alveolus or an area of the lung receives no ventilation, all the blood that flows through it
is returned to the circulation on the left side without being oxygenated. This condition is known as "shunt." At the other extreme, if an alveolus is ventilated but totally unperfused, the condition known as "dead space" exists. In a healthy 70-kg
man, the normal alveolar ventilation at rest is approximately 4 L/min and the total
perfusion is approximately 5 L/min. Therefore, the VQ ratio is approximately 4:5
or 0.8. In the ideal lung this ratio would be similar for each individual alveolus. It
is a fact, however, that ventilation per cross-sectional area of the lung increases
slowly from the top to the bottom in the upright lung while blood flow increases much
more rapidly due to gravitational effects. The V/Q ratio ranges from 3 at the apex
of the lung (which shows an overabundance of ventilation) to a minimum of 0.63 at
the base of the lung (which shows a relative overabundance of perfusion or blood
flow). During exercise blood flow is more evenly distributed. In the supine individual, V/Q differences are not as marked; the anterior lung assumes the characteristics of the apical lung of the upright patient. The difference in PAO_2 from the apex
(130) to the base of the lung (90) in the upright lung is 40 torr. Those alveoli which
are relatively overventilated cannot aid underventilated alveoli by overloading the
blood with O_2. This is due to the O_2 dissociation curve of hemoglobin. Even at a
PO_2 of approximately 90, hemoglobin is nearly 100% saturated. Additional O_2 taken
in by the blood going past overventilated alveoli (in which the PO_2 is 140-150) can
only be dissolved into the serum, since the hemoglobin is already saturated. The
situation with CO_2 is similar but less critical because the dissociation curve of
CO_2 and blood is nearly linear in the physiologic range. Therefore, alveoli which
are relatively overventilated can remove a proportionately higher quantity of CO_2
(almost enough to compensate for the relatively underventilated areas at the base of
the lung which cannot remove as much CO_2). In diseased states in which the VQ ratio for the overall lung changes drastically, both O_2 delivery and CO_2 removal are
greatly affected. An increase in arterial CO_2, however, triggers the compensatory
mechanism of hyperventilation. This increase in ventilation is very effective in decreasing arterial CO_2 but not in delivering O_2 because of the differences in the O_2
and CO_2 transport noted above.

VENTILATION, SPONTANEOUS: The natural rate and depth of breathing set by a
physiologic requirement and performance of an individual.

VENTILATOR: A device to assist or control the respiration of a patient. Ventilators can be mechanical or powered by a compressed gas supply. There are two basic types of ventilators: the pressure-limited and volume-limited. In the pressure
limited device, gas is delivered to the patient by increasing pressure until some arbitrary pressure limit is reached, at which point the patient is allowed to passively
exhale. In volume-limited ventilators, pressure is built up during inspiration until
the selected volume of gas has been pushed out of the machine. When this volume is
reached, the machine recycles and expiration is allowed to take place. Essentially
all of the modern sophisticated ventilators are volume-limited. Volume-limited machines are considered superior to pressure-limited machines in every parameter
except compensating for leaks. An older type of ventilator is the flow-generator or
flow-limited machine. The machine was set by flow rate in liters per minute for a

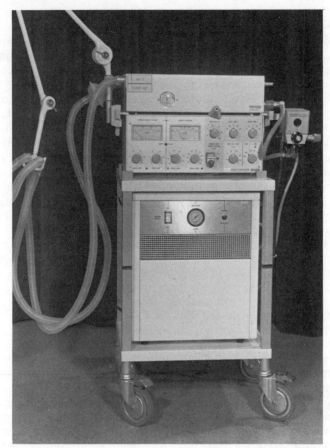

Ventilator: An electrically driven multistage ventilator with gas-mixing
options.

variable period of inspiratory time. Some intraoperative, pneumatically driven anesthesia machine-mounted units still use this system. See Fig. See Compression
volume.

VENTIMASK: A face mask which delivers precise quantities of O_2 (24, 28, 35, 40%)
via a high flow of room air as the O_2 passes through a Venturi tube (a flowmeter device with two flared ends and a constricted center). As the velocity of flow of a fluid
or gas increases in the constricted area, the pressure decreases.

VENTRICULAR FIBRILLATION: The nonrhythmic, irregular, and uncoordinated
contraction of segments of the ventricular walls. See Fig.

VENTRICULAR SEPTAL DEFECT: Most commonly a congenital cardiac anomaly
in which there is a persistent communication between the right and left ventricle in
either the muscular or fibrous portions. Corrective surgery performed during in-
fancy or childhood offers the patient an excellent prognosis. Ventricular septal defects may occur as the only abnormality or may be associated with other malforma-
tions. Sometimes ventricular septal defects can occur because of myocardial infarct damage. See Atrial septal defect.

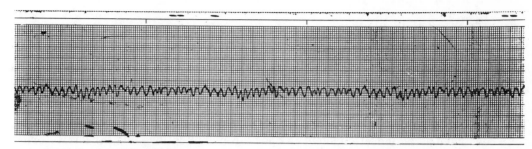

Ventricular Fibrillation.

VENTRICULOGRAPHY: The radiographic examination of the ventricles of the brain with the aid of an injection of air or dye as a contrast medium. (A small amount of cerebrospinal fluid is removed and is replaced by the contrast medium.) If air is used as a medium for filling the ventricles, general anesthesia employing N_2O would be extremely hazardous for a variable period following the ventriculography because if diffuses into the air in the ventricles faster than N_2 diffuses out, causing swelling, brain injury, and possibly death. See Nitrous oxide.

VENTRICULOSTOMY CATHETER: A small cannula which is inserted into the skull (via a burr hole) and is directed through brain tissue into the ventricles of the brain. It is used to measure cerebrospinal fluid pressure, withdraw fluid for sampling, and reduce pressure, e.g., in hydrocephalus.

VENTURI EFFECT: A physical phenomenon describing fluid flow in a tube which has a constriction. Upstream of the constriction, pressure is elevated. Downstream, a partial vacuum and turbulence can be created near the walls of the tube. This effect is useful to dilute O_2 with room air in the Ventimask. In addition, the Venturi effect is evident in the mixture of gasoline and air in a carburetor. See Ventimask.

VENTURI TUBE: See Bernoulli law, Ventimask.

VERNITROL: A bubble-through, out-of-system, multiagent vaporizer manufactured by Ohio Medical Products. Its mode of operation is similar to that of the copper kettle vaporizer. Passive temperature compensation is accomplished by the mass of metal surrounding the vaporizing chamber. See Copper kettle, Vaporizer.

VERONAL: A trade name for barbital. See Barbiturate.

VESSEL-RICH GROUP (VRG), VESSEL-POOR GROUP (VPG): The major subgroups of a circulatory model based on percentage of cardiac output received. The VRG includes highly perfused organs such as brain, heart, kidney, liver, and endocrine glands. The VRG comprises only 9% of the body mass but receives 75% of the cardiac output. The other divisions of the model are the muscle group, which comprises 50-55% of the body mass but receives only 18% of the cardiac output; the VPG (bones, ligaments, and cartilage), which comprises 22% of the body mass but receives only 1.5% of the cardiac output; and the fat group, which comprises 19% of the body mass but receives approximately 5% of the cardiac output.

VESTIBULAR FOLDS: See Laryngospasm.

VINAMAR: See Ethyl vinyl ether.

VINETHENE: See Vinyl ether.

VINETHENE ANESTHETIC MIXTURE (VAM): A general anesthetic (no longer available in the United States) composed of 75% diethyl ether and 25% vinyl ether. It has a rapid onset of action due to the vinyl ether and a decreased toxicity (compared to vinyl ether alone) due to diethyl ether. See Vinyl ether.

VINYL ETHER (DIVINYL ETHER): An extremely volatile ether preparation which had been used as an induction agent in open-drop applications and for short-term general anesthesia. It can cause liver damage depending on the dose and the duration of administration. Vinyl ether is flammable, explosive, and, because of its high volatility, can cause freezing of tissues if dripped on the face. Vinethene is a trade name for an inhalation anesthetic agent composed of 96% vinyl ether and 4% absolute alcohol. The alcohol renders the product less likely to produce ice formation on the face mask.

VISCERA: The organs within the body cavities (especially in the abdomen). See Splanchnic.

VISCOSITY: The resistance to the flow of fluid caused by cohesion of the molecules within the fluid. The unit of absolute viscosity in the CGS system is the poise (P) in which $1P = 1$ dyne sec/cm^2. The viscosity of water at 20 degrees Celsius is 1 cP. The viscosity of whole blood is 2.7 cP. A viscosimeter is the apparatus used to measure viscosity. See Reynolds number.

VISTARIL: See Hydroxyzine.

VITAL CAPACITY: The maximal expiratory volume following maximal inspiration. See Lung volumes and capacities.

VITALOGRAPH: A device for measuring the vital capacity and the forced expiratory volume per second (FEV_1). The patient exhales forcefully into a tube which is connected to the device. This produces expansion of a bellows which drives a pen to record on a calibrated chart. The chart is moved by an appropriate system during the patient's exhalation so that an X-Y plot is obtained.

VMA (4-HYDROXY-3-METHOXYMANDELIC ACID): The principal metabolite (found in urine) of norepinephrine and epinephrine. Abnormally high levels of VMA may be found in the urine of patients with the adrenal medulla tumor pheochromocytoma, the cells of which can secrete excessive amounts of epinephrine and norepinephrine.

V_{max}: See Force-velocity relations.

VOCAL CORDS: See Larynx.

VOID SPACE: The intergranular space in a CO_2 absorber. The void space of fresh soda lime absorbent is approximately 47% of the gross volume. Therefore, a CO_2 canister of 1000 ml will have 470 ml of void space. As the fresh soda lime is progressively converted to carbonate by the absorption of CO_2, the void space is filled with water (a byproduct of the hydroxide-carbonate reaction).

VOLATILE ACID: An acid in solution the concentration of which depends on the concentration of one of its components in the gas in contact with the solution. For practical purposes, the only volatile acid of clinical importance is carbonic acid (H_2CO_3), and its concentration depends on the amount of CO_2 in equilibrium with the blood. This, in turn, is dependent on the ability of the lungs to dispose of the CO_2 produced by metabolism.

VOLT: The unit of electric potential difference and electromotive force necessary to produce 1 amp of current through a resistance of 1 ohm.

VOLTAGE: The potential energy difference between two points in a circuit expressed in volts.

VOLTAGE DROP: The voltage difference measured across the input and output of a device or circuit element. A device offering high resistance to current flow has a high voltage drop measured across its input and output side. See Ohm law.

VOLTMETER: A device which measures voltage. Voltmeters can be either analog or digital instruments and can display information via dials, number displays, or cathode-ray tube displays.

VOLUME-LIMITED VENTILATOR: See Ventilator.

VOLUMES PERCENT: The concentration of a specific gas in a mixture of gases in terms of its percentage of the total volume.

VOMITING: See Esophageal reflux.

VON WILLEBRAND DISEASE: A familial (autosomal dominant) hemorrhagic disorder which classically has three constituents: prolonged bleeding time, reduced factor VIII levels, and altered in vitro platelet function. See Platelet.

WAGNER NEEDLE: See Epidural needle.

WALTON-BRODIE STRAIN GAUGE ARCH: A device which can be sutured directly to the ventricular surface to measure contractile force. It is obviously not a technique to be done casually as a thoracotomy must be performed.

WARBURG APPARATUS: A laboratory device which provides controlled conditions necessary for precise manometric determination of O_2 consumption by tissue. The pressure drop caused by O_2 uptake when CO_2 is absorbed is measured in a sealed chamber.

WARRANTY: A promise that goods or services meet an agreed upon standard. In medicolegal terms a prudent health practitioner does not warrant or guarantee results but only that the standard of care for his or her level of skill will not be violated.

WASHOUT: A continuous process by which a given constituent of a mixture is removed. Lung or alveolar washout of an inhalation anesthetic refers to the gradual removal of the anesthetic by continued respiration after administration of the anesthetic ceases. Washout rate of an inhalation anesthetic is determined by the initial concentration in the lungs, respiratory rate and volume, and "resupply" of the lung from anesthetic previously dissolved in the blood. This resupply from the blood continues for a relatively long period of time as fat can store a significant amount of halogenated hydrocarbon anesthetics. These are gradually released into the circulation as the amount dissolved in the blood falls.

WASTE GAS SYSTEM: See Scavenger system.

WATER BALANCE: The sum total of water ingressing and egressing from the body in a designated time period (usually calculated for 24 hr). In the normal adult, water leaves the body through a number of routes, including kidneys, respiratory tract, skin, and, to a lesser extent, gastrointestinal tract. The average water loss through the kidneys is approximately 1.5 L/day whereas the loss through the skin and the respiratory tract is approximately 1 L/day. The loss of water via the respiratory tract increases with an increase in respiratory rate. Water loss through the skin increases (1) in a hot, dry environment, (2) when the patient's body temperature rises, or (3) when the skin is injured, e.g., by burns or large abrasions. Kidney

Water Balance: Routine water exchange in the adult patient.

	Average Daily Volume (ml)	Maximal Daily Volume (ml)
WATER GAIN:		
Ingestion		
Fluids	1500-2000	1500/hr
Solids	500-600	1500/hr
Body metabolism	250	1000
WATER LOSSES:		
Insensible		
Skin	700	1500
Lung	200	
Sensible		
Urine	1000-1200	2000+/hr
Intestinal	200	8000
Sweat	0	2000+/hr

water loss varies with the solute load and with the level of antidiuretic hormone. When the solute load increases, e.g., as in the case of diabetes mellitus when excess glucose is excreted in the urine, the kidney is obligated to excrete sufficient urine to carry the solutes into the bladder. Replacement of water loss is normally accomplished in two major ways: by ingestion (the average water content of food is between 60 and 97%) or by body metabolism. (The metabolism of approximately 100 cal releases approximately 14 ml water.) Water balance is best measured by accurate daily weights (1 L water weighs 1 kg or 2.2 lb). See Fig.

WATER DEPRESSION FLOWMETER: See Bernoulli law.

WATERSTON SHUNT: A surgical procedure in which the ascending aorta is anastomosed side-to-side with the right pulmonary artery. This palliative procedure is performed to increase pulmonary blood flow by shunting blood from the systemic circulation to the pulmonary circulation. The Waterston shunt operation is performed on smaller infants than Blalock-Taussig shunt patients. See Blalcock-Taussig shunt.

WATT: The standard international unit of power equal to the dissipation of 1 joule of energy/sec. It also equals 1 amp X 1 V and is equivalent to 1/746 hp.

WAVE: A curve of alternating quantity when it is plotted against time. A wave can also be a continuous or transient disturbance which travels through a medium due to the elastic or inertia factors of the medium. When the disturbance is eliminated, the motion ceases.

WAVEFORM: The shape of a curve generated by plotting the instantaneous values of a variable against time, e.g., amplitude versus frequency.

WAVEGUIDE: A hollow metal conducting tube which is used to direct an ultrahigh-frequency electromagnetic wave. The wave reflects off the internal surfaces of the guide.

WAVELENGTH: The distance between two points of corresponding phase on two con-
secutive wave cycles, represented by the Greek letter lambda. The relationship between wavelength, wave velocity, and wave frequency can be stated as lambda = ve-
locity/frequency.

WEANING: The process by which a patient is gradually allowed to resume spontaneous ventilation after controlled mechanical ventilation. Many protocols for weaning exist. The length of the weaning period is dependent on the chronicity of the respiratory failure, length of time mechanical ventilation is needed, age of the patient,
and presence of other body system failures. See Fig. See Intermittent mandatory
ventilation, Mandatory minute volume.

Weaning: Criteria for weaning from controlled ventilation. Several
schemes exist.

A. ADEQUATE VENTILATION

$PaCO_2$	< 50 mmHg
Tidal Volume	5 ml/kg
Respiration	< 30/mm
Vital Capacity	> 0.12 ml/kg
Inspire Force	> 25 ml H_2O

B. ADEQUATE OXYGENATING

PaO_2 (100% O_2)	> 300 mmHg
PaO_2 (40% O_2)	> 100 mmHg
PAO_2-PaO_2	< 350 torr
Pul. Shunt	$< 25\%$

WEDENSKY EFFECT (THRESHOLD BLOCK): A fleeting phenomenon seen precisely at the time when the minimum anesthetic concentration (C_m) for local anesthetic
is reached at a particular nerve fiber. Repeated stimulation of the nerve distal to
the local anesthetic block appears to cause summation of the impulses at the site of
the block so that every second or third impulse is conducted through the blocked
area. What apparently occurs is that the first and second impulses facilitate the
passage of the third impulse. The Wedensky effect multiplies the frequency of the
train of impulses by one-half, one-third, or one-quarter. As the anesthetic concentration around the nerve rises above C_m, the block becomes increasingly more profound and total block ensues. The Wedensky effect is most frequently seen clinically during recovery from a block because the gradients of local anesthetic concentration change much more slowly.

WEDENSKY INHIBITION (WEDENSKY FADE): The characteristic fade or decrease
in muscle movement seen at both slow and fast rates of nerve stimulation during

partial paralysis with a nondepolarizing relaxant such as curare. This fade, seen with either repeated single twitches or a "train of four," is characteristic of a non-depolarizing agent and may be useful in distinguishing a nondepolarizing from a de-polarizing agent. However, this issue is not clear because some "fade" can be observed during the early stages of recovery from total paralysis with a depolarizing agent. This disappears, however, as the block continues to decrease. See Neuro-muscular blockade, assessment of.

WEDGE PRESSURE: See Pulmonary capillary wedge pressure.

WELLS, HORACE: See Morton, William T. G.

WET AND DRY BULB HYDROMETER: An instrument used to measure relative humidity. It consists of two adjacent thermometers with the bulb of one surrounded by fibers soaking in water. Evaporation of the water from the fibers cools the wet bulb. The rate of evaporation depends on the relative humidity of the surrounding air. The relative humidity is based on the difference in temperature readings of the two thermometers.

WETTING AGENT: A substance which becomes adsorbed thereby decreasing the surface tension of a material. This enables solids and liquids to mix and aids in dispersing a liquid on the surface of a solid. See Surface tension.

WHEATSTONE BRIDGE: A network of known resistors arranged in a square pattern and used to determine the resistance of an unknown electric element. A conductor joins two branches of a circuit.

WHITEOUT: An end point radiologic finding in the completely opaque lung. It can be caused by multiple and diverse conditions (infection, tumor, atelectasis, or pulmonary edema).

WINDKESSEL EFFECT: A phenomenon of cardiac function, dependent on the elastic recoil of the aorta, in which part of the systolic pulse pressure rise is absorbed by dilatation of the vessel. The systolic pressure rise is never as high as it would be if the vessel walls were rigid; the recoil provides augmentation of diastolic pressure and helps to continue flow along the system.

WINDOW: A selected subrange in a range of values. For example, in liquid scintil-lation counting, energy windows are selected to detect the emission of particles of a particular energy band, differentiating them from all particles emitted by the radio-isotope.

WORK: The magnitude of force times the distance moved, measured in joules. One joule equals the work done when a force of 1 newton moves through a distance of 1 m.

WORK OF BREATHING: The total energy required to ventilate the lungs and defined in terms of the O_2 uptake necessary to perform this work. Work is done in expand-ing the elastic tissues of the lung and chest wall, in displacing the ribs, and in over-coming the resistance to gas flow down the trachea and airways. In various disease states, any or all of these factors may be affected. In normal circumstances, the work of breathing uses between 2 and 5% of the O_2 consumed/min. In severe res-piratory disease, the work increases three- to fivefold.

WORLD FEDERATION OF SOCIETIES OF ANESTHESIOLOGISTS (WFSA): An inter-national anesthesia society initiated in 1951. The WFSA promotes the specialty of anesthesiology by disseminating scientific information and recommending standards of training for anesthesiologists on a worldwide basis. The WFSA members are from the major anesthesia societies. A World Congress of Anesthesiologists and regional congresses are sponsored by the WFSA every 4 years.

WRIGHT RESPIROMETER: A device for measuring the minute volume and vital capacity. It consists of a gas inlet which directs gas flow to strike a small propeller. This propeller spins in the gas stream and is connected to a direct-reading dial by a gear train. The device tends to overread high flow rates and underread low flow rates.

WYAMINE: See Mephentermine.

XENON-133: A gamma ray-emitting isotope, which is a gas at normal temperature and pressure, used to determine regional perfusion in the lung and brain. The xenon is injected intravenously and its patterns of distribution are determined based on detection of gamma radiation by external scintillation counters.

XEROGRAPHY: An x-ray technique of imaging body tissues, e.g., breast, on selenium-coated metal plates. Xerography is also a copying process in which light passes through the document to be copied and falls on an electrostatically charged plate. This electrostatic charge is dissipated depending on the intensity of the light. A powder with an electric charge is added to the plate. It adheres to the dark areas where the plate has not been discharged. The powder is then transferred to a charged paper where it is heat-fixed. In this manner areas of light and dark can be transferred from one sheet of paper to another.

X-RAY (ROENTGEN RAY): The portion of the electromagnetic spectrum of a short wavelength between ultraviolet and gamma rays. X-rays are able to penetrate most substances.

XYLOCAINE: A brand name for lidocaine. See Local anesthetic.

YAWNING: An involuntary, deep inspiration done with the mouth open, and often accompanied by stretching. Yawning is a poorly understood phenomenom but it has been postulated that it is an automatic reflex operating to reexpand underventilated alveoli after a period of quiet, rhythmic respirations.

YOKE BLOCK: A device which connects a gas source to the yoke of an anesthesia machine by means of a flexible hose. The yoke block takes the place of a small cylinder valve stem. It usually contains holes for the Pin-Index Safety System.

YOKE, HANGER: A device which supports a gas cylinder and connects it to an anesthesia machine. It allows gas to be piped into the gas delivery system. The hanger yoke usually contains an orifice (which mates up against the gas port of the cylinder valve), a retaining screw, a check-valve assembly, and the pins of the Pin-Index Safety System which mate into appropriate holes on the cylinder valve.

Y-PIECE: A tube with two inflow ports and one outflow port used to connect the two sides of the anesthesia circle to the endotracheal tube or mask.

Z-79: A set of standards formulated by the American National Standards Institute (ANSI) to evaluate anesthesia equipment and materials for the purpose of lowering costs and enhancing patient safety. It is necessary to test items such as endotracheal tubes for potential tissue toxicity. All pieces of equipment that pass inspection are labeled Z-79 or IT (implant tested).

ZENER DIODE: A bilayered semiconductor usually used as a voltage regulator.

ZERO END EXPIRATORY PRESSURE: A technique of mechanical respiration in which the alveolar pressure is allowed to drop to the atmospheric pressure at the end of expiration. See Continuous positive airway pressure, Positive end expiratory pressure.

Z LINE: See Actomyosin.

Credits

The illustrations in this book were borrowed through the courtesy of the following:

ACID-BASE BALANCE I: Borrow, M. 1983. Body Functions in Health and Disease. p. 68. New York: Medical Examination Publishing Company, Inc.

ACTION POTENTIAL I: Ganong, W. F. 1983. Review of Medical Physiology. In press. Los Altos: Lange Medical Publications.

ACTION POTENTIAL II: Malamed, S. F. 1980. Handbook of Local Anesthesia. p. 6. St. Louis: The C. V. Mosby Co.

ACTOMYOSIN I: Ganong, W. F. 1983. Review of Medical Physiology, 11th ed. In press. Los Altos: Lange Medical Publications.

ACTOMYOSIN IIa: Ganong, W. F. 1983. Review of Medical Physiology, 11th ed. In press. Los Altos: Lange Medical Publications.

ACTOMYOSIN IIb: Ganong, W. F. 1983. Review of Medical Physiology, 11th ed. In press. Los Altos: Lange Medical Publications.

ACTOMYOSIN III: Ganong, W. F. 1983. Review of Medical Physiology, 11th ed. In press. Los Altos: Lange Medical Publications.

ACTOMYOSIN IV: Ganong, W. F. 1983. Review of Medical Physiology, 11th ed. In press. Los Altos: Lange Medical Publications.

ACUPUNCTURE: Matsumoto, T. 1974. Acupuncture for Physicians. pp. 42-44. Springfield: Charles C Thomas, Publisher.

ADENOSINE TRIPHOSPHATE: Ganong, W. F. 1977. Review of Medical Physiology, 9th ed. p. 212. Los Altos: Lange Medical Publications.

ALPHANUMERIC DISPLAY: Courtesy of Texas Instruments Incorporated.

ALVEOLAR END CAPILLARY DIFFERENCE: West, J. B. 1974. Respiratory Physiology - the Essentials. p. 27. Baltimore: The Williams & Wilkins Company.

ALVEOLUS: Weibel, E.R. 1970. Morphometric estimation of pulmonary diffusion capacity. J. Appl. Physiol. 11:57.

ANESTHESIA CHART: Reproduced with the permission of The University of Iowa Hospitals and Clinics.

ANESTHESIA SYSTEM, OPEN: Dorsch, J.A., Dorsch, S.E. 1975. Understanding Anesthesia Equipment: Construction, Care and Complications. p. 154. Baltimore: The Williams & Wilkins Company.

ANTICOAGULANTS: From Matsumoto, T. 1979. Pre- and Postoperative Evaluation of Surgical Patients. p. 14. New York: Medical Examination Publishing Company, Inc.

ARNOLD-CHIARI DEFORMITY: From Pryse-Phillips, W. 1978. Essential Neurology. p. 219. New York: Medical Examination Publishing Company, Inc.

ARRHYTHMIA: From the personal collection of D. Brown, M.D., The University of Iowa Hospitals and Clinics.

ARTERIALIZATION OF BLOOD: Kinney, J.M. 1960. Transport of carbon dioxide in blood. Anesthesiology. 21:615.

ARTERIOLE: Ganong, W.F. 1977. Review of Medical Physiology, 9th ed. p. 449. Los Altos: Lange Medical Publications.

ATELECTASIS: Kent, T.H., Hart, M.N., Shires, T.K. 1979. Introduction to Human Disease. p. 89. New York: Appleton-Century-Crofts.

ATRIAL FIBRILLATION: From the personal collection of D. Brown, M.D., The University of Iowa Hospitals and Clinics.

ATRIAL FLUTTER: From the personal collection of D. Brown, M.D., The University of Iowa Hospitals and Clinics.

AUTONOMIC NERVOUS SYSTEM I: From Daly, B. 1980. Intensive Care Nursing. p. 473. New York: Medical Examination Publishing Company, Inc.

AUTONOMIC NERVOUS SYSTEM II: Goth, A. 1981. Medical Pharmacology, 10th ed. p. 119. St. Louis: The C.V. Mosby Co. Reproduced with permission of Sandoz Pharmaceuticals, Division of Sandoz, Inc.

AYRE T-PIECE I: Dorsch, J.A., Dorsch, S.E. 1975. Understanding Anesthesia Equipment: Construction, Care and Complications. pp. 160-161. Baltimore: The Williams & Wilkins Company.

AYRE T-PIECE II: Dorsch, J.A. Dorsch, S.E. 1975. Understanding Anesthesia Equipment: Construction, Care and Complications. pp. 162-163. Baltimore: The Williams & Wilkins Company.

BARBITURATE II: From Goth, A. 1981. Medical Pharmacology, 10th ed. p. 304. St. Louis: The C.V. Mosby Co.

BARIUM SULFATE: From Matsumoto, T. 1979. Pre- and Postoperative Evaluation of Surgical Patients. p. 132. New York: Medical Examination Publishing Company, Inc.

BLALOCK-HANLON PROCEDURE: From Doty, D.B.: Cardiac surgery. In Liechty, R.D., Sopor, R.T.: Synopsis of Surgery, 4th ed. 1980. St. Louis: The C.V. Mosby Co.

BLALOCK-TAUSSIG: From Doty, D.B.: Cardiac surgery. In Liechty, R.D., Sopor, R.T.: Synopsis of Surgery, 4th ed. 1980. St. Louis: The C.V. Mosby Co.

BLOOD-BRAIN BARRIER: Seigel, G. 1981. Basic Neurochemistry, 3rd ed. p. 500. Boston: Little, Brown and Company.

BLOOD COAGULATION I: Ellison, N., Jobes, D.R. 1979. Diagnosis of disorder of hemostasis. 30th Annual Refresher Course Lectures in Anesthesiology. 7:91.

BLOOD COAGULATION II: Barrer, M.J., Ellison, N. 1977. Platelet function. Anesthesiology. 46:205.

BLOOD-GAS MACHINE: Photo courtesy of Radiometer America, Inc.

BLOOD TYPES I: Greendyke, P.M. 1980. Introduction to Blood Banking, 3rd ed. p. 99. New York: Medical Examination Publishing Company, Inc.

BLOOD TYPES II: Greendyke, P.M. 1980. Introduction to Blood Banking, 3rd ed. p. 101. New York: Medical Examination Publishing Company, Inc.

BODY FLUID COMPARTMENT I: Talbot, N.B., Richie, R.H., Crawford, J.D. 1959. Metabolic Homeostasis. Cambridge: Harvard University Press.

BODY FLUID COMPARTMENT II: Gamble, J.L. 1954. Chemical Anatomy, Physiology, and Pathology of Extracellular Fluid, 6th ed. Boston: Harvard University Press.

BOYLE BOTTLE: Courtesy of the Medishield Corporation Limited.

BRACHIAL PLEXUS BLOCK I: Cousins, M.J., Bridenbaugh, P.O. Neural Blockade in Clinical Anesthesia & Management of Pain. p. 306. Philadelphia: Lippincott (Harper Medical).

BRACHIAL PLEXUS BLOCK II: Labat, G.L. 1928. Regional Anesthesia. 1928. 2nd ed. Philadelphia: W.B. Saunders Company.

BRACHIAL PLEXUS BLOCK III: Cousins, M.J., Bridenbaugh, P.O. Neural Blockade in Clinical Anesthesia & Management of Pain. P. 307. Philadelphia: Lippincott (Harper Medical).

BREATHING BAG: Courtesy of Dryden Corporation.

BRONCHOSCOPE, FLEXIBLE: Photo courtesy of Olympus Corporation.

BRONCHOSCOPE, RIGID: Courtesy of Pilling Company, Fort Washington, PA.

CALOMEL ELECTRODE: Wellard, Merritt, Dean, 1951. Instrumental Analysis. Princeton: Van Nostrand Reinhold, Company.

CARBON DIOXIDE ELECTRODE: Courtesy of Radiometer A/S, Copenhagen NV, Denmark.

CARDIAC CATHETERIZATION: Nadas, A.S. 1957. Pediatric Cardiology, 3rd ed. p. 116. Philadelphia: W.B. Saunders Company.

CARDIAC CYCLE: Guyton, A. 1981. Textbook of Medical Physiology, 6th ed. p. 154. Philadelphia. W.B. Saunders Company.

CARDIAC OUTPUT: Guyton, A.C. 1973. Circulatory Physiology: Cardiac Output and Its Regulation. 2nd ed. p. 9. Philadelphia: W.B. Saunders Company.

CARDIOPULMONARY BYPASS: From Doty, D.B. Cardiac Surgery. In Liechty, R.D., Soper, R.T. Synopsis of Surgery, 4th ed. 1980. St. Louis: The C.V. Mosby Co.

CARDIOPULMONARY RESUSCITATION: 1979 National Conference on Cardiopulmonary Resuscitation and Emergency Care. 1980. Standards and guidelines for cardiopulmonary resuscitation (CPR) and emergency cardiac care (ECC). JAMA 244:453-509.

CAUDAL ANESTHESIA: Fox, G. (Hunter, A.R., Marx, G.F., Bassell, G.M., eds.) 1980. Monographs in Anaesthesiology. Vol. 7. p. 239. Amsterdam: Elsevier Biomedical Press B.V.

CENTRAL GAS SUPPLY: Reprinted with permission from NFPA 56F-1977. Standard for Nonflammable Medical Gas Systems, Copyright © 1977, National Fire Protection Association, Quincy, MA 02269. This reprinted material is not the complete and official position of the NFPA on the referenced subject, which is represented only by the standard in its entirety.

CENTRAL NERVOUS SYSTEM: Chusid, J.G. 1979. Correlative Neuroanatomy & Functional Neurology. p. 112. Los Altos: Lange Medical Publications.

CENTRAL VENOUS PRESSURE: Kaplan, J.A. 1979. Cardiac Anesthesia. p. 79. New York: Grune & Stratton, Inc. By permission.

CEREBRAL ANGIOGRAPHY: Courtesy of The University of Iowa Hospitals and Clinics, Department of Radiology.

CEREBRAL BLOOD FLOW I: Shapiro, H. 1979. Lecture 214. Physiologic and pharmacologic regulation of cerebral blood flow. 1979 Annual Refresher Course Lectures in Anesthesiology. p. 2. Chicago: American Society of Anesthesiology.

CEREBRAL BLOOD FLOW II: Lassen, N.A., Tweed, W.A. 1979. Monographs in Anaesthesiology. Vol. 2. A Basis and Practice of Neuroanaesthesia. p. 118. Amsterdam: Elsevier Biomedical Press B.V.

CEREBRAL BLOOD FLOW III: Lassen, N.A., Tweed, W.A. 1979. Monographs in Anaesthesiology. Vol. 2. A Basis and Practice of Neuroanaesthesia. p. 119. Amsterdam: Elsevier Biomedical Press B.V.

CEREBROSPINAL FLUID: Reproduced from: Gilman, S. and Winans, S.S.: Manter and Gatz's Essentials of Clinical Neuroanatomy and Neurophysiology, 6th ed. F.A. Davis Co., Philadelphia, 1982.

CHIP: Courtesy of Texas Instruments Incorporated.

CIRCLE OF WILLIS (CIRCULUS ARTERIOSUS): Reproduced from: Gilman, S. and Winans, S.S.: Manter and Gatz's Essentials of Clinical Neuroanatomy and Neurophysiology, 6th ed. F.A. Davis Co., Philadelphia, 1982.

CIRCLE SYSTEM: Dorsch, J.A., Dorsch, S.E. 1975. Understanding Anesthesia Equipment Construction, Care and Complications. p. 204. Baltimore: The Williams & Wilkins Company.

CLOSING CAPACITY: Nunn, J.F. 1977. Applied Respiratory Physiology, 2nd ed. p. 118. London: Butterworth Publishers Inc.

COMA I: Marsh, M.L., Marshall, L.F., Shapiro, H.M. 1977. Neurosurgical intensive care. Anesthesiology. 47:159-163.

COMA II: Marsh, M.L., Marshall, L.F., Shapiro, H.M. 1977. Neurosurgical intensive care. Anesthesiology. 47:149-163.

COMPUTERIZED AXIAL TOMOGRAPHY: Courtesy of The University of Iowa Hospitals and Clinics, Department of Radiology.

CONDUCTING AIRWAYS I: West, J.B. 1974. Respiratory Physiology – the Essentials. p. 5. Baltimore: The Williams & Wilkins Company.

CONDUCTING AIRWAYS II: West, J.B. 1974. Respiratory Physiology – the Essentials. p. 7. Baltimore: The Williams & Wilkins Company.

CONGESTIVE HEART FAILURE: Kent, T.H., Hart, M.N., Shires, T.K. 1979. Introduction to Human Disease. p. 134. New York: Appleton-Century-Crofts.

CONSENT FORM: Reproduced with the permission of The University of Iowa Hospitals and Clinics.

CONTINUOUS FLOW ANESTHESIA MACHINE: Courtesy of Puritan-Bennett Corporation, Foregger Medical Division.

CONTINUOUS POSITIVE AIRWAY PRESSURE: From Levin, R. 1976. Pediatric Respiratory Intensive Care Handbook. p. 92. New York: Medical Examination Publishing Company, Inc.

COPPER KETTLE: Courtesy of Puritan-Bennett Corporation, Foregger Medical Division.

CORTICOSTEROID: Goth, A. 1981. Medical Pharmacology, 10th ed. p. 547. St. Louis: The C.V. Mosby Co.

CRANIAL NERVES: Chusid, J.G. 1979. Correlative Neuroanatomy & Functional Neurology. p. 86. Los Altos: Lange Medical Publications.

CYLINDER, GAS: Dorsch, J.A., Dorsch, S.E. 1975. Understanding Anesthesia Equipment: Construction, Care and Complications. p. 4. Baltimore: The Williams & Wilkins Company.

DEFIBRILLATION: Courtesy of Physio-Control Corporation, Redmond, WA.

DEHYDRATION: Dell, R.B. (Winters, R.W., ed.) 1973. The Body Fluids in Pediatrics. p. 142. Boston: Little, Brown and Company.

DERMATOME: Chusid, J.G. 1979. Correlative Neuroanatomy & Functional Neurology. pp. 205-206. Los Altos: Lange Medical Publications.

DIABETES INSIPIDUS: From Mazzaferri, E. 1980. Endocrinology, 2nd ed. p. 63. New York: Medical Examination Publishing Company, Inc.

DIFFUSION CONSTANT: West, J.B. 1974. Respiratory Physiology - the Essentials. p. 24. Baltimore: The Williams & Wilkins Company.

DINAMAPtm: DINAMAP^{tm} Vital Signs Monitor, Criticon, Inc.

DISC DRIVE: Courtesy of Digital Equipment Corporation.

DISPERSIVE ELECTRODE: Courtesy of Bovie® Products - by Castle - Division of Sybron Corp., Rochester, NY.

DISSEMINATED INTRAVASCULAR COAGULATION: From Matsumoto, T. 1979. Pre- and Postoperative Evaluation of Surgical Patients. p. 13. New York: Medical Examination Publishing Company, Inc.

DISSOCIATION CONSTANT: Malamed, S.F. 1980. Handbook of Local Anesthesia. p. 13. St. Louis: The C.V. Mosby Co.

DOPPLER EFFECT: Reprinted by permission of the publisher, from Saidman/ Smith: Monitoring in Anesthesia. New York: John Wiley & Sons, 1978; Woburn: Butterworth Publishers, 1981.

DOUBLE-LUMEN TUBE: From Stark, D.C. 1980. Practical Points in Anesthesiology. p. 297. New York: Medical Examination Publishing Company, Inc.

DRUG DISTRIBUTION: Price, H.L. 1960. The uptake of thiopental by body tissues and its relation to the duration of narcosis. Clin. Pharmacol. Ther. 1:21.

EINTHOVEN TRIANGLE: Reprinted by permission of the publisher from electrocardiography, by Kuida, H., Fundamental Principles of Circulation Physiology for Physicians. p. 45. Copyright © 1979 by Elsevier Science Publishing Co., Inc.

ELECTROCARDIOGRAM: From Daly, B. 1980. Intensive Care Nursing, p. 109. New York: Medical Examination Publishing Company, Inc.

ELECTROMAGNETIC SPECTRUM: Pitt, V. The Penguin Dictionary of Science. London: Usasov and Isaacs.

ENDOTRACHEAL TUBE I: Courtesy of Shiley Corporation, Irvine, CA.

ENDOTRACHEAL TUBE II: Dorsch, J.A., Dorsch, S.E. 1975. Understanding Anesthesia Equipment: Construction, Care and Complications. p. 253. Baltimore: The Williams & Wilkins Company.

EQUIVALENT SYSTEM OF MEASUREMENT: Courtesy of Abbott Laboratories. p. 12. Fluid and Electrolytes.

EVOKED POTENTIAL: Courtesy of Nicolet Biomedical, A Division of Nicolet Instrument Corporation.

FACE MASK: Courtesy of Dryden Corporation.

FAIL-SAFE DEVICE: Courtesy of Puritan-Bennett Corporation, Foregger Medical Division.

FETAL CIRCULATION: Brown, T.C.K., Fisk, G.C. 1979. Anesthesia for Children Including Aspects for Intensive Care. p. 8. Oxford: Blackwell Scientific.

FETAL HEART RATE TERMINOLOGY: American College of Obstetricians and Gynecologists: Fetal Heart Rate Monitoring (ACOG Technical Bulletin 32). Washington, D.C., 1975.

FIBEROPTICS: Courtesy of AO Scientific Instrument Division of Warner Lambert, Southbridge, MA 01550.

FLOW CONTROL VALVE: Courtesy of Puritan-Bennett Corporation, Foregger Medical Division.

FLOWMETER I: Courtesy of Puritan-Bennett Corporation, Foregger Medical Division.

FLOWMETER II: Courtesy of Puritan-Bennett Corporation, Foregger Medical Division.

FORCE-VELOCITY RELATIONS: Shimasato, S. 1973. Effect of halothane on altered contractility of isolated heart muscle obtained from cats with experimentally produced ventricular hypertrophy and failure. Br. J. Anaesth. 45:2-9.

FOURIER TRANSFORM: Stockard, J., Bickford, R. (Hunter, A.R., Gordon, E., eds.) 1975. Monographs in Anaesthesiology. Vol. 2. A Basis and Practice of Neuroanaesthesia. p. 19. Amsterdam: Elsevier Biomedical Press B.V.

GATE THEORY OF PAIN: Melzack, R., Wall, P.D. 1965. Pain mechanisms. A new theory. Science 150:971-979.

HEMOSTASIS I: Ellison, N., Jobes, D.R. 1979. Diagnosing disorders of hemostasis. ASA Refresher Courses in Anesthesiology. 7:95.

HEMOSTASIS II: Ellison, N., Jobes, D.R. 1979. Diagnosing disorders of hemostasis. ASA Refresher Courses in Anesthesiology. 7:100.

HISTAMINE II: From Goth, A. 1981. Medical Pharmacology, 10th ed. p. 235. St. Louis: The C.V. Mosby Co.

HISTOGRAM: Klein, S.L., Klein, V.L. 1979. The electroencephalogram under fentanyl - nitrous oxide anesthesia. Anesthesiology 51:53.

HYDROCEPHALUS: Courtesy of The University of Iowa Hospitals and Clinics, Department of Radiology.

HYPNOTIC DRUGS: Goodman, A.G., Goodman, L.S., Gilman, A. 1980. Goodman and Gilman's The Pharmacological Basis of Therapeutics, 6th ed. pp. 350-351. New York: Macmillan Publishing Co., Inc.

HYPOXIA: Siesjo, B., et al. 1974. Brain Dysfunction in Metabolic Disorder. p. 72. New York: Raven Press.

HYSTERESIS, LUNG: Scarpelli, E. 1968. The Surfactant System of the Lung. p. 16. Philadelphia: Lea & Febiger.

INTENSIVE CARE UNIT: Courtesy of The University of Iowa Hospitals and Clinics.

INTERCOSTAL BLOCK I: Lichtiger, M., Moya, F. 1978. Introduction to the Practice of Anesthesia, 2nd ed. p. 200. New York: Lippincott (Harper Medical).

INTERCOSTAL BLOCK II: Lichtiger, M., Moya, F. 1978. Introduction to the Practice of Anesthesia, 2nd ed. p. 200. New York: Lippincott (Harper Medical).

INTRACRANIAL HYPERTENSION: Shapiro, H. 1979. Lecture 214-Physiologic and pharmacologic regulation of cerebral blood flow. p. 4. 1979 Annual Refresher Course Lectures in Anesthesiology. Chicago: American Society of Anesthesiologists.

JACKSON-REES APPARATUS: From Levin, R. 1980. Pediatric Anesthesia Handbook, 2nd ed. p. 49. New York: Medical Examination Publishing Company, Inc.

JUGULAR VEINS: From Daly, B. 1980. Intensive Care Nursing. p. 54. New York: Medical Examination Publishing Company, Inc.

KIDNEY: From Daly, B. 1980. Intensive Care Nursing. p. 258. New York: Medical Examination Publishing Company, Inc.

LABOR: Reprinted with permission from The American College of Obstetricians and Gynecologists. Obstetrics and Gynecology 6:569, 1975.

LAMINAR FLOW: Reprinted by permission of the publisher from General aspects of circulation physiology, by Kuida, H., Fundamental Principles of Circulation Physiology for Physicians. p. 20. Copyright © 1979 by Elsevier Science Publishing Co., Inc.

LARYNX: Romanes, G.J. 1964. Cunningham's Textbook of Anatomy, 10th ed. p. 454. London: Oxford University Press.

LIQUID-CRYSTAL DISPLAY: From Modern Dictionary of Electronics, 5th ed. 1977, by Rudolf F. Graff. Howard W. Sams & Co., Inc. Used with the permission of the publisher.

LUMBAR PUNCTURE: Cousins, M. J., Bridenbaugh, P.O. 1980. Neural Blockade in Clinical Anesthesia and Management of Pain. p. 166. Philadelphia: Lippincott (Harper Medical).

LUNG VOLUMES AND CAPACITIES I: Reproduced with permission from Comroe, J.H., Jr., et al.: The Lung, Clinical Physiology and Pulmonary Function Tests, 2nd ed. Copyright © 1962 by Year Book Medical Publishers, Inc., Chicago.

LUNG VOLUMES AND CAPACITIES II: From Levin, R. 1980. Pediatric Anesthesia Handbook, 2nd ed. p. 320. New York: Medical Examination Publishing Company, Inc.

MANDIBLE: Illustration reprinted with permission from Anesthesiology Review, Vol. VII, No. 7, July, 1980.

MASS SPECTROMETER: Courtesy of Perkin-Elmer, Aerospace Division, Pomona, CA 91769.

MYELIN SHEATH: Malamed, S. F. 1980. Handbook of Local Anesthesia. p. 5. St. Louis: The C.V. Mosby Co.

NARCOTIC: Goodman, A. G., Goodman, L.S., Gilman, A. 1980. Goodman and Gilman's The Pharmacological Basis of Therapeutics, 6th ed. p. 507. New York: Macmillan Publishing Co., Inc.

NEUROMUSCULAR JUNCTION: Sokoll, M.D., Gergis, S.D. 1977. Neuromuscular transmission: anatomy, physiology and pharmacology. 1977 Refresher Courses in Anesthesiology. 5:180.

NOMOGRAM: Reprinted by the permission of The New England Journal of Medicine, 251:877, 1954.

OSCILLOTONOMETER: Oscillotonometer® (oscillometer-Von Recklinghausen) Propper Manufacturing Co., Inc., Long Island City, NY 11101.

OXIDATIVE PHOSPHORYLATION: Guyton, A. 1976. Textbook of Medical Physiology, 5th ed. p. 911. Philadelphia: W.B. Saunders Company.

OXYGEN ANALYZER I: Reprinted with permission from Respiratory Care 21:410, 1975.

OXYGEN ANALYZER II: Courtesy of Safety Products, Malvern, PA.

OXYGEN ANALYZER III: Courtesy of Beckman Industries.

OXYGEN ELECTRODE: Courtesy of Radiometer A/S, Copenhagen NV, Denmark.

OXYGEN-HEMOGLOBIN DISSOCIATION CURVE: From Levin, R. 1980. Pediatric Anesthesia Handbook, 2nd ed. p. 333. New York: Medical Examination Publishing Company, Inc.

PARACERVICAL BLOCK: Fox, G. (Hunter, A. R., Marx, G. F., Bassell, G. M., eds.) Monographs in Anesthesiology. Vol. 7, p. 233. Amsterdam: Elsevier Biomedical Press.

PARENTERAL INFUSION: Dunphy, J. E. 1973. Current Surgical Diagnosis and Treatment. p. 158. Los Altos: Lange Medical Publications.

PATENT DUCTUS ARTERIOSUS: From Doty, D. B.: Cardiac surgery. In Liechty, R. D., Soper, R. T.: Synopsis of Surgery, 4th ed. 1980. St. Louis: The C. V. Mosby Co.

PATIENT POSITIONING II: From Stark, D. C. 1980. Practical Points in Anesthesiology, 2nd ed. pp. 37-38. New York: Medical Examination Publishing Company, Inc.

PATIENT POSITIONING III: From Poland, J. L., Hobart, D. J., Payton, O. D. 1981. The Musculoskeletal System, 2nd ed. p. 83. New York: Medical Examination Publishing Company, Inc.

PERIPHERAL NERVE STIMULATOR: From Levin, R. 1976. Pediatric Respiratory Intensive Care Handbook. p. 112. New York: Medical Examination Publishing Company, Inc.

PERIODIC TABLE: Reprinted from Weast, R. C. 1974. CRC Handbook of Chemistry and Physics. Copyright CRC Press, Inc.

pH I: From Levin, R. 1976. Pediatric Respiratory Intensive Care Handbook. p. 61. New York: Medical Examination Publishing Company, Inc.

pH II: From Levin, R. 1976. Pediatric Respiratory Intensive Care Handbook. p. 61. New York: Medical Examination Publishing Company, Inc.

pH ELECTRODE: Courtesy of Radiometer A/S. Copenhagen NV, Denmark.

PHEOCHROMOCYTOMA: From Matsumoto, T. 1979. Pre- and Postoperative Evaluation of Surgical Patients. p. 213. New York: Medical Examination Publishing Company, Inc.

PHOTOVOLTAIC EFFECT: From Modern Dictionary of Electronics, 5th ed, 1977, by Rudolf F. Graff. Howard W. Sams & Co., Inc. Used with permission of the publisher.

PNEUMOTHORAX: Reproduced by kind permission from Wylie & Churchill-Davidson, 1978. A Practice of Anesthesia, 4th ed., edited by H. C. Churchill-Davidson, M. D. London: Lloyd-Luke (Medical Books).

POTASSIUM: Matsumoto, T. 1979. Pre- and Postoperative Evaluation of Surgical Patients. p. 20. New York: Medical Examination Publishing Company, Inc.

PROSTHETIC HEART VALVES: From Doty, D. B.: Cardiac surgery. In Liechty, R. D., Sopor, R. T.: Synopsis of Surgery, 4th ed. 1980. St. Louis: The C. V. Mosby Co.

PULMONARY PERFUSION, ZONES OF: West, J.B., Dollery, C.T., Naimark, A. 1964. Distribution of blood flow in isolated lung; relation to vascular and alveolar pressures. J. Appl. Physiol. 19:723.

PULMONARY PHYSIOLOGY SYMBOLS: Reproduced with permission from Comroe, J.H., Jr., et al.: The Lung, Clinical Physiology and Pulmonary Function Tests, 2nd ed. Copyright © 1962 by Year Book Medical Publishers, Inc., Chicago, as modified from: 1950. Standardization of definitions and symbols in respiratory physiology. Fed. Proc. 9:602-605.

PULSUS ALTERNANS: Used with permission of Hurst, J.W., Logue, R.B., Schlant, R.C., Wenger, N.K. 1978. The Heart - Arteries and Veins, 4th ed. p. 190. New York: McGraw-Hill Book Company.

PUMPING EFFECT; PRESSURE EFFECT I, III: Modified from Dorsch, J.A., Dorsch, S.E. 1975. Understanding Anesthesia Equipment: Construction, Care and Complications. p. 98. Baltimore: The Williams & Wilkins Company.

RECEPTOR/RECEPTOR SITE: From Jastak, J.T., Yagiela, J.A. Regional Anesthesia of the Oral Cavity. p. 62. St. Louis: The C.V. Mosby Co.

RENDELL-BAKER-SOUCEK MASK: From Levin, R. 1976. Pediatric Respiratory Care Handbook. p. 86. New York: Medical Examination Publishing Company, Inc.

REYE SYNDROME: From Levin, R. 1976. Pediatric Respiratory Intensive Care Handbook. p. 187. New York: Medical Examination Publishing Company, Inc. Data from Lovejoy, F.H., Jr. et al. Clinical Staging in Reye Syndrome. Am. J. Dis. Child. 128:36. EEG data from Lovejoy, F.H., Jr., Bresnan, M.J., Lombroso, C.T., Smith, A.L. Anticerebral oedema therapy in Reye's syndrome. Arch. Dis. Child. 50:933-937.

SANDERS INJECTOR: Courtesy of Pilling Company, Fort Washington, PA.

SHIFT REGISTER: Reproduced with permission from Handbook of Blood Pressure Monitoring by John M.R. Bruner, © 1978 by John Wright PSG Inc., Littleton, MA.

SHOCK: From Daly, B. 1980. Intensive Care Nursing. p. 524. New York: Medical Examination Publishing Company, Inc.

SHUNT: West, J.B. 1974. Respiratory Physiology - the Essentials. p. 56. Baltimore: The Williams & Wilkins Company.

SIGGAARD-ANDERSEN ALIGNMENT NOMOGRAM: Courtesy of Radiometer A/S, Copenhagen NV, Denmark, Radiometer©.

SIGNAL AVERAGING: Cooper, R., Osselton, J.W., Shaw, J.C. 1980. EEG Technology, 3rd ed. p. 193. London: Butterworth Publishers, Inc.

SODIUM: From Matsumoto, T. 1979. Pre- and Postoperative Evaluation of Surgical Patients. p. 20. New York: Medical Examination Publishing Company, Inc.

SPINAL NEEDLES: Lund, P.C. 1966. Peridural Analgesia and Anesthesia. p. 147. Springfield: Charles C Thomas.

STAGES AND PLANES OF ANESTHESIA: Reproduced with kind permission from Wylie & Churchill-Davidson, 1978. A Practice of Anaesthesia, 4th ed. edited by H. C. Churchill-Davidson, M. D. London: Lloyd-Luke (Medical Books).

SWAN-GANZ CATHETER: Courtesy of American Edwards Laboratories, Division of American Hospital Supply Corporation. Santa Ana, CA.

TEMPERATURE BLANKET: Photo courtesy of American Medical Systems. A Division of American Hospital Supply. 134 Merchant Street, Suite 200, Cincinnati, OH 45246, (513) 772-7778.

TO-AND-FRO CARBON DIOXIDE ABSORPTION: Courtesy of Puritan-Bennett Corporation, Foregger Medical Division.

TOOTH: Illustration reprinted with permission from Anesthesiology Review, Vol. VII, No. 7, July, 1980.

TRACHEOESOPHAGEAL FISTULA: From Levin, R. 1980. Pediatric Anesthesia Handbook, 2nd ed. p. 139. New York: Medical Examination Publishing Company, Inc.

TRANSDUCER: Courtesy of Gould Inc., Medical Products Division. Overland Park, KA 66212.

VAPORIZER: Courtesy of Puritan-Bennett Corporation, Foregger Medical Division.

VENTILATOR: Courtesy of Siemens-Elema Ventilator Systems, Elk Grove Village, IL.

VENTRICULAR FIBRILLATION: From the personal collection of D. Brown, M. D., The University of Iowa Hospitals and Clinics.

WATER BALANCE: From Borrow, M. 1983. Body Functions in Health and Disease. p. 10. New York: Medical Examination Publishing Company, Inc.

WEANING: From Borrow, M. 1983. Body Functions in Health and Disease. p. 109. New York: Medical Examination Publishing Company, Inc.

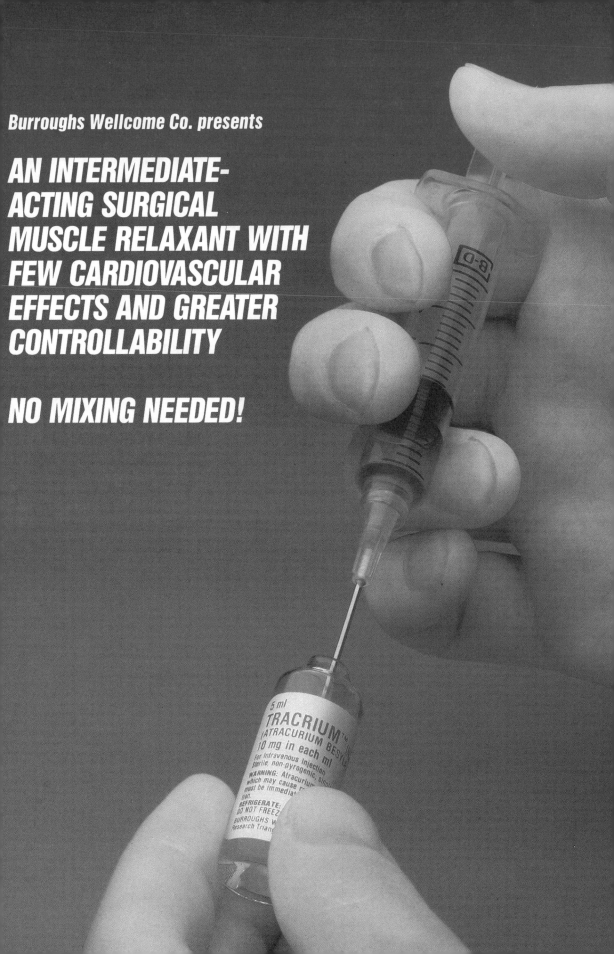

UNIQUE METABOLISM PROVIDES BETTER PREDICTABILITY, ALLOWING BETTER CONTROL

DUAL PATHWAYS

ESTER HYDROLYSIS
Catalyzed by nonspecific esterases

HOFMANN ELIMINATION
At normal body temperature (37°C) and pH (7.4)

Quaternary Acid

Quaternary Alcohol

Monoacrylate

Laudanosine

□ Tracrium® Injection (atracurium besylate) is inactivated by two nonoxidative pathways that are not dependent on kidney or liver function:

① Hofmann elimination—a nonenzymatic process that occurs at physiologic temperature and pH

② Ester hydrolysis—catalyzed by nonspecific esterases; normal levels of plasma cholinesterase are not required

These attributes make Tracrium a more flexible surgical muscle relaxant—it may be tailored to a wide variety of surgical cases.

"Atracurium has the special feature of being broken down to inactive products by the Hofmann elimination reaction. This means that the active drug can be removed from the biophase by other means not totally dependent on enzyme action, redistribution or excretion."[1]

"At present, no other available muscle relaxant undergoes this kind of degradation at physiologic pH."[2]

Convenient and Ready to Use
Tracrium is easily administered—requires no premixing.

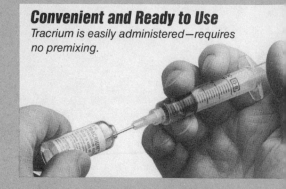

ew Cardiovascular Effects
t Recommended Dosages

] *Tracrium* (atracurium besylate) produces virtually
o clinically significant cardiovascular hemodynamic
*hanges when administered at recommended dosage
vels—a significant benefit in patients with compro-
ised cardiac ability or cardiac risk.

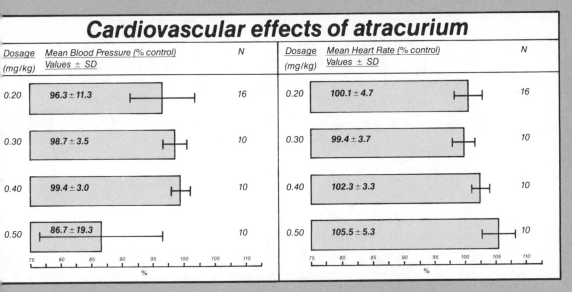

Cardiovascular effects of atracurium

Dosage (mg/kg)	Mean Blood Pressure (% control) Values ± SD	N	Dosage (mg/kg)	Mean Heart Rate (% control) Values ± SD	N
0.20	96.3 ± 11.3	16	0.20	100.1 ± 4.7	16
0.30	98.7 ± 3.5	10	0.30	99.4 ± 3.7	10
0.40	99.4 ± 3.0	10	0.40	102.3 ± 3.3	10
0.50	86.7 ± 19.3	10	0.50	105.5 ± 5.3	10

dapted from Basta et al.[3]

lo Cumulative Effects Upon Recovery, After Multiple Doses

] Repeated equipotent doses of Tracrium, admin-
*tered at equal points of recovery, have no cumulative
ffect on recovery time

] Once recovery begins, it is relatively rapid and
*dependent of dose

] This means that you do not have to calculate pro-
*ressively smaller doses for repeat administration, and
*hat recovery is more consistent and predictable

One patient received 12 successive doses of
*tracurium after recovering completely from the initial
*ose, yet the 25%-75% recovery times were 10.0 and
2.2 min, respectively. This may indicate that
*tracurium is not cumulative...."[1]

Minimal Histamine Release

□ Tracrium is a less potent histamine releaser than
d-tubocurarine or metocurine

□ Clinically significant histamine release occurs well
within the clinical dosage range (at ED_{95}) for curare,
at the upper limits of the clinical dosage range
(at $2 \times ED_{95}$) for metocurine and outside the clinical
dosage range (at $3 \times ED_{95}$) for atracurium[4]

□ The lack of hemodynamic changes due to
Tracrium suggests minimal histamine release

Please see brief summary of prescribing information on the following page.

REFERENCES:
1. Ali HH, Savarese JJ, Basta SJ, et al: Clinical pharmacology of atracurium: A new intermediate acting nondepolarizing relaxant. Seminars in Anesthesia 1982; 1:57-62.
2. Katz RL, Stirt J, Murray AL, et al: Neuromuscular effects of atracurium in man. Anesth Analg 1982; 61:730-734.
3. Basta SJ, Ali HH, Savarese JJ, et al: Clinical pharmacology of atracurium besylate (BW 33A): A new non-depolarizing muscle relaxant. Anesth Analg 1982; 61:723-729.
4. Basta SJ, Savarese JJ, Ali HH, et al: Histamine-releasing potencies of atracurium besylate (BW 33A), metocurine, and d-tubocurarine. Anesthesiology 1982;57:A261.

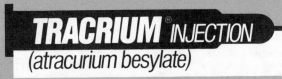

TRACRIUM® INJECTION
(atracurium besylate)

TRACRIUM® INJECTION
(atracurium besylate)

DESCRIPTION: Tracrium (atracurium besylate) is an intermediate-duration, nondepolarizing, skeletal muscle relaxant for intravenous administration.

INDICATIONS AND USAGE: Tracrium is indicated, as an adjunct to general anesthesia, to facilitate endotracheal intubation and to provide skeletal muscle relaxation during surgery or mechanical ventilation.

CONTRAINDICATIONS: Tracrium is contraindicated in patients known to have a hypersensitivity to it.

WARNINGS: TRACRIUM SHOULD BE USED ONLY BY THOSE SKILLED IN AIRWAY MANAGEMENT AND RESPIRATORY SUPPORT.

DO NOT GIVE TRACRIUM BY INTRAMUSCULAR ADMINISTRATION.

Tracrium has no known effect on consciousness, pain threshold, or cerebration. It should be used only with adequate anesthesia.

Tracrium Injection should not be mixed with alkaline solutions (e.g., barbiturate solutions) in the same syringe or administered simultaneously during intravenous infusion through the same needle. Depending on the resultant pH of such mixtures, Tracrium may be inactivated and a free acid may be precipitated.

PRECAUTIONS:

General: Tracrium is a less potent histamine releaser than d-tubocurarine or metocurine. The possibility of substantial histamine release in sensitive individuals must be considered however. Special caution should be exercised in administering Tracrium to patients in whom substantial histamine release would be especially hazardous (e.g., patients with clinically significant cardiovascular disease) and in patients with any history (e.g., severe anaphylactoid reactions or asthma) suggesting a greater risk of histamine release. In these patients, the recommended initial Tracrium dose is lower (0.3 to 0.4 mg/kg) than for other patients and should be administered slowly or in divided doses over one minute.

Since Tracrium has no clinically significant effects on heart rate in the recommended dosage range, it will not counteract the bradycardia produced by many anesthetic agents or vagal stimulation. As a result, bradycardia during anesthesia may be more common with Tracrium than with other muscle relaxants.

Tracrium may have profound effects in patients with myasthenia gravis, Eaton-Lambert syndrome or other neuromuscular diseases or in patients with severe electrolyte disorders or carcinomatosis.

The safety of Tracrium has not been established in patients with bronchial asthma.

Drug Interactions: The neuromuscular blocking action of Tracrium may be enhanced by enflurane; isoflurane; halothane; certain antibiotics, especially the aminoglycosides and polymyxins; lithium; magnesium salts; procainamide; or quinidine.

If other muscle relaxants are used during the same procedure, the possibility of a synergistic or antagonist effect should be considered.

Prior administration of succinylcholine does not enhance the duration, but quickens the onset and may increase the depth of neuromuscular blockade induced by Tracrium. Tracrium should not be administered until a patient has recovered from succinylcholine-induced neuromuscular blockade.

Pregnancy: *Teratogenic Effects:* Pregnancy Category C. There are no adequate and well-controlled studies in pregnant women. Tracrium should be used during pregnancy only if the potential benefit justifies the potential risk to the fetus.

Labor and Delivery: It is not known whether muscle relaxants administered during vaginal delivery have immediate or delayed adverse effects on the fetus or increase the likelihood that resuscitation of the newborn will be necessary. The possibility that forceps delivery will be necessary may increase.

Tracrium (0.3. mg/kg) has been administered to 26 pregnant women during delivery by cesarean section. No harmful effects were attributable to Tracrium in any of the newborn infants, although small amounts of Tracrium were shown to cross the placental barrier. The possibility of respiratory depression in the newborn infant should always be considered following cesarean section during which a neuromuscular blocking agent has been administered. In patients receiving magnesium sulfate, the reversal of neuromuscular blockade may be unsatisfactory and Tracrium dose should be lowered as indicated.

Nursing Mothers: It is not known whether this drug is excreted in human milk. Caution should be exercised when Tracrium is administered to a nursing woman.

Pediatric Use: Safety and effectiveness in children below the age of 2 years have not been established.

ADVERSE REACTIONS: Tracrium produced few adverse reactions during extensive clinical trials, most of which were suggestive of histamine release (see PRECAUTIONS section). The overall incidence of clinically important adverse reactions was 7/875 or 0.8%.

In the United Kingdom, where Tracrium has been marketed since December, 1982, the most frequent adverse reactions reported in association with the use of Tracrium are cutaneous histamine-like reactions, bronchospasm, and bradycardia. These have been reported to occur in about one in 10,000 patients. Less frequent adverse reactions are hypotension, heart arrest, tachycardia, cyanosis, and apnea, which have been reported to occur in approximately one in 100,000 patients.

DOSAGE AND ADMINISTRATION: Tracrium should be administered intravenously. DO NOT GIVE TRACRIUM BY INTRAMUSCULAR ADMINISTRATION.

A Tracrium dose of 0.4 to 0.5 mg/kg, given as an intravenous bolus injection, is the recommended initial dose for most patients. With this dose, good or excellent conditions for nonemergency intubation can be expected in 2 to 2.5 minutes in most patients, with maximum neuromuscular blockade achieved approximately 3 to 5 minutes after injection. Clinically acceptable neuromuscular blockade under balanced anesthesia generally lasts 20 to 35 minutes; recovery to 25% of control is achieved approximately 35 to 45 minutes after injection, and recovery is usually 95% complete approximately 60 minutes after injection.

An initial Tracrium dose of 0.3 to 0.4 mg/kg is recommended following the use of succinylcholine for intubation under balanced anesthesia.

Tracrium is potentiated by isoflurane or enflurane anesthesia. The same initial Tracrium dose of 0.4 to 0.5 mg/kg may be used for intubation prior to administration of these inhalation agents; however, if Tracrium is first administered under steady state of isoflurane or enflurane, the initial Tracrium dose should be reduced by approximately one-third, i.e., to 0.25 to 0.35 mg/kg; with halothane, which has only a marginal (approximately 20%) potentiating effect on Tracrium, smaller dosage reductions may be considered.

Tracrium doses of 0.08 to 0.10 mg/kg are recommended for maintenance of neuromuscular blockade during prolonged surgical procedures. The first maintenance dose will generally be required 20 to 45 minutes after the initial Tracrium injection, but the need for maintenance doses should be determined by clinical criteria. Maintenance doses may be administered at relatively regular intervals for each patient, ranging approximately from 15 to 25 minutes under balanced anesthesia, slightly longer under isoflurane or enflurane.

An initial Tracrium dose of 0.3 to 0.4 mg/kg, given slowly or in divided doses over one minute, is recommended for patients with significant cardiovascular disease and for patients with any history (e.g., severe anaphylactoid reactions or asthma) suggesting a greater risk of histamine release.

Dosage reductions must be considered also in patients with neuromuscular disease, severe electrolyte disorders, or carcinomatosis in which potentiation of neuromuscular blockade or difficulties with reversal have been demonstrated.

No Tracrium dosage adjustments are required for patients with renal disease or for pediatric patients two years of age or older. In pediatric patients, maintenance doses may be required with slightly greater frequency than in adults.

HOW SUPPLIED: Tracrium Injection, 10 mg atracurium besylate in each ml. Ampuls of 5 ml (50 mg atracurium besylate per ampul). Box of 10 ampuls (NDC-0081-0940-10).
Store under refrigeration at 2° to 8°C (36° to 46°F); DO NOT FREEZE.

U.S. Patent No. 4179507   Printed in U.S.A.   84-TRA-4

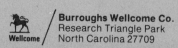

Burroughs Wellcome Co.
Research Triangle Park
North Carolina 27709

TRACRIUM® INJECTION
(atracurium besylate)